Study Guide for
PIMA MEDICAL INSTITUTE

Medical Assistant & Medical Administrative Assistant

CUSTOM EDITION 2

CUSTOM EDITION 2

Study Guide for
PIMA MEDICAL INSTITUTE

Medical Assistant & Medical Administrative Assistant

Judy Kronenberger, PhD, RN, CMA(AAMA)
Associate Professor and Program Director, Medical Assistant Program
University of Cincinnati Blue Ash
Blue Ash, Ohio

Julie Ledbetter, CMA(AAMA), CMRS, CPC
Adjunct Faculty, Medical Assistant Technology
Sinclair Community College
Dayton, Ohio

Wolters Kluwer

Philadelphia • Baltimore • New York • London
Buenos Aires • Hong Kong • Sydney • Tokyo

Acquisitions Editor: Jay Campbell
Senior Product Development Editor: Amy Millholen
Editorial Assistant: Tish Rodgers
Marketing Manager: Shauna Kelley
Production Project Manager: David Saltzberg
Design Coordinator: Joan Wendt
Manufacturing Coordinator: Margie Orzech
Prepress Vendor: SPi Global

5th Edition

9 8 7 6 5 4 3 2

Printed in China

Custom ISBN: 978-1-4963-7333-5
Standard ISBN: 978-1-4963-0249-6

LWW.com

Preface

Welcome to the *Study Guide for Lippincott Williams & Wilkins' Comprehensive Medical Assisting, Fifth Edition.* In this edition, we have aligned the exercises and activities with the most current (2015) Medical Assisting Education Review Board (MAERB) of the American Association of Medical Assistants (AAMA) curriculum standards. Program directors, instructors, and students will know which activities in this *Study Guide* support comprehension of knowledge from the textbook (cognitive domain), which support the practice and skills needed to become a competent entry-level medical assistant (psychomotor domain), and which exercises encourage critical thinking and professional behaviors in the medical office (affective domain). This *Study Guide* is unique in a number of ways and offers features that are not found in most Medical Assisting study guides.

The *Study Guide* is divided into sections that coincide with the textbook: Administrative, Clinical, Laboratory, and Career Strategies. Parts I to IV include exercises that reinforce the knowledge and skills required of all Medical Assistants. Part V includes activities to "put it all together" as a potential medical office employee. All chapters have been updated and revised and we believe the extensive revision of the Clinical Laboratory chapters will be especially helpful.

Each chapter includes the following:

- **Learning Outcomes**—Learning outcomes are listed at the beginning of the chapter and are divided into AAMA/CAAHEP categories (Cognitive, Psychomotor, Affective) and ABHES competencies.
- **A Variety of Question Formats**—To meet the needs of a variety of learning styles and to reinforce content and knowledge, each chapter of the *Study Guide* includes multiple choice, matching, short answer, completion, and where applicable, calculation-type questions. These formats will help you retain new information, reinforce previously learned content, and build confidence.
- **Case Studies for Critical Thinking**—These scenarios and questions are designed with real-world situations in mind and are intended to promote conversation about possible responses, not just one correct answer! These questions will be valuable to students who confront these types of situations during externship and graduates who encounter similar situations after employment.
- **Procedure Skill Sheets**—Every procedure in the textbook has a procedure skill sheet in the *Study Guide.* These procedures have been updated and revised in this edition and include steps on interacting with diverse patients, such as those who are visually or hearing impaired, those who do not speak English or who speak English as a second language (ESL), and patients who may have developmental challenges.
- **Putting It All Together**—Chapter 47 in the textbook allows students in the final stages of their educational program to take a comprehensive examination, and Chapter 47 in the *Study Guide* gives students the opportunity to reinforce information learned throughout their program. This final *Study Guide* chapter includes documentation skills practice for a multitude of situations and active learning activities to engage students with previously learned knowledge.

This *Study Guide* has been developed in response to numerous requests from students and instructors for a concise, understandable, and interactive resource that covers the skills necessary to become a successful Medical Assistant. We hope you find the exercises and tools in this book productive and useful toward your goal of becoming the best Medical Assistant possible!

Contents

PART 6

Study Guide Addendum: Lab Skills for Medical Administrative Assistant and Medical Assistant

Study Guide for
PIMA MEDICAL INSTITUTE

Medical Assistant & Medical Administrative Assistant

CUSTOM EDITION 2

PART

1

Introduction to Medical Assisting

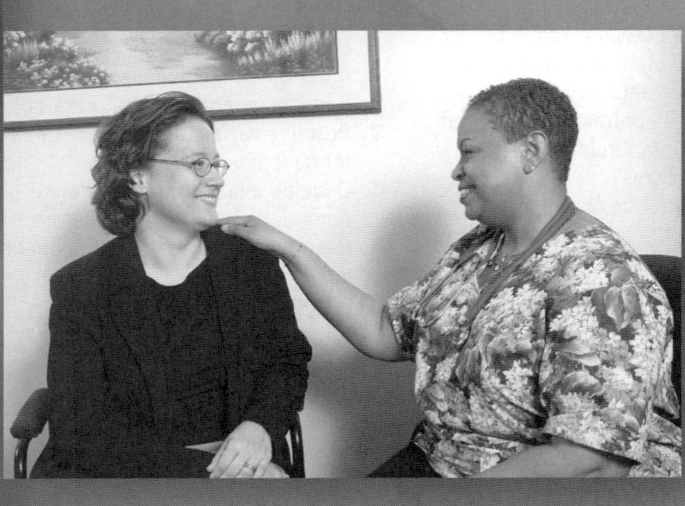

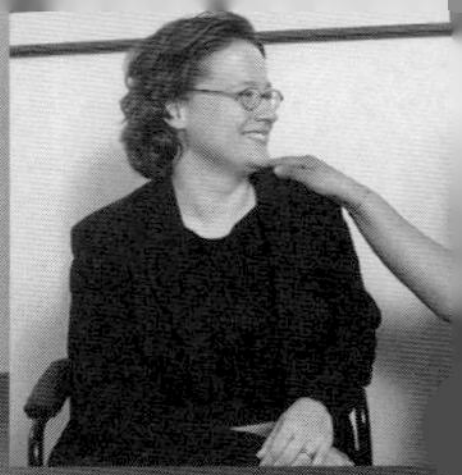

UNIT ONE UNDERSTANDING THE PROFESSION

CHAPTER 1 Medicine and Medical Assisting

Learning Outcomes

COG Cognitive Domain

1. Spell and define the key terms
2. Summarize a brief history of modern medicine
3. Explain the system of health care in the United States
4. Discuss the typical medical office
5. List medical specialties a medical assistant may encounter
6. List settings in which medical assistants may be employed
7. List the duties of a medical assistant
8. Describe the desired characteristics of a medical assistant
9. Differentiate between scope of practice and standards of care for medical assistants
10. Compare and contrast provider and medical assistant roles in terms of standard of care
11. Recognize the role of patient advocacy in the practice of medical assisting
12. Define a patient-centered medical home
13. Define the principles of self boundaries
14. Differentiate between adaptive and nonadaptive coping mechanisms
15. Identify members of the health care team
16. Explain the pathways of education for medical assistants
17. Discuss the importance of program accreditation
18. Name and describe the two nationally recognized accrediting agencies for medical assisting education programs
19. Explain the benefits and avenues of certification for the medical assistant
20. Discuss licensure and certification as it applies to health care providers
21. List the benefits of membership in a professional organization
22. Identify the effect personal morals may have on professional performance

PSY Psychomotor Domain

1. Locate a state's legal scope of practice for medical assistants
2. Perform within scope of practice
3. Practice within the standard of care for a medical assistant
4. Develop a plan for separation of personal and professional ethics
5. Respond to issues of confidentiality

AFF Affective Domain

1. Demonstrate awareness of the consequences of not working within the legal scope of practice
2. Apply ethical behaviors, including honesty and integrity in performance of medical assisting practice
3. Recognize the impact personal ethics and morals have on the delivery of health care
4. Demonstrate the principles of self-boundaries

ABHES Competencies

1. Comprehend the current employment outlook for the medical assistant
2. Compare and contrast the allied health professions and understand their relation to medical assisting
3. Understand medical assistant credentialing requirements and the process to obtain the credential. Comprehend the importance of credentialing
4. Have knowledge of the general responsibilities of the medical assistant
5. Define scope of practice for the medical assistant, and comprehend the conditions for practice within the state that the medical assistant is employed
6. Demonstrate professionalism by:
   a. *Exhibiting dependability, punctuality, and a positive work ethic*
   b. *Exhibiting a positive attitude and a sense of responsibility*
   c. *Maintaining confidentiality at all times*
   d. *Being cognizant of ethical boundaries*
   e. *Exhibiting initiative*
   f. *Adapting to change*
   g. *Expressing a responsible attitude*
   h. *Being courteous and diplomatic*
   i. *Conducting work within scope of education, training, and ability*
7. Comply with federal, state, and local health laws and regulations
8. Analyze the effect of hereditary, cultural, and environmental influences

51. You are a CMA in a busy Ob/Gyn practice. You have been asked to orient a high school student who was hired to help up front and in medical records in the afternoons. She wants a career in health care but is unsure if she would be happier in a doctor's office or a hospital. She is debating between becoming a CMA or an RN but is confused about the difference. She asks for your help in deciding what profession to choose. How would you explain the difference in the two careers?

____

____

____

52. Why is the ability to respect patient confidentiality essential to the role of the medical assistant?

____

____

____

53. The medical office in which you work treats a variety of patients, from all ages and backgrounds. Why should you work with a multidisciplinary health care team? What are the benefits to the patients?

____

____

____

WHAT WOULD YOU DO?

Grade: ________

54. You are preparing a patient for his or her examination, but the physician is running behind schedule. The patient is becoming anxious and asks you to perform the examination, instead of the physician. You tell his or her that you will go check how much longer the physician will be. But she or he responds, "Can't you just perform the exam? Aren't you like a nurse?" How should you respond?

____

____

____

55. The patient who asked you to perform the examination now refuses to wait for the physician. Even though he or she has a serious heart condition requiring monthly checkups, he or she leaves without being treated by the physician. You need to write a note that will be included in his or her chart and in an incident report. What would you say?

____

____

____

COG AFF PSY ACTIVE LEARNING

Grade: _______

56. Review the list of specialists who employ medical assistants in textbook Table 1-3. Choose one specialty that interests you. Perform research on what kinds of procedures the specialist performs. Then consider what kinds of tasks a medical assistant employed by this specialist might perform. Write a letter to this specialist explaining why you would want to work in this kind of office. Be sure to include specific references to the tasks and procedures that interest you based on your research.

____

____

____

57. Scope of practice for medical assistants can vary from state to state. In some states, CMAs are not allowed to perform invasive procedures, such as injections or phlebotomy. Go to the Web site for your state and research the laws in your state regarding the medical assistant's scope of practice. Why is it important to understand your scope of practice before beginning work in a new medical office?

____

____

____

AFF CASE STUDY FOR CRITICAL THINKING A

Grade: _______

You are a CMA in a family practice where many of your friends and neighbors are patients. One of them is being treated for breast cancer. It seems as though everywhere you go, someone asks about her condition. They are just concerned, and so are you. You really want to give them an update on her treatment, but you know that is prohibited.

58. What is your best action? Choose all appropriate actions from the list below.

a. Ask the patient if she minds letting you give updates to their mutual friends.
b. Tell them that you would be violating a federal law if you discuss her care, but they should call her to find out.
c. Tell them what they want to know. After all, they are asking because they care.
d. Offer to help your friend/patient join a Web site that will allow her to update her friends.

AFF CASE STUDY FOR CRITICAL THINKING B

Grade: _______

You start your new position as a CMA for a busy pediatric practice. You are unsure of your job responsibilities, but the office manager expects you to "hit the ground running." Your first day is busy, and you are asked to handle the phones. Your first caller is a mother who is worried about his or her child's fever.

59. Your best response is:

a. Don't worry. I'm sure he or she will be fine.
b. Let me check the office protocol for children with fever. I will call you back.
c. Today is my first day; I don't know, but I think he or she will be fine.
d. You will need to make an appointment.
e. I'll put you through to the doctor immediately.

60. What action could have prevented this uncomfortable situation?
a. Having the opportunity to observe the office for a few weeks before starting
b. Having read the policy and procedure manual before starting work
c. Having more experience in the medical assisting field
d. Paying better attention in class
e. Refusing to answer the phone

61. You ask another CMA what you should do, and her response is, "I thought you were a CMA; you should know what to do." What is your next best action?
a. Go immediately to your supervisor for guidance.
b. Tell another coworker what she said and ask what she thinks you should do.
c. Start looking for another job.
d. Tell her that if the facility had trained you properly, you would have known what to do.
e. Tell her that you are doing your best, and you are sure you will get up to speed soon.

AFF CASE STUDY FOR CRITICAL THINKING C

Grade: ___________

Mrs. Esposito approaches Jan, a medical assistant, at the front desk. Jan has recently treated Mrs. Esposito's son, Manuel, for a foot injury. Mrs. Esposito has just arrived in the United States and, with broken English, asks Jan if she may have her son's medical records to show Manuel's soccer coach that he will be unable to play for the rest of the season. Jan tries to explain to Mrs. Esposito that because her son is 18 years old and legally an adult, she must have his permission to release his medical records. Mrs. Esposito is frustrated and angry. Using Spanish translating software, Jan calmly attempts to explain that the physician would be happy to write a note for Manuel to give to his soccer coach explaining his injuries. After a great deal of time and effort, Mrs. Esposito thanks her for this information and apologizes for becoming angry.

62. From the list below, choose the characteristic of a professional medical assistant that Jan exhibited in the above scenario.
a. Accuracy
b. Proper hygiene
c. The ability to respect patient confidentiality
d. Honesty

63. What was the best action for Jan when she learned that Mrs. Esposito did not speak much English?
a. Look in the Yellow Pages for a translator
b. Try to find a Spanish translating software online
c. Enlist the assistance of a fellow employee who speaks fluent Spanish
d. Tell Mrs. Esposito to come back when she can bring a translator

64. When dealing with an angry person such as Mrs. Esposito, the most important action is to:
a. Raise your voice so he or she will hear you
b. Treat his or her as he or she is treating you
c. Remain calm
d. Notify the office manager of a problem

65. When responding to a request for the release of medical information, your first action should be to:
a. explain the policy to the patient.
b. check for the patient's signed authorization.
c. ask the physician.
d. copy the records.

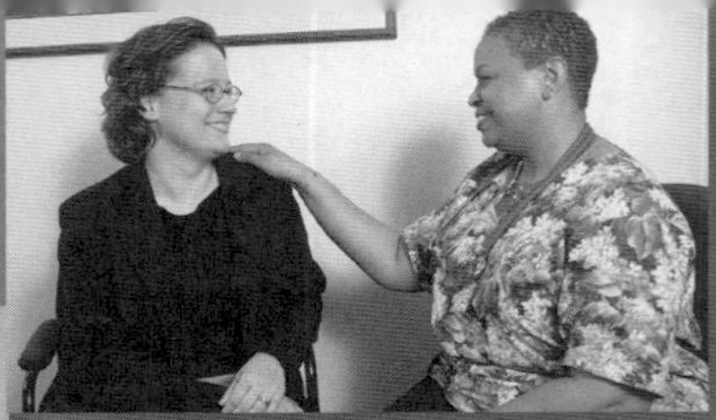

CHAPTER

2 Law and Ethics

Learning Outcomes

COG Cognitive Domain

1. Spell and define the key terms
2. Discuss all levels of governmental legislation and regulation as they apply to medical assisting practice, including the Food and Drug Administration and the Drug Enforcement Agency
3. Compare criminal and civil law as it applies to the practicing medical assistant
4. Provide an example of tort law as it would apply to a medical assistant
5. List the elements and types of contractual agreements and describe the difference in implied and express contracts
6. List four items that must be included in a contract termination or withdrawal letter
7. List six items that must be included in an informed consent form and explain who may sign consent forms
8. List five legally required disclosures that must be reported to specified authorities
9. Describe the four elements that must be proven in a medical legal suit
10. Describe four possible defenses against litigation for the medical professional
11. Explain the theory of respondeat superior, or law of agency, and how it applies to the medical assistant
12. Outline the laws regarding employment and safety issues in the medical office
13. Identify:
    a. Genetic Information Nondiscrimination Act of 2008 (GINA)
    b. Americans with Disabilities Act Amendments Act (ADAAA)
14. Differentiate between legal, ethical, and moral issues affecting health care
15. Define:
    a. Negligence
    b. Malpractice
    c. Statute of limitations
    d. Good Samaritan Act
    e. Uniform Anatomical Gift Act
    f. Living will/advanced directives
    g. Medical durable power of attorney
    h. Patient Self-Determination Act (PSDA)
16. List the seven American Medical Association principles of ethics
17. List the five ethical principles of ethical and moral conduct outlined by the American Association of Medical Assistants
18. Define patient navigator
19. Describe the role of the medical assistant as the patient navigator
20. Describe the purpose of the Self-Determination Act
21. Explore issue of confidentiality as it applies to the medical assistant
22. Describe components of the Health Information Portability & Accountability Act (HIPAA)
23. Describe the implications of the Health Insurance Portability and Accountability Act for the medical assistant in various medical settings
24. Summarize the Patients' Bill of Rights
25. Discuss licensure and certification as it applies to health care providers
26. Describe the following types of insurance: liability, professional (malpractice), and personal injury

COG IDENTIFICATION

Grade: ________

66. Which of the following must be included in a patient consent form? Circle all that apply.

a. Name of the physician performing the procedure

b. Alternatives to the procedure and their risks

c. Date the procedure will take place

d. Probable effect on the patient's condition if the procedure is not performed

e. Potential risks from the procedure

f. Patient's next of kin

g. Any exclusions that the patient requests

h. Success rate of the procedure

67. Dr. Janeway has decided to terminate his patient, Mrs. King. The office manager drafted the following letter to Mrs. King. However, when you review the letter, you find that there are errors. Read the letter below and then explain the three problems with this letter in the space below.

Dear Mrs. King,

Because you have consistently refused to follow the dietary restrictions and to take the medication necessary to control your high blood pressure, I feel I am no longer able to provide your medical care. This termination is effective immediately.

Because you do not seem to take your medical condition seriously, I'm not sure that any other physician would want to treat you either. I will hold on to your medical records for 30 days and then they will be destroyed.

Sincerely,
Anthony Janeway, MD

a. ____

b. ____

c. ____

COG PSY ACTIVE LEARNING

Grade: ________

68. Research two recent medical malpractice cases on the Internet. Write a brief outline of each case and make a record of whether the tort was intentional or unintentional, and what the outcome of the case was. Compare the cases to see if there is a common theme.

69. Visit a physician's office and make a list of steps that have been taken to comply with the law. For example, if the physician charges for canceling appointments without notice, there is probably a sign by the reception desk to warn patients of the fee. How many other legal requirements can you find? Are there any that are missing?

70. As technology develops, new laws have to be written to protect the rights of patients who use it. Stem cell research is a particularly gray area and has raised many interesting ethical dilemmas. Research some recent legal cases regarding stem cell research, and write a report on some of the ethical issues the cases have raised.

71. You are a medical assistant in a busy office, and the physician has been called away on an emergency. Some of the patients have been waiting for over 2 hours, and one of them urgently needs a physical checkup for a job application. Although you are not officially qualified, you feel confident that you are able to carry out the examination by yourself. Six months later, the patient files a malpractice suit because you failed to notice a lump in her throat that turned out to be cancerous. Describe the law of agency and explain whether it would help you in the lawsuit.

AFF WHAT WOULD YOU DO?

Grade: ___________

72. A family member calls to inquire about a patient's condition. You know that the patient has not given written consent for information to be passed on, but you recognize the person's voice and remember that she came in with the patient the previous day. Explain what you would say and why.

COG IDENTIFICATION

Grade: ___________

73. Mrs. Stevens visits Dr. Johnson's office with neck pain. Dr. Johnson examines her and recommends that she see a specialist. Several months later, Mrs. Stevens sues Dr. Johnson for malpractice, claiming that when he examined her, he made her neck pain worse. In court, she provides pictures of her neck that show severe bruising. A specialist confirms that muscle damage has restricted Mrs. Stevens from going about her daily life. Which of the four elements needed in a medical lawsuit has Mrs. Stevens failed to prove? Circle all that apply.

a. Duty

b. Dereliction of duty

c. Direct cause

d. Damage

AFF PATIENT EDUCATION

Grade: ___________

74. You have a patient who has just been diagnosed with a sexually transmitted disease. After the physician leaves the office, the patient turns to you and begs you to keep the information confidential. It is obvious that the patient is worried and embarrassed. Explain how you would inform the patient about legally required disclosures and what you would say.

____

____

____

____

AFF CASE STUDY FOR CRITICAL THINKING A

Grade: ___________

Pamela Dorsett is a patient at Highland Oaks Family Practice. She is a 40-year-old woman who has five children and a house full of cats. She brings her children in for immunizations, but otherwise you rarely see them. She walks into the office on a busy Monday morning with all five children. They are surrounded by a pungent smell of cat feces. The children are dirty, and it appears are being neglected. All five of them have runny noses. She wants the doctor to see them now because she has transportation problems. You are the receptionist that day. Remember, pick the BEST answer.

75. The doctor is legally obligated to see the children at some point because:

a. the children look neglected.

b. there is a legal contract in place.

c. medical ethics dictate it.

d. all of the above.

76. If child neglect is suspected, the physician is required by federal law to:

a. talk to the mother about her care.

b. try to contact a family member.

c. do nothing, as mandated by HIPAA.

d. report the suspicions to authorities.

77. What would your first action be?

a. Try to work the five children into the busy schedule.

b. Consult with the providers.

c. Make future appointments as soon as possible.

d. Have them wait until the end of the day after all scheduled patients have been seen.

COG AFF CASE STUDY FOR CRITICAL THINKING B

Grade: _______

As a medical assistant, you will be involved in some administrative issues. Read the following scenarios and assess whether the American Medical Association standards for office management are being met. Place a check mark in the appropriate box.

Scenario	Standards Met	Standards Not Met
78. Dr. Benson tells his medical assistant to cancel Mrs. Burke's tests because she recently lost her job and will be unable to pay for them.		
79. Mr. Grant canceled his appointment with less than 24 hours' notice. He was charged a fee as noted in a sign by the receptionist's desk.		
80. Mrs. O'Malley asks Dr. Jones to help her fill out an insurance form. The form is a four-page document that takes Dr. Jones an hour to fill out. Dr. Jones charges Mrs. O'Malley $15 for filling out the form.		
81. Dr. Harris dies suddenly, and his staff tell patients that the office will close and that copies of their medical records will be transferred to another physician.		
82. Mr. Davies owes the physician's office several thousand dollars. He is moving and asks the office to transfer his medical records to his new physician. The office refuses on the grounds that Mr. Davies has not paid his bill.		
83. Mrs. Jones comes into the office for a vaccination. The physician tells the medical assistant to charge her $10 less than other patients because she is elderly and cannot afford the standard charges.		

PSY PROCEDURE 2-1 Obtaining an Informed Consent for Treatment

Name: ______________________ **Date:** __________ **Time:** __________ **Grade:** __________

EQUIPMENT: Computer, Internet connection, search engine, or Web site list

KEY: 4 = Satisfactory 0 = Unsatisfactory NA = This step is not counted

PROCEDURE STEPS	SELF	PARTNER	INSTRUCTOR
1. Using a search engine, go to the CDC's Web site to download and print the most recent Vaccine Information Statement for the inactivated influenza vaccine.	❑	❑	❑
2. Complete an Informed Consent form for the inactivated influenza vaccine.	❑	❑	❑
3. File the Informed Consent in the patient's medical record after obtaining the patient's signature.	❑	❑	❑
4. AFF Explain what you would say to a fellow employee who responds to a change in a current law with, "I will just keep doing it the old way. Who is going to care?"	❑	❑	❑

____

____

____

____

CALCULATION

Total Possible Points: __________

Total Points Earned: __________ Multiplied by 100 = __________ Divided by Total Possible Points = __________ %

PASS ❑ **FAIL** ❑ **COMMENTS:**

Student's signature ____________________ Date __________

Partner's signature ____________________ Date __________

Instructor's signature ____________________ Date __________

Great Falls Medical Center Physician Offices

INFORMED CONSENT FOR INACTIVATED INFLUENZA VACCINE

Complete ALL of the following information and sign the acknowledgment for consent to receive an inactivated influenza vaccine.

PATIENT INFORMATION:

Last name, First Name, Middle Initial	Date of Birth	Age:
Street Address:	Gender: M F (circle)	Email:
City, State, Zip	Cell Phone Number:	Work Phone Number:

INSURANCE/RESPONSIBLE PARTY INFORMATION:

Name of Financially Responsible Person:	Name of Policy Holder (Last, First, MI)	Date of Birth:
Address if different from patient:	Insurance Company:	
Relationship to Patient:	Member ID Number:	Group Number:

HEALTH QUESTIONNAIRE *(check yes or no):*

Place a check mark next to the questions below for the person receiving the vaccine:	Yes	No
1. Do you feel sick today or are you experiencing a high fever, vomiting or diarrhea?		
2. Have you ever had a serious reaction after receiving an immunization?		
3. Do you have any allergies to **medication, latex, or food** including eggs, yeast, or gelatin?		
4. Do you have a weakened immune system due to a disease such as cancer, HIV/AIDS, etc.?		
5. Have you ever had a seizure disorder for which you are on medications?		
6. Have you ever had a nervous system problem?		
7. Do you have any chronic health condition such as heart, lung, kidney, or blood disorder?		
8. Are you pregnant?		

CONSENT FOR TREATMENT:

A copy of the **most recent Vaccine Information Statement dated _______ has been provided to me about the inactivated influenza vaccine.**

I have read information and have been given an opportunity to ask questions that have been answered to my satisfaction about the disease and the vaccine to be administered. I understand the benefits and risks of the vaccine and hereby **consent and authorization for the administration of the inactivated influenza vaccine.**

Signature of Patient *(Parent or Guardian, if minor)*	**Date:**

PSY PROCEDURE 2-2 Reporting an Infectious Disease

Name: ____________________ **Date:** __________ **Time:** __________ **Grade:** __________

EQUIPMENT: Computer, Internet connection, search engine, or Web site list

KEY: 4 = Satisfactory 0 = Unsatisfactory NA = This step is not counted

PROCEDURE STEPS	SELF	PARTNER	INSTRUCTOR
1. Using a search engine, go to the Department of Health for your state and search for reporting requirements for hepatitis B.	❑	❑	❑
2. Input keywords such as: Reportable disease, hepatitis B, etc.	❑	❑	❑
3. Interpret your state's requirement and circulate information gathered to all appropriate employees with an avenue for sharing information.	❑	❑	❑
4. AFF Explain how you can protect the patient's private health information in the medical record from being accessed by others.	❑	❑	❑

____

____

____

____

CALCULATION

Total Possible Points: __________

Total Points Earned: __________ Multiplied by 100 = __________ Divided by Total Possible Points = __________ %

PASS **FAIL** **COMMENTS:**

❑ ❑

Student's signature ____________________ Date __________

Partner's signature ____________________ Date __________

Instructor's signature ____________________ Date __________

PSY PROCEDURE 2-3 Monitoring Federal and State Regulations, Changes, and Updates

Name: ______________ **Date:** ________ **Time:** ________ **Grade:** ________

EQUIPMENT: Computer, Internet connection, search engine, or Web site list

KEY: 4 = Satisfactory 0 = Unsatisfactory NA = This step is not counted

PROCEDURE STEPS	SELF	PARTNER	INSTRUCTOR
1. Using a search engine, go to the homepage for your state government (Example: http://www.nc.gov) and/or other related sites such as: Centers for Disease Control and Prevention (CDC), Occupational Safety and Health Act (OSHA), your state medical society, and the American Medical Association (AMA).	❑	❑	❑
2. Input keywords such as: Health care finances, allied health professionals, outpatient medical care, Medicare, etc.	❑	❑	❑
3. Create and enforce a policy for timely dissemination of information received by fax or e-mail from outside agencies.	❑	❑	❑
4. Circulate information gathered to all appropriate employees with an avenue for sharing information. Any information obtained should be shared.	❑	❑	❑
5. Post changes in policies and procedures in a designated area of the office.	❑	❑	❑
6. AFF Explain what you would say to a fellow employee who responds to a change in a current law with, "I will just keep doing it the old way. Who is going to care?"	❑	❑	❑

____

____

____

____

CALCULATION

Total Possible Points: ________

Total Points Earned: ________ Multiplied by 100 = ________ Divided by Total Possible Points = ________ %

PASS ❑ **FAIL** ❑ **COMMENTS:**

Student's signature ______________ Date ________

Partner's signature ______________ Date ________

Instructor's signature ______________ Date ________

PSY PROCEDURE 2-4 Create an Office Policy to Report an Illegal Activity

Name: ______________________ **Date:** __________ **Time:** __________ **Grade:** __________

EQUIPMENT: Computer, Internet connection, search engine, or Web site list

KEY: 4 = Satisfactory 0 = Unsatisfactory NA = This step is not counted

PROCEDURE STEPS	SELF	PARTNER	INSTRUCTOR
1. Using a search engine, locate your state's law that defines reportable child abuse and find your Health and Human Services Department for contact information to report cases of suspected child abuse and/or neglect.	❑	❑	❑
2. Write an office policy listing the steps for documenting the action taken and follow-up as directed by the child welfare agency.	❑	❑	❑
3. Identify the name and title of the employee who will be responsible for contacting the child welfare or law enforcement member when directed by a physician in the office policy.	❑	❑	❑
4. Distribute the policy to every employee obtaining signatures of acknowledgment of receipt and of their understanding of the policy and/or revisions.	❑	❑	❑

____

____

____

____

CALCULATION

Total Possible Points: __________

Total Points Earned: __________ Multiplied by 100 = __________ Divided by Total Possible Points = __________ %

PASS ❑ **FAIL** ❑ **COMMENTS:**

Student's signature ____________________ Date __________

Partner's signature ____________________ Date __________

Instructor's signature ____________________ Date __________

PSY PROCEDURE 2-5 Create an Office Policy to Protect Patient's Private Health Information

Name: ______________________ **Date:** __________ **Time:** __________ **Grade:** __________

EQUIPMENT: Computer, Internet connection, search engine, or Web site list

KEY: 4 = Satisfactory 0 = Unsatisfactory NA = This step is not counted

PROCEDURE STEPS	SELF	PARTNER	INSTRUCTOR
1. Using a search engine, locate your state's law that defines reportable child abuse and find your Health and Human Services Department for contact information to report cases of suspected child abuse and/or neglect.	❑	❑	❑
2. Write an office policy listing the steps for documenting the action taken and follow-up as directed by the child welfare agency.	❑	❑	❑
3. Identify the name and title of the employee who will be responsible for contacting the child welfare or law enforcement member when directed by a physician in the office policy.	❑	❑	❑
4. Distribute the policy to every employee obtaining signatures of acknowledgment of receipt and of their understanding of the policy and/or revisions.	❑	❑	❑

____

____

____

____

CALCULATION

Total Possible Points: __________

Total Points Earned: __________ Multiplied by 100 = __________ Divided by Total Possible Points = __________ %

PASS ❑ **FAIL** ❑ **COMMENTS:**

Student's signature ____________________ Date __________

Partner's signature ____________________ Date __________

Instructor's signature ____________________ Date __________

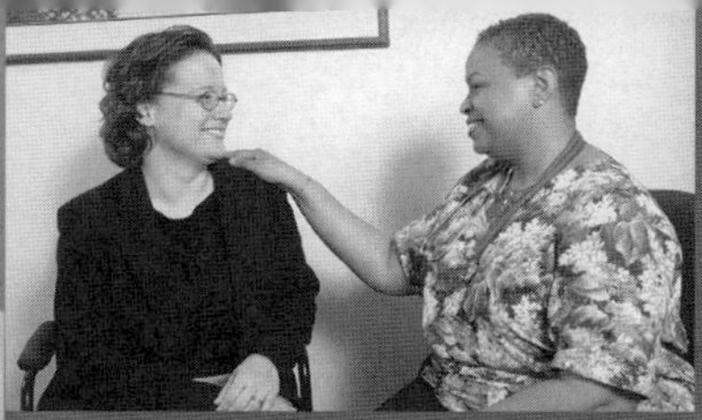

CHAPTER

3 Communication Skills

Learning Outcomes

COG Cognitive Domain

1. Spell and define the key terms
2. List two major forms of communication
3. Identify styles and types of verbal communication
4. Identify types of nonverbal communication
5. Recognize barriers to communication
6. Identify techniques for overcoming communication barriers
7. Recognize the elements of oral communication using a sender–receiver process
8. Identify resources and adaptations that are required based on individual needs, that is, culture and environment, developmental life stage, language, and physical threats to communication
9. Discuss examples of diversity: cultural, social, and ethnic
10. Discuss the role of cultural, social, and ethic diversity in ethical performance of medical assisting practice
11. Discuss the role of assertiveness in effective professional communication. Relate the following behaviors to professional communications: assertive, aggressive, and passive
12. Discuss the theories of Erik Erikson and Kübler-Ross
13. Explain how various components of communication can affect the meaning of verbal messages
14. Define active listening
15. List and describe the six interviewing techniques
16. Give an example of how cultural differences may affect communication
17. Discuss how to handle communication problems caused by language barriers
18. List two methods that you can use to promote communication among hearing-, sight-, and speech-impaired patients
19. Discuss how to handle an angry or distressed patient
20. List five actions that you can take to improve communication with a child
21. Discuss your role in communicating with a grieving patient or family member
22. Discuss the key elements of interdisciplinary communication
23. Explore issue of confidentiality as it applies to the medical assistant

PSY Psychomotor Domain

1. Respond to nonverbal communication (Procedure 3-1)
2. Use feedback techniques to obtain patient information, including reflection, restatement, and clarification (Procedure 3-1)
3. Coach patients appropriately considering cultural diversity, developmental life stage, and communication barriers (Procedure 3-2)

AFF Affective Domain

1. Demonstrate empathy, active listening, and nonverbal communication
2. Demonstrate respect for individual diversity including gender, race, religion, age, economic standing, and appearance
3. Use appropriate body language and other nonverbal skills in communicating with patients, family, and staff
4. Demonstrate awareness of the territorial boundaries of the person with whom you are communicating
5. Demonstrate sensitivity appropriate to the message being delivered
6. Demonstrate awareness of how an individual's personal appearance affects anticipated responses
7. Demonstrate recognition of the patient's level of understanding in communications
8. Analyze communication in providing appropriate responses/feedback
9. Demonstrate the principles of self-boundaries
10. Respond to issues of confidentiality

Learning Outcomes (continued)

ABHES Competencies

1. Identify and respond appropriately when working with/caring for patients with special needs
2. Use empathy when treating terminally ill patients
3. Identify common stages that terminally ill patients go through and list organizations/support groups that can assist patients and family members of patients struggling with terminal illness
4. Advocate on behalf of family/patients, having the ability to deal and communicate with family
5. Analyze the effect of hereditary, cultural, and environmental influences
6. Locate resources and information for patients and employers
7. Be attentive, listen, and learn
8. Be impartial and show empathy when dealing with patients
9. Communicate on the recipient's level of comprehension
10. Serve as liaison between physician and others
11. Recognize and respond to verbal and nonverbal communication

PSY PROCEDURE 4-1 Document Patient Education

Name: ______________________ **Date:** __________ **Time:** __________ **Grade:** __________

EQUIPMENT/SUPPLIES: Patient's chart, pen

STANDARDS: Given the needed equipment and a place to work, the student will perform this skill with _______ % accuracy in a total of _______ minutes. *(Your instructor will tell you what the percentage and time limits will be before you begin.)*

KEY: 4 = Satisfactory 0 = Unsatisfactory NA = This step is not counted

PROCEDURE STEPS	SELF	PARTNER	INSTRUCTOR
1. Record the date and time of teaching.	❑	❑	❑
2. Record the information taught.	❑	❑	❑
3. Record the manner in which the information was taught.	❑	❑	❑
4. Record your evaluation of your teaching.	❑	❑	❑
5. Record any additional teaching planned.	❑	❑	❑
6. AFF Explain what you would do if you forgot to document an action you took during the patient education process.	❑	❑	❑

____

____

____

Note: The medical assistant may sign his or her name in the patient record using only the "CMA" credential if the office has a signature log denoting the entire credential as "CMA(AAMA)."

CALCULATION

Total Possible Points: __________

Total Points Earned: __________ Multiplied by 100 = __________ Divided by Total Possible Points = __________ %

PASS ❑ **FAIL** ❑ **COMMENTS:**

Student's signature ____________________ Date __________

Partner's signature ____________________ Date __________

Instructor's signature ____________________ Date __________

PSY PROCEDURE 4-2 Advocating on Behalf of Patients

Name: ______________________ **Date:** __________ **Time:** __________ **Grade:** __________

EQUIPMENT/SUPPLIES: Computer with Internet access

STANDARDS: Given the needed equipment and a place to work, the student will perform this skill with ________ % accuracy in a total of ________ minutes. *(Your instructor will tell you what the percentage and time limits will be before you begin.)*

KEY: 4 = Satisfactory 0 = Unsatisfactory NA = This step is not counted

PROCEDURE STEPS	SELF	PARTNER	INSTRUCTOR
1. Assess the patient's needs for the following: **a.** Education **b.** Health insurance coverage **c.** Financial information **d.** Support groups **e.** Home health needs	❑	❑	❑
2. Using a search engine, research available resources to have available for patients and to be prepared with materials on hand to give to patients	❑	❑	❑
3. Give the patient the contact information in writing.	❑	❑	❑
4. Document actions and the information given to the patient.	❑	❑	❑
5. Instruct the patient to contact the office if he has any difficulty.	❑	❑	❑
6. AFF Explain what suggestions or assistance you would offer to a patient who would benefit from online patient education resources but does not own a computer.	❑	❑	❑

____

____

____

CALCULATION

Total Possible Points: __________

Total Points Earned: __________ Multiplied by 100 = __________ Divided by Total Possible Points = __________ %

PASS ❑ **FAIL** ❑ **COMMENTS:**

Student's signature ______________________ Date __________

Partner's signature ______________________ Date __________

Instructor's signature ______________________ Date __________

PART

2

The Administrative Medical Assistant

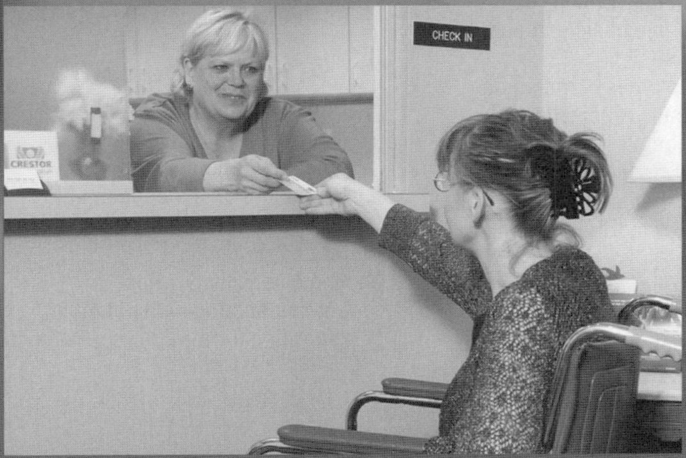

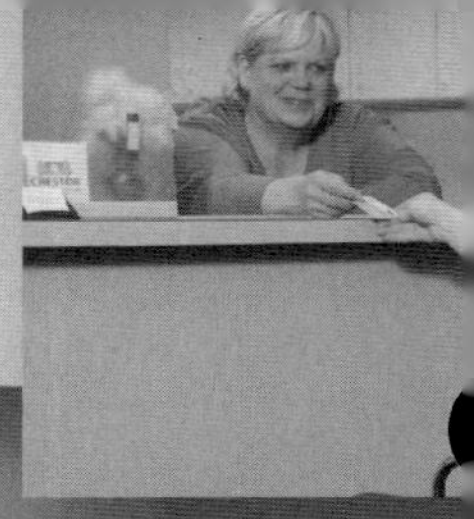

CHAPTER 5 The First Contact: Telephone and Reception

Learning Outcomes

COG Cognitive Domain

1. Spell and define the key terms
2. Explain the importance of displaying a professional image to all patients
3. List six duties of the medical office receptionist
4. List four sources from which messages can be retrieved
5. Discuss various steps that can be taken to promote good ergonomics
6. Describe the basic guidelines for waiting room environments
7. Describe the proper method for maintaining infection control standards in the waiting room
8. Discuss the five basic guidelines for telephone use
9. Describe the types of incoming telephone calls received by the medical office
10. Discuss how to identify and handle callers with medical emergencies
11. Describe how to triage incoming calls
12. List the information that should be given to an emergency medical service dispatcher
13. Describe the types of telephone services and special features
14. Discuss applications of electronic technology in effective communication

PSY Psychomotor Domain

1. Handle incoming calls (Procedure 5-1)
   - Demonstrate professional telephone techniques (Procedures 5-1 and 5-2)
2. Coach patients regarding office policies (Procedure 5-3)
3. Report relevant information concisely, succinctly, and accurately (Procedure 5-1)

AFF Affective Domain

1. Demonstrate empathy, active listening, and nonverbal communication
2. Implement time management principles to maintain effective office function
3. Show sensitivity when communicating with patients regarding third-party requirements
4. Demonstrate awareness of the consequences of not working within the legal scope of practice
5. Demonstrate sensitivity in communicating with both providers and patients
6. Demonstrate sensitivity to patient rights
7. Protect the integrity of the medical record
8. Recognize the physical and emotional effects on persons involved in an emergency situation
9. Demonstrate self-awareness in responding to an emergency situation

ABHES Competencies

1. Use proper telephone technique
2. Receive, organize, prioritize, and transmit information expediently
3. Apply electronic technology

37. A patient comes into the office with a severe bloody nose. He or she leaves bloody tissues in the waiting room and got blood on a magazine and a chair. Your supervisor says to you, "Come on! Get some gloves. We've got to clean this right away." Why do you need gloves? Why is it important that the waiting room be cleaned immediately?

____

____

____

____

COG TRUE OR FALSE?

Grade: ____________

As a receptionist, you'll be answering incoming calls. Review the statements below and place a check in the "True" column for those that are true and place a check in the "False" column for those that are false.

Incoming Calls	True	False
38. Always ask new patients for their phone number in case you need to call them back.		
39. Always give patients an exact quote for services if asked.		
40. Patient information cannot be given to anyone without the patient's consent.		
41. All laboratory results phoned into the office must be immediately brought to the physician's attention.		
42. When a nursing home calls with a satisfactory report about a patient, you should take the information down, record it in the patient's chart, and place it on the physician's desk for review.		
43. Never discuss unsatisfactory test results with a patient unless the doctor directs you to do so.		
44. Medical assistants are not allowed to take care of prescription refill requests.		

PSY TRIAGE

Grade: ____________

45. Triage the following calls by writing the letters in the proper order. ____________

a. Line 1: A school nurse calls with a question about a medical form.

b. Line 2: A mother calls about her child who is having an asthma attack.

c. Line 3: A father calls with a question about his daughter's medication.

d. Line 4: A patient calls complaining about a sore throat.

COG SHORT ANSWER

Grade: ______

46. A woman calls the office frantic because she thinks she is having a heart attack. What information should you try to get first from the caller?

______

47. A patient in your office is having trouble breathing. You have been asked to call EMS. What five pieces of information will you need before you make the call?

______

48. Dr. Porter is in a meeting, but he has instructed you to communicate with him via cell phone when you get the test results back for a certain patient. However, he does not like to have his cell phone ring while he is in meetings. How will you communicate with him?

______

49. It is an exceptionally hot day in the spring. Because the air conditioner is not on yet, you take a chair from the waiting room and prop the door open with it. You also move the boxes that were delivered earlier away from the window so the air comes in. How is this a violation of the Americans with Disabilities Act?

______

50. You receive a call from a patient who complains of being short of breath. What questions will you ask to determine whether this is an emergency?

______

AFF PSY ACTIVE LEARNING

Grade: ___________

51. Working with two classmates, role-play a medical emergency in the physician's office waiting room. Have one person play the role of the patient, the second person play the role of the receptionist, and the third person play the role of the EMS call operator. The patient should describe his or her condition, and the receptionist is responsible for conveying these details to EMS. Switch roles so that everyone gets a chance to play each role.

____

____

____

____

WHAT WOULD YOU DO?

Grade: ___________

52. Your office shows videos about healthy living, exercise, and nutrition throughout the day. It seems that most of the adults watch and enjoy the programming. One crowded afternoon, a patient comes up to the desk to complain that the programming is distracting and he would prefer having the television turned off. However, there are people in the room watching the television. What would you say to the upset patient?

____

____

____

____

53. Mrs. Gonzalez calls to schedule her annual checkup. She is put on hold, and when the receptionist comes back to her call, she is upset that she was placed on hold. When she comes in for her appointment, she says that the receptionist should deal with every call individually and that no one should be placed on hold. How would you explain the phone call triage system to her?

____

____

____

____

AFF CASE STUDY FOR CRITICAL THINKING

Grade: ___________

You are working for a pediatrician. A mother arrives carrying an 18-month-old child with symptoms of a respiratory illness. You ask for her insurance card and she yells, "take care of my child first." You are willing to rearrange the usual order of things, but when you direct her to sit in the sick-child area, as per office protocol, the mother refuses, stating, "I don't want my child to get sicker." Circle the appropriate response from the lists below each question.

54. What might you say to make the mother give you the insurance information?

a. I am required to update your chart, including your insurance information, at each visit *before* you see the physician.

b. The physician will not see your child until I see your card.

c. You are being very difficult. Can we start over?

d. I'll hold the child while you get your card out.

55. What is your best action regarding the waiting area?
a. Tell the physician.
b. Calmly explain the policy and why you have it.
c. Even though you will be putting her ahead of others, put the child in an open exam room.
d. Ask the mother to leave.
e. Tell her to take the child to the emergency room.

56. What is the most important thing you can do to make difficult situations like this better?
a. Place signs in the waiting area about behavior.
b. Make sure your work area is clean and neat.
c. Make sure you always have someone else with you in the reception area.
d. Remain calm and act professionally.
e. Stand your ground with the angry person.

PSY PROCEDURE 5-1 Handling Incoming Calls

Name: ______________________ **Date:** __________ **Time:** __________ **Grade:** __________

EQUIPMENT/SUPPLIES: Telephone, telephone message pad, writing utensil (pen or pencil), headset (if applicable)

STANDARDS: Given the needed equipment and a place to work, the student will perform this skill with _____ % accuracy in a total of _____ minutes. *(Your instructor will tell you what the percentage and time limits will be before you begin.)*

KEY: 4 = Satisfactory 0 = Unsatisfactory NA = This step is not counted

PROCEDURE STEPS	SELF	PARTNER	INSTRUCTOR
1. Gather the needed equipment.	❑	❑	❑
2. Answer the phone within three rings.	❑	❑	❑
3. Greet caller with proper identification (your name and the name of the office).	❑	❑	❑
4. Identify the nature or reason for the call in a timely manner.	❑	❑	❑
5. Triage the call appropriately.	❑	❑	❑
6. Communicate in a professional manner and with unhurried speech.	❑	❑	❑
7. Clarify information as needed.	❑	❑	❑
8. Record the message on a message pad. Include the name of caller, date, time, telephone number where the caller can be reached, description of the caller's concerns, and person to whom the message is routed.	❑	❑	❑
9. Give the caller an approximate time for a return call.	❑	❑	❑
10. Ask the caller whether he or she has any additional questions or needs any other help.	❑	❑	❑
11. Allow the caller to disconnect first.	❑	❑	❑
12. Put the message in an assigned place.	❑	❑	❑
13. Complete the task within 10 minutes.	❑	❑	❑
14. AFF Explain how you would respond to a patient who is obviously angry.	❑	❑	❑

____

____

____

____

PSY PROCEDURE 5-1 Handling Incoming Calls (continued)

CALCULATION

Total Possible Points: __________

Total Points Earned: __________ Multiplied by 100 = __________ Divided by Total Possible Points = __________ %

PASS ❑ **FAIL** ❑ **COMMENTS:**

Student's signature ____________________ Date __________

Partner's signature ____________________ Date __________

Instructor's signature ____________________ Date __________

PSY PROCEDURE 5-2 Calling Emergency Medical Services

Name: ______________________ **Date:** __________ **Time:** __________ **Grade:** __________

EQUIPMENT/SUPPLIES: Telephone, patient information, writing utensil (pen, pencil)

STANDARDS: Given the needed equipment and a place to work, the student will perform this skill with _____ % accuracy in a total of _____ minutes. *(Your instructor will tell you what the percentage and time limits will be before you begin.)*

KEY: 4 = Satisfactory 0 = Unsatisfactory NA = This step is not counted

PROCEDURE STEPS	SELF	PARTNER	INSTRUCTOR
1. Obtain the following the information before dialing: patient's name, age, sex, nature of medical condition, type of service the physician is requesting, any special instructions or requests the physician may have, your location, and any special information for access.	❑	❑	❑
2. Dial 911 or other EMS number.	❑	❑	❑
3. Calmly provide the dispatcher with the above information.	❑	❑	❑
4. Answer the dispatcher's questions calmly and professionally.	❑	❑	❑
5. Follow the dispatcher's instructions, if applicable.	❑	❑	❑
6. End the call as per dispatcher instructions.	❑	❑	❑
7. Complete the task within 10 minutes.	❑	❑	❑
8. AFF Explain how you would respond to a family member who is getting in the way of performing this task.	❑	❑	❑

____

____

____

____

CALCULATION

Total Possible Points: __________

Total Points Earned: __________ Multiplied by 100 = __________ Divided by Total Possible Points = __________ %

PASS **FAIL** **COMMENTS:**

❑ ❑

Student's signature ____________________ Date __________

Partner's signature ____________________ Date __________

Instructor's signature ____________________ Date __________

PSY PROCEDURE 5-3 Searching on the Internet

Name: ______________________ **Date:** __________ **Time:** __________ **Grade:** __________

EQUIPMENT/SUPPLIES: Patient's chart, office brochure

STANDARDS: Given the needed equipment and a place to work, the student will perform this skill with _____ % accuracy in a total of _____ minutes. *(Your instructor will tell you what the percentage and time limits will be before you begin.)*

KEY: 4 = Satisfactory 0 = Unsatisfactory NA = This step is not counted

PROCEDURE STEPS	SELF	PARTNER	INSTRUCTOR
1. Assess the patient's level of understanding.	❑	❑	❑
2. Review important areas and highlight these in the office brochure.	❑	❑	❑
3. Ask the patient if he or she understands or has any questions.	❑	❑	❑
4. Give the patient the brochure to take home.	❑	❑	❑
5. Put in place a procedure for updating information and letting patients know of changes.	❑	❑	❑
6. AFF Explain how you would instruct a hearing-impaired patient about office procedures.	❑	❑	❑

____

____

____

____

CALCULATION

Total Possible Points: __________

Total Points Earned: __________ Multiplied by 100 = __________ Divided by Total Possible Points = __________ %

PASS ❑ **FAIL** ❑ **COMMENTS:**

Student's signature ____________________ Date __________

Partner's signature ____________________ Date __________

Instructor's signature ____________________ Date __________

41. When calling another physician's office for an appointment for your patient, you'll need to provide certain information. List the seven pieces of information that you should provide to another physician's office.

____

____

____

____

42. List three items usually included in preadmission testing for surgery.

____

____

____

____

COG TRUE OR FALSE?

Grade: ________

Determine whether the following statements are true or false. If false, explain why.

43. Fixed scheduling is the most commonly used method.

____

44. A medical office that operates with open hours for patient visits is open 24 hours a day, 7 days a week.

____

45. Most appointments for new patients are made in person.

____

46. Patients with medical emergencies need to be seen immediately.

____

COG PSY ACTIVE LEARNING

Grade: ________

47. The appointment book below is divided into half-hour increments. The spaces below each time slot are empty. Fill in the appointment book with the following information: Dr. Brown has hospital rounds from 8:00 AM to 9:00 AM. He has the following appointments: Cindy Wallis at 9:30 AM; Bill Waters at 10:00 AM; Rodney Kingston at 10:30 AM.

8:00	8:30	9:00	9:30	10:00	10:30

Draw a line from the service to the appropriate time allotment.

Service	Estimated Time
48. blood pressure check	**a.** 5 minutes
49. complete physical exam	**b.** 10 minutes
50. dressing change	**c.** 15 minutes
51. recheck	**d.** 30 minutes
52. school physical	**e.** 1 hour

COG IDENTIFICATION

Grade: ________

Identify each type of scheduling system in the chart below.

Description	Type of Scheduling System
53. Several patients are scheduled for the first 30 minutes of each hour.	
54. Appointments are given based on the needs of individual patients.	
55. Each hour is divided into increments of 15, 30, 45, or 60 minutes for appointments depending on the reason for the visit.	
56. Patients are grouped according to needs or problems.	
57. Two patients are scheduled for the same period with the same physician.	

COG PSY CORRECT OR INCORRECT?

Grade: ________

Below are the steps for making a return appointment. Some of the steps are false or incomplete. Review each step and then decide if it is correct or incorrect. If incorrect, rewrite the statement to make it true and complete.

58. Carefully check your appointment book or screen before offering an appointment time. If a specific examination, test, or x-ray is to be performed on the return visit, avoid scheduling two patients for the same examination at the same time.

____

59. Ask the patient when he or she would like to return.

____

60. Write the patient's name and telephone number in the appointment book or enter the information in computer.

____

61. Transfer the information to an appointment card that you will mail out to the patient at a later date.

____

62. Double-check your book or screen to be sure there are no errors.

____

63. End your conversation with a pleasant word and a smile.

____

AFF WHAT WOULD YOU DO?

Grade: ___________

64. An older adult patient walks into the medical office. His constellation of symptoms includes chest discomfort, shortness of breath, and nausea. He doesn't have an appointment. Explain what you would do.

____

____

____

____

65. Sometimes, a patient may neglect to keep an appointment. When this happens, you should call the patient. What should you do if you are unable to reach the patient by phone?

____

____

____

____

66. Maria has just called into the office to cancel her appointment for today. Explain what you should do.

____

____

____

____

67. If diagnostic testing requires preparation from the patient, what should you do?

____

____

____

____

AFF PATIENT EDUCATION

Grade: ___________

68. Juan is consistently late for appointments. You've spoken with him several times. What should you do next? Explain what you will you say to him and the information you will provide him with.

____

____

____

____

AFF CASE STUDY FOR CRITICAL THINKING A

Grade: ___________

You are the RMA at the front desk of a busy family practice. The success of the day depends on how smoothly the schedule runs. It is your responsibility to check patients in as they arrive. Your office uses a sign-in sheet. Mr. Simpson is always late for his appointments and today is no exception.

69. Regarding the sign-in sheet, what other methods could you use that would limit the potential for invasion of patient privacy?
- **a.** Have patients give their name to the receptionist as they arrive.
- **b.** Periodically walk through the waiting area to see who is there.
- **c.** Post a sign asking patients to whisper when they speak.
- **d.** Use a sign-in clipboard that has a sliding shield to prevent seeing other names.

70. You notice that patients typically wait 30 to 45 minutes past their scheduled appointment times because the physician is chronically behind schedule. How would you handle the situation? Circle the best answer.
- **a.** Tell the office manager to talk to him or you will find other employment.
- **b.** Ask the office manager to put the issue of running behind on the next office meeting agenda.
- **c.** Ask to speak with him or her in private and explain how his running behind affects the entire office.
- **d.** Tease him or her about running behind in front of the patients and employees.

71. Circle the best strategy to handle Mr. Simpson's chronic tardiness.
- **a.** Schedule him for the last appointment of the day.
- **b.** Dismiss him from the physician's care.
- **c.** Call his family and ask if they can get him there on time.
- **d.** Tell him that he is messing up your whole day and he MUST stop being late.
- **e.** Do not worry about it. No matter what you do, he will still be late.

PSY PROCEDURE 6-1 Scheduling an Appointment for a New Patient

Name: ______________________________ **Date:** __________ **Time:** __________ **Grade:** __________

EQUIPMENT/ITEMS NEEDED: Patient's demographic information, patient's chief complaint, appointment book or computer with appointment software, information found in Activity #1

STANDARDS: Given the needed equipment and a place to work, the student will perform this skill with ________ % accuracy in a total of __________ minutes. *(Your instructor will tell you what the percentage and time limits will be before you begin.)*

KEY: 4 = Satisfactory 0 = Unsatisfactory NA = This step is not counted

PROCEDURE STEPS	SELF	PARTNER	INSTRUCTOR
1. Obtain as much information as possible from the patient, such as: • Full name and correct spelling • Mailing address (not all offices require this) • Day and evening telephone numbers • Reason for the visit • Name of the referring person	❑	❑	❑
2. Determine the patient's chief complaint or the reason for seeing the physician.	❑	❑	❑
3. Enter the appointment on a date and for the amount of time established by office policies for a new patient appointment			
4. Explain the cancellation and financial policies of the practice. Instruct patients to bring all pertinent insurance information.	❑	❑	❑
5. Give concise directions if needed.	❑	❑	❑
6. Ask the patient if it is permissible to call at home or at work.	❑	❑	❑
7. Confirm the time and date of the appointment.	❑	❑	❑
8. Check your appointment book to be sure that you have placed the appointment on the correct day in the right time slot.	❑	❑	❑
9. If the patient was referred by another physician, call that physician's office before the appointment for copies of laboratory work, radiology, pathology reports, and so on. Give this information to the physician prior to the patient's appointment.	❑	❑	❑
10. AFF Explain how you would respond in a situation in which a patient does NOT give permission to phone him or her at work.	❑	❑	❑

____

____

____

____

PSY PROCEDURE 6-1 Scheduling an Appointment for a New Patient (continued)

CALCULATION

Total Possible Points: __________

Total Points Earned: __________ Multiplied by 100 = __________ Divided by Total Possible Points = __________ %

PASS **FAIL** **COMMENTS:**

❑ ❑

Student's signature ____________________ Date __________

Partner's signature ____________________ Date __________

Instructor's signature ____________________ Date __________

PSY PROCEDURE 6-2 Scheduling an Appointment for an Established Patient

Name: ______________________ **Date:** __________ **Time:** __________ **Grade:** __________

EQUIPMENT: Appointment book or computer with appointment software, appointment card, information found in Activity #1

STANDARDS: Given the needed equipment and a place to work, the student will perform this skill with _______ % accuracy in a total of _________ minutes. *(Your instructor will tell you what the percentage and time limits will be before you begin.)*

KEY: 4 = Satisfactory 0 = Unsatisfactory NA = This step is not counted

PROCEDURE STEPS	SELF	PARTNER	INSTRUCTOR
1. Determine what will be done at the return visit. Check your appointment book or computer system before offering an appointment.	❏	❏	❏
2. Offer the patient a specific time and date. Avoid asking the patient when he or she would like to return, as this can cause indecision.	❏	❏	❏
3. Write the patient's name and telephone number in the appointment book or enter it in the computer.	❏	❏	❏
4. Transfer the pertinent information to an appointment card and give it to the patient. Repeat aloud the appointment day, date, and time to the patient as you hand over the card.	❏	❏	❏
5. Double-check your book or computer to be sure you have not made an error.	❏	❏	❏
6. End your conversation with a pleasant word and a smile.	❏	❏	❏
7. AFF Explain how you would respond to a patient who insists on coming for a return appointment at a time when their doctor is in surgery.	❏	❏	❏

____

____

____

____

CALCULATION

Total Possible Points: __________

Total Points Earned: __________ Multiplied by 100 = __________ Divided by Total Possible Points = __________ %

PASS ❏ **FAIL** ❏ **COMMENTS:**

Student's signature ______________________ Date __________

Partner's signature ______________________ Date __________

Instructor's signature ______________________ Date __________

PSY PROCEDURE 6-3 Scheduling an Appointment for a Referral to an Outpatient Facility

Name: ______________________ **Date:** __________ **Time:** __________ **Grade:** __________

EQUIPMENT: Patient's chart with demographic information; physician's order for services needed by the patient and reason for the services; patient's insurance card with referral information, referral form, and directions to office, information found in Activity #3

STANDARDS: Given the needed equipment and a place to work, the student will perform this skill with _______ % accuracy in a total of __________ minutes. *(Your instructor will tell you what the percentage and time limits will be before you begin.)*

KEY: 4 = Satisfactory 0 = Unsatisfactory NA = This step is not counted

PROCEDURE STEPS	SELF	PARTNER	INSTRUCTOR
1. Make certain that the requirements of any third-party payers are met.	❑	❑	❑
2. Refer to the patient's insurance to determine if the outpatient facility and the physician performing the procedure participate with the patient's insurance.	❑	❑	❑
3. Have the following information available when you make the call to schedule the procedure: • Physician's name and telephone number • Patient's name, address, and telephone number • Reason for the call • Degree of urgency • The patient's insurance information and precertification number, if necessary • Whether the patient is being sent for consultation or referral	❑	❑	❑
4. Advise the patient verbally and in writing of the following information as soon as possible: • The date, time, and location of the procedures • Any specific restrictions or requirements to prepare for the procedure	❑	❑	❑
5. Record in the patient's chart the time and date of the call and the name of the person who received your call.	❑	❑	❑
6. Tell the person you are calling that you wish to be notified if your patient does not keep the appointment. If this occurs, be sure to tell your physician and enter this information in the patient's record.	❑	❑	❑
7. AFF Explain how you would handle the following situation: There are two physicians listed for a certain specialty in a patient's managed care's preferred provider list. The patient asks you who she should choose.	❑	❑	❑

PSY PROCEDURE 6-3 Scheduling an Appointment for a Referral to an Outpatient Facility (continued)

____

____

____

____

CALCULATION

Total Possible Points: __________

Total Points Earned: __________ Multiplied by 100 = __________ Divided by Total Possible Points = __________ %

PASS ❑ **FAIL** ❑ **COMMENTS:**

Student's signature ____________________ Date __________

Partner's signature ____________________ Date __________

Instructor's signature ____________________ Date __________

PSY PROCEDURE 6-4 Arranging for Admission to an Inpatient Facility

Name: ______________________ **Date:** __________ **Time:** __________ **Grade:** __________

EQUIPMENT: Physician's order with diagnosis, patient's chart with demographic information, contact information for inpatient facility, information found in Activity #2

STANDARDS: Given the needed equipment and a place to work, the student will perform this skill with ________ % accuracy in a total of __________ minutes. *(Your instructor will tell you what the percentage and time limits will be before you begin.)*

KEY: 4 = Satisfactory 0 = Unsatisfactory NA = This step is not counted

PROCEDURE STEPS	SELF	PARTNER	INSTRUCTOR
1. Determine the place patient and/or physician wants the admission arranged.	❑	❑	❑
2. Gather information for the other facility, including demographic and insurance information.	❑	❑	❑
3. Determine any precertification requirements. If needed, locate contact information on the back of the insurance card and call the insurance carrier to obtain a precertification number.	❑	❑	❑
4. Obtain from the physician the diagnosis and exact needs of the patient for an admission.	❑	❑	❑
5. Call the admissions department of the inpatient facility and give information from step 2.	❑	❑	❑
6. Obtain instructions for the patient and call or give the patient instructions and information.	❑	❑	❑
7. Provide the patient with the physician's orders for their hospital stay, including diet, medications, bed rest, etc.	❑	❑	❑
8. Document time, place, etc. in patient's chart, including any pre-certification requirements completed.	❑	❑	❑
9. AFF Explain how you would respond to a patient who is visibly shaken about finding out that he is being admitted to the hospital.	❑	❑	❑

____

____

____

____

PROCEDURE 6-4 Arranging for Admission to an Inpatient Facility (continued)

CALCULATION

Total Possible Points: __________

Total Points Earned: __________ Multiplied by 100 = __________ Divided by Total Possible Points = __________ %

PASS ❑ **FAIL** ❑ **COMMENTS:**

Student's signature ____________________ Date __________

Partner's signature ____________________ Date __________

Instructor's signature ____________________ Date __________

Activity #1: Scheduling New and Returning Patients

Place the patients on the appointment book page provided. In order to make this activity more realistic, imagine that the patients are calling the office in the order they are listed. You will need to determine the time needed for the visit and the urgency of the patient's problem in assigning slots. Refer to Box 6-1 in the textbook for suggested time allotment.

Set up the page and establish the matrix: Providers and availability:

Dr. Jones sees patients from 2:00 PM to 5:00 PM. In surgery until 12:00.
Dr. Smith sees patients from 8:00 AM to 3:00 PM. No lunch.
Dr. Stowe sees patients from 8:00 AM to 5:00 PM with lunch from 12:00 to 1:30 PM.

Jessica Marshall, CMA (AAMA), can give injections and do blood pressure checks. Lunch 1:00 to 2:00 PM. Use the lab column for patients who can see her.

Patient Name	Reason	Telephone #
1. Jeremy Cole	Stepped on rusty nail	570-7890
2. Cheryl Jennings (New)	Needs college physical	765-9087
3. Patty Cook	Sore throat	799-7225
4. Susan Stills	Woke up feeling dizzy	836-8765
5. Pamela Jones (New)	Wants to talk about weight reduction	765-0123
6. Steve Elliott	Hand laceration at work (supv. called)	799-4391
7. Amy Quarrels	Vomiting and diarrhea × 3 days	571-5923
8. Layla Harris	Nosebleed that won't stop	799-0127
9. Sharon Morris	Needs refill on pain meds	836-2100
10. Jared Davis	Blood pressure check	792-8333
11. Ginger Parks	Knee injury last week, still swelling	791-4752
12. Landon Smythe	Coughing up blood	414-6787
13. Raymond Gray	Confused and foggy, per son	922-8641
14. Seth Etchison	Skin rash	266-0999
15. Raji Omar	Allergy injection	607-9125
16. Marilyn Easley	Shortness of breath and nausea	903-8957
17. Stephanie Lewis	Frequent urination and burning	792-1480
18. Shannon Mitchell	Pregnancy test	799-0731
19. Shantina Branch (New)	Kindergarten physical	792-4500
20. Lee Davis	Recheck on strep throat	799-4800

What might you do differently with the new patients?

___

___

___

___

THURSDAY, APRIL 11

HOUR		Dr. Jones	Dr. Smith	Dr. Stowe	Lab
8	00				
8	15				
8	30				
8	45				
9	00				
9	15				
9	30				
9	45				
10	00				
10	15				
10	30				
10	45				
11	00				
11	15				
11	30				
11	45				
12	00				
12	15				
12	30				
12	45				
1	00				
1	15				
1	30				
1	45				
2	00				
2	15				
2	30				
2	45				
3	00				
3	15				
3	30				
3	45				
4	00				
4	15				
4	30				
4	45				
5	00				
5	15				
5	30				
5	45				
6	00				
6	15				
6	30				
6	45				
7	00				
N					
O					
T					
E					
S					

Activity #2: Scheduling Inpatient Admission

You work for Dr. James Gibbs, whose office is at 102 South Hawthorne Road, Winston-Salem, NC 27103. The office phone number is 336-760-4216.

Stella Walker is a 42-year-old female patient with diabetes. She has Blue Cross Blue Shield of NC. Her date of birth is 5/6/64. Her subscriber ID# is 260-21-5612. Her group # is 26178. She is the policyholder.

Dr. Gibbs instructs you to arrange admission to Forsyth Medical Center for Stella Walker for tomorrow. Her admitting diagnosis is uncontrolled diabetes. Her insurance requires that you precertify her for this admission. The doctor gives you his written orders and instructs you to give them to the patient to hand carry to the hospital.

You call the insurance company using the phone number on the back of her insurance card. The insurance company gives you the precertification number 1238952-1 and tells you that she is certified to stay in the hospital for 3 days. She has a $100.00 co-pay for a hospital stay.

Complete the form provided.

Hospital Admission

Patient Name: ______________________________

Patient Insurance Company: ______________________________

Patient Date of Birth: ______________________________

Patient Subscriber ID#: ______________________________

Patient Group #: ______________________________

Insurance Policy Holder: ______________________________

Precertification #: ______________________________

Reason for Admission: ______________________________

Admitting Physician Name and Address ______________________________

____

Approved Length of Stay: ______________________________

Inpatient Co-Pay: ______________________________

Activity #3: Scheduling an Outpatient Procedure

Using the information on the physician's order below, record the dates and times for appointments made for Grace Woods to have arthroscopy of the left knee and physical therapy at Miracle Rehabilitation before and after surgery. Read the information carefully!

Physician's Order:

Hinged knee brace fitting for use after surgery at Miracle Rehabilitation.

Left knee arthroscopy with medial meniscal repair. Follow-up with me in office 5 days post-op.

Physical Therapy at Miracle Rehabilitation for eight sessions beginning 1 week after surgery.

Date of surgery: ______________________________

Date of Miracle Rehab appointment for fitting of brace: ______________________________

Dates of Miracle Rehab physical therapy appointments: ______________________________

____

____

Date of postoperative visit in your office: ______________________________

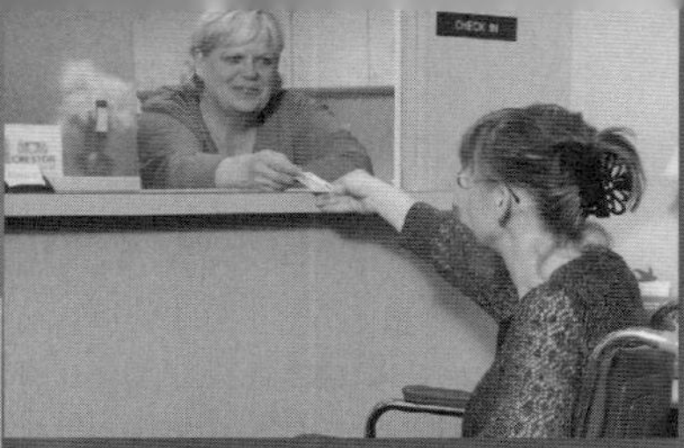

CHAPTER

7 Written Communications

Learning Outcomes

COG Cognitive Domain

1. Spell and define the key terms
2. Recognize elements of fundamental writing skills
3. Discuss the basic guidelines for grammar, punctuation, and spelling in medical writing
4. Organize technical information and summaries
5. Discuss the 11 key components of a business letter
6. Describe the process of writing a memorandum
7. List the items that must be included in an agenda
8. Identify the items that must be included when typing minutes
9. Cite the various services available for sending written information
10. Discuss the various mailing options
11. Identify the types of incoming written communication seen in a physician's office
12. Explain the guidelines for opening and sorting mail
13. Discuss applications of electronic technology in effective communication

PSY Psychomotor Domain

1. Compose a professional correspondence utilizing electronic technology (Procedure 7-1)
2. Open and sort mail (Procedure 7-2)
3. Report relevant information concisely and accurately (Procedure 7-1)

AFF Affective Domain

1. Use language/verbal skills that enable patient's understanding
2. Demonstrate empathy in communicating with patients, family, and staff
3. Demonstrate sensitivity appropriate to the message being delivered
4. Demonstrate recognition of the patient's level of understanding in communications

ABHES Competencies

1. Perform fundamental writing skills including correct grammar, spelling, and formatting techniques when writing prescriptions, documenting medical records, etc.
2. Apply electronic technology
3. Adapt communications to individual's ability to understand
4. Respond to and initiate written communications
5. Utilize electronic technology to receive, organize, prioritize, and transmit information
6. Use correct grammar, spelling, and formatting techniques in written word

COG IDENTIFICATION

Grade: ____

Review the list of terms below and place a check mark to indicate whether each term must always be capitalized.

Name	Always	Not Always
49. Streptococcus		
50. Tylenol		
51. Benadryl		
52. Diagnosis		
53. Analgesic		
54. Merck		
55. Antihistamine		
56. Tampax		

COG PSY ACTIVE LEARNING

Grade: ____

57. Dr. Bruce Mosley asks you to prepare a memorandum for distribution to the entire office. He hands you a note to use as the body of the memo. It reads as follows:
On May 9, Jerry Henderson, a representative of Conrad Insurance, will be visiting the office during the morning. Please extend him the utmost courtesy and introduce yourself if you have not yet met him. Jerry is a wonderful man who has been very helpful to our practice. I will be unavailable during the morning as a result of his visit. Please direct questions to Shelly or Dr. Garcia. Of course, I may be contacted in case of an emergency. Using the sample memorandum format in Figure 7-5 of your text, construct the memo.

COG IDENTIFICATION

Grade: ____

58. You have been asked to send a summary of a patient's recent visit to a specialist. Review the list of forms of written communication below and place a check mark to indicate whether it is an appropriate means of written communication.

Form	Appropriate	Not Appropriate
a. A formal letter labeled confidential		
b. An e-mail marked urgent		
c. A memorandum		
d. A fax with a confidentiality statement		
e. A memorandum labeled urgent		

59. You always take the minutes at the staff meeting, but you'll be on vacation during the next meeting. Identify and list for your coworker what information belongs in the minutes.

____

____

____

60. Dr. Shadrick is at a week-long conference in another state. She needs a patient's complete history to present to the conference one day from now, but has forgotten it at the office. Name three suitable delivery options.

a. ______________________________

b. ______________________________

c. ______________________________

61. Which of the following is/are good practice(s) in regard to handling mail? Place a check mark in the correct box below to answer "Yes" or "No."

Practice	Yes	No
a. Handling promotional materials last		
b. Opening mail addressed to a physician marked "confidential"		
c. Asking a physician or office manager about a piece of mail you are unsure about		
d. Leaving patient correspondence in an external mailbox		
e. Disposing of a physician's personal mail if he or she is away		
f. Informing a covering physician about mail requiring urgent attention		
g. Prioritizing patient care-related mail over pharmaceutical samples		

AFF PSY WHAT WOULD YOU DO?

Grade: __________

62. You are asked to open the mail today. There is a variety of material including several letters addressed to the physician marked "Urgent," "Confidential," and "Personal." Some of the other mail is from patients, but it is not marked in any unusual fashion. Other letters are from insurance companies with which your office is associated. There are also several advertisements and promotional mailings from medical supply companies, pharmaceutical companies, and insurance companies. In addition, there are pieces of mail that do not include a return address. Explain the procedure you would follow in dealing with this mail.

____

____

____

____

PSY PATIENT EDUCATION

Grade: __________

63. The office's policy is to mail a welcome letter to new patients. Make a list of information that should be included in this letter so the patient is prepared for her first visit.

____

____

____

____

AFF CASE STUDY FOR CRITICAL THINKING

Grade: _____

The office manager has asked you to compose a letter to every patient in the practice explaining why their physician will be out of the office for 10 months. The physician is having extensive cosmetic surgery and is taking a medical leave of absence.

64. Your letter should _____ should not _____ include the reason for the absence.

65. Circle the more appropriate sentence for your letter from the two choices below:

a. This letter is to tell you that Dr. Smith will not be here for the next ten months, effective October 1, 2012.

b. This letter is to inform you that Dr. William Smith will be taking a ten-month leave of absence beginning October 1, 2012.

66. Circle the more appropriate sentence for your letter from the two choices below:

a. We hope you will continue to receive medical care from our office. We have 12 other providers who will be available to handle your health care needs.

b. Dr. Smith wants you to see one of our other many excellent providers in the interim

PSY PROCEDURE 7-1 Composing a Business Letter

Name: ______________________ **Date:** __________ **Time:** __________ **Grade:** __________

EQUIPMENT/SUPPLIES: Computer with word processing software, 8 1/2 × 11 white paper, #10 sized envelope

STANDARDS: Given the needed equipment and a place to work, the student will perform this skill with _____ % accuracy in a total of _____ minutes. *(Your instructor will tell you what the percentage and time limits will be before you begin.)*

KEY: 4 = Satisfactory 0 = Unsatisfactory NA = This step is not counted

PROCEDURE STEPS	SELF	PARTNER	INSTRUCTOR
1. Move cursor down two lines below the letterhead and enter today's date, flush right.	❑	❑	❑
2. Flush left, move cursor down two lines and enter the inside address using the name and address of the person to whom you are writing.	❑	❑	❑
3. Enter a reference line.	❑	❑	❑
4. Double space and type the salutation followed by a colon.	❑	❑	❑
5. Double space between paragraphs.	❑	❑	❑
6. Double space and flush right, enter the complimentary close.	❑	❑	❑
7. Move cursor down four spaces and enter the sender's name.	❑	❑	❑
8. Double space and enter initials of the sender in all caps.	❑	❑	❑
9. Enter a slash and your initials in lower case letters.	❑	❑	❑
10. Enter c: and names of those who get copies of the letter.	❑	❑	❑
11. Enter Enc: and the number and description of each enclosed sheet.	❑	❑	❑
12. Print on letterhead.	❑	❑	❑
13. Proofread the letter.	❑	❑	❑
14. Attach the letter to the patient's chart.	❑	❑	❑
15. Submit to the sender of the letter for review and signature.	❑	❑	❑
16. Make a copy of the letter for the patient's chart.	❑	❑	❑
17. Address envelopes using all caps and no punctuation.	❑	❑	❑
18. AFF Explain how you would respond in this situation: your physician receives the letter you prepared and asks you to insert a comma where you know a comma is not required.	❑	❑	❑

PSY PROCEDURE 7-1 Composing a Business Letter (continued)

____

____

____

____

CALCULATION

Total Possible Points: __________

Total Points Earned: __________ Multiplied by 100 = __________ Divided by Total Possible Points = __________ %

PASS ❑ **FAIL** ❑ **COMMENTS:**

Student's signature ____________________ Date __________

Partner's signature ____________________ Date __________

Instructor's signature ____________________ Date __________

PSY PROCEDURE 7-2 Opening and Sorting Incoming Mail

Name: ______________________ **Date:** __________ **Time:** __________ **Grade:** __________

EQUIPMENT/SUPPLIES: Letter opener, paper clips, directional tabs, date stamp

STANDARDS: Given the needed equipment and a place to work, the student will perform this skill with _______ % accuracy in a total of _________ minutes. *(Your instructor will tell you what the percentage and time limits will be before you begin.)*

KEY: 4 = Satisfactory 0 = Unsatisfactory NA = This step is not counted

PROCEDURE STEPS	SELF	PARTNER	INSTRUCTOR
1. Gather the necessary equipment.	❑	❑	❑
2. Open all letters and check for enclosures.	❑	❑	❑
3. Paper clip enclosures to the letter.	❑	❑	❑
4. Date-stamp each item.	❑	❑	❑
5. Sort the mail into categories and deal with it appropriately. Generally, you should handle the following types of mail as noted: • Correspondence regarding a patient: Use a paper clip to attach letters, test results, etc., to the patient's chart; place the chart in a pile for the physician to review • Payments and other checks: Record promptly all insurance payments and checks and deposit them according to office policy; account for all drug samples and appropriately log them into the sample book	❑	❑	❑
6. Dispose of miscellaneous advertisements unless otherwise directed.	❑	❑	❑
7. Distribute the mail to the appropriate staff members (physician, office manager, billing manager, etc.)	❑	❑	❑
8. AFF Explain how you would handle a letter marked "Personal and confidential."	❑	❑	❑

____

____

____

____

PSY PROCEDURE 7-2 Opening and Sorting Incoming Mail (continued)

CALCULATION

Total Possible Points: __________

Total Points Earned: __________ Multiplied by 100 = __________ Divided by Total Possible Points = __________ %

PASS ❑ **FAIL** ❑ **COMMENTS:**

Student's signature ____________________ Date __________

Partner's signature ____________________ Date __________

Instructor's signature ____________________ Date __________

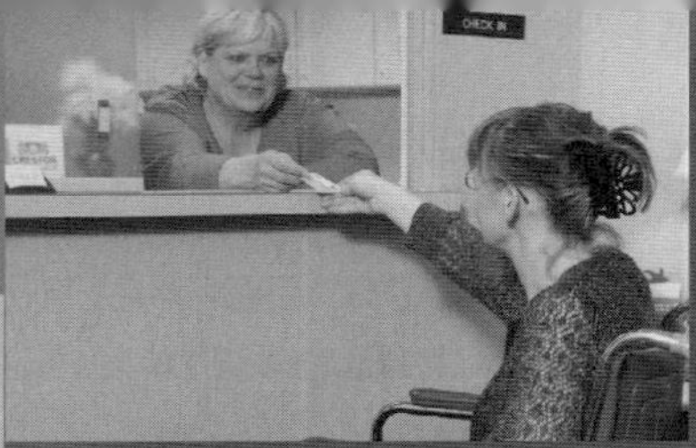

CHAPTER

8 Health Information Management and Protection

Learning Outcomes

COG Cognitive Domain

1. Spell and define the key terms
2. Explain the requirements of the Health Insurance Portability and Accountability Act relating to the sharing and saving of personal and protected health information
3. Identify types of records common to the health care setting
4. Describe standard and electronic health record systems
5. Explain the process for releasing medical records to third-party payers and individual patients
6. Discuss principles of using an electronic medical record
7. Define and describe types of information contained in the patient's medical record
8. Identify methods of organizing the patient's medical record based on problem-oriented medical record (POMR) and source-oriented medical record (SOMR).
9. Explain how to make an entry in a patient's medical record, using abbreviations when appropriate
10. Explain how to make a correction in a standard and electronic health record
11. Discuss pros and cons of various filing methods
12. Describe filing indexing rules
13. Discuss filing procedures
14. Identify equipment and supplies needed for medical records in order to create, maintain, and store.
15. Explain the guidelines of sound policies for record retention
16. Describe the proper disposal of paper and electronic protected health information (PHI)
17. Explore issue of confidentiality as it applies to the medical assistant
18. Describe the implications of HIPAA for the medical assistant in various medical settings
19. Explain the importance of data backup
20. Explain meaningful use as it applies to EMR

PSY Psychomotor Domain

1. Create and organize a patient's medical record (Procedure 8-1)
2. File patient medical records (Procedure 8-2)
3. Maintain organization by filing (Procedure 8-2)
4. Respond to issues of confidentiality (Procedure 8-3)
5. Apply HIPAA rules in regard to privacy/release of information (Procedure 8-3)

AFF Affective Domain

1. Demonstrate sensitivity to patient rights
2. Demonstrate awareness of the consequences of not working within the legal scope of practice
3. Recognize the importance of local, state, and federal legislation and regulations in the practice setting
4. Protect the integrity of the medical record

ABHES Competencies

1. Perform basic clerical functions
2. Prepare and maintain medical records
3. Receive, organize, prioritize, and transmit information expediently
4. Apply electronic technology
5. Institute federal and state guidelines when releasing medical records or information
6. Efficiently maintain and understand different types of medical correspondence and medical reports

52. Your medical office uses an alphabetic filing system. Place the following names in the correct order to show how you would place each record in a filing system.

Brandon P. Snow	Kristen F. Darian-Lewes	Shante L. Dawes	Emil S. Faqir, Jr.
Shaunice L. DeBlase	Juan R. Ortiz	Kim Soo	Fernando P. Vasquez, D.O.

a. ______________________________

b. ______________________________

c. ______________________________

d. ______________________________

e. ______________________________

f. ______________________________

g. ______________________________

h. ______________________________

COG IDENTIFICATION

Grade: __________

53. HIPAA has privacy rules that protect your personal health information. Under HIPAA, covered entities must take certain safety measures to protect patients' information. Read the paragraph below. For each blank, there are two choices. Circle the correct word or phrase for each sentence.

Covered entities must designate a (a) (HIPAA officer, privacy officer) to keep track of who has access to health information. They must also adopt written (b) (privacy, health care) procedures. Under HIPAA, patients have the right to decide if they provide (c) (permission, marketing) before their health information can be used or shared for certain purposes. They also have the right to get a (d) (narrative, report) on when and why their health care information was shared for certain purposes.

COG PSY IDENTIFICATION

Grade: __________

The rules for releasing medical records and authorization are meant to protect patients' privacy rights. Read the questions below regarding the release of medical records and circle "Yes" or "No" for each question.

54. May an 18-year-old patient get copies of his or her own medical records? Yes No

55. May all minors seek treatment for sexually transmitted diseases and birth control without parental knowledge or consent? Yes No

56. When a patient requests copies of his or her own records, does the doctor make the decision about what to copy? Yes No

57. Must the authorization form give the patient the opportunity to limit the information released? Yes No

58. When a patient authorizes the release of information, may he request that the physician leave out information pertinent to the situation? Yes No

COG FILL IN THE BLANKS

Grade: ______

HIPAA requirements provide guidelines and suggestions for safe computer practices when storing or transferring patient information. The following is a list of guidelines that medical facilities are urged to follow. Complete each sentence with the appropriate word from the word bank below.

59. Store _____ in a bank safe deposit box.

60. Change log-in _____ and passwords every 30 days.

61. Turn _____ away from areas where information may be seen by patients.

62. Use _____ with _____ other than letters.

63. Prepare a backup _____ for use when the computer system is down.

Word Bank

characters	plan	disks	information
codes	passwords	template	terminals

Note: Not all words will be used.

MATCHING

Grade: ______

A standard medical record in an outpatient facility, known as a chart or file, contains clinical information as well as billing and insurance information. In the clinical section of the file, you will often find certain types of information. In the columns below, draw a diagonal line to match the clinical type of information with its correct description.

Name of Clinical Information	Description
64. Chief complaint	**a.** Documentation of each patient encounter
65. Family and personal history	**b.** Provider's opinion of the patient's problem
66. Progress notes	**c.** Symptoms that led the patient to seek the physician's care
67. Diagnosis or medical impression	**d.** Letters or memos generated in the facility and sent out
68. Correspondence pertaining to patient	**e.** Review of major illnesses of family members

TRUE OR FALSE?

Grade: ______

69. True or False? Determine whether the following statements are true or false. If false, explain why.

a. HIPAA allows patients to ask to see and get a copy of their health records.

____

b. To maintain secure files, you should change log-in codes and passwords every 10 days.

____

c. Medical history forms are commonly used to gather information from the patient before the visit with the physician.

____

d. Before treating a patient for a possible workers' compensation case, you must first obtain verification from the employer unless the situation is life threatening.

____

WHAT WOULD YOU DO?

Grade: ___________

70. A mother is accused of physically abusing her 16-year-old daughter, a patient with your facility. A police officer who has been asked to investigate visits the medical office and asks for the patient's medical records. What would you do?

____

____

____

____

71. You're in the medical office and you suddenly realize that you've forgotten to document a telephone conversation you had with a patient 2 days ago. What would you do?

____

____

____

____

CASE STUDY FOR CRITICAL THINKING A

Grade: ___________

You are tasked with creating the office policy for the retention of records for your facility.

72. Circle any appropriate actions from the list below.
  a. Research federal law that mandates how long you must keep records.
  b. Research the state legislature to determine the statute of limitations for your state.
  c. Make sure the time limit for retaining records includes inactive and closed files.
  d. Set the time limits for retaining children's records from their 18th birthday.
  e. Set the time limits for retaining the records of adults and children the same for ease of remembering.
  f. Have the policy approved by the physician and/or appropriate employee.

73. This task is not in your job description, and you feel that you are not qualified to set policy for the facility. Circle the appropriate actions from the list below.
  a. Tell your supervisor of your concerns and ask for his or her guidance.
  b. Consider this a great opportunity to show your employer your skills.
  c. Ask the attorney for the facility to create the policy for you.
  d. Ask the attorney not to tell your supervisor that he helped you.
  e. Do the task, but make sure everyone in the office knows who did it.
  f. Do the task without assistance and ask for a promotion and/or raise when finished.

74. What is the statute of limitations for patients to file malpractice or negligence suits in your state? ___________

AFF CASE STUDY FOR CRITICAL THINKING B

Grade: ___________

Your mother's best friend is a patient in the office where you work. You have known her all of your life. She has just been seen for a suspicious lump in her breast. She is very nervous and calls you at home that night to see if you know the results of her test. You saw the stat biopsy report before you left work and you know that the lump is malignant. She was given an appointment in 2 days for the physician to give her the results.

75. Circle all appropriate actions from the list below.
- **a.** Tell her that it is not in your scope of practice to give patients results without specific instructions from a provider, even if they are friends.
- **b.** To minimize the time she must anxiously wait, try to move her appointment to tomorrow as soon as you get to work in the morning.
- **c.** Tell her that the report was not good and to bring someone with her to the visit.
- **d.** Call the physician at home to ask if you can tell her.
- **e.** Tell her that you do not know the results of the test, but even if you did you could not tell her.
- **f.** Call your mother, tell her the situation, and ask for her advice.

76. Let's say you tell the patient that you cannot give test results, and she replies, "I have a right to know what is wrong with me." Circle all of the appropriate responses below.
- **a.** Only a provider can give test results in my office unless they specifically direct an employee to do so.
- **b.** I am a professional, and I don't really care about your rights.
- **c.** I know you are my mother's friend, but I am a CMA, and I follow the rules.
- **d.** Giving you the results of your biopsy may have caused me to get fired. I'm not getting fired for you or anybody.
- **e.** You do have that right, but I do not have the right to tell you.
- **f.** Talk to the physician about it.

77. Why is it important for the physician to give test results such as the one in the case study?

____

____

____

____

PSY PROCEDURE 8-1 Establishing, Organizing, and Maintaining a Medical File

Name: ______________________ **Date:** __________ **Time:** __________ **Grade:** __________

EQUIPMENT/SUPPLIES: File folder; metal fasteners; hole punch; five divider sheets with tabs, title, year, and alphabetic or numeric labels

STANDARDS: Given the needed equipment and a place to work, the student will perform this skill with _____ % accuracy in a total of _____ minutes. *(Your instructor will tell you what the percentage and time limits will be before you begin.)*

KEY: 4 = Satisfactory 0 = Unsatisfactory NA = This step is not counted

PROCEDURE STEPS	SELF	PARTNER	INSTRUCTOR
1. Place the label along the tabbed edge of the folder so that the title extends out beyond the folder itself. (Tabs can be either the length of the folder or tabbed in various positions, such as left, center, and right.)	❑	❑	❑
2. Place a year label along the top edge of the tab before the label with the title. This will be changed each year the patient has been seen. *Note:* Do not automatically replace these labels at the start of a new year; remove the old year and replace with a new one only when the patient comes in for the first visit of the new year.	❑	❑	❑
3. Place the appropriate alphabetic or numeric labels below the title.	❑	❑	❑
4. Apply any additional labels that your office may decide to use.	❑	❑	❑
5. Punch holes and insert demographic and financial information on the left side of the chart using top fasteners across the top.	❑	❑	❑
6. Make tabs for: Ex. H&P, Progress Notes, Medication Log, Correspondence, and Test Results.	❑	❑	❑
7. Place pages behind appropriate tabs.	❑	❑	❑
8. AFF Explain what you would do when you receive a revised copy correcting an error on a document already in a patient's chart.	❑	❑	❑

____

____

____

____

PSY PROCEDURE 8-1 Establishing, Organizing, and Maintaining a Medical File (continued)

CALCULATION

Total Possible Points: __________

Total Points Earned: __________ Multiplied by 100 = __________ Divided by Total Possible Points = __________ %

PASS ❑ **FAIL** ❑ **COMMENTS:**

Student's signature ____________________ Date __________

Partner's signature ____________________ Date __________

Instructor's signature ____________________ Date __________

PSY PROCEDURE 8-2 Filing Medical Records

Name: ______________________ **Date:** __________ **Time:** __________ **Grade:** __________

EQUIPMENT/SUPPLIES: Simulated patient file folder, several single sheets to be filed in the chart, file cabinet with other file

STANDARDS: Given the needed equipment and a place to work, the student will perform this skill with _____ % accuracy in a total of _____ minutes. *(Your instructor will tell you what the percentage and time limits will be before you begin.)*

KEY: 4 = Satisfactory 0 = Unsatisfactory NA = This step is not counted

PROCEDURE STEPS	SELF	PARTNER	INSTRUCTOR
1. Double check spelling of names on the chart and any single sheets to be placed in the folder.	❑	❑	❑
2. Condition any single sheets, etc.	❑	❑	❑
3. Place sheets behind proper tab in the chart.	❑	❑	❑
4. Remove guide.	❑	❑	❑
5. Place the folder between the two appropriate existing folders, taking care to place the folder between the two charts.	❑	❑	❑
6. Scan color coding to ensure none of the charts in that section are out of order.	❑	❑	❑
7. AFF Explain what you would do when you find a chart out of order. Should you bring it to the attention of your supervisor?	❑	❑	❑

____

____

____

____

CALCULATION

Total Possible Points: __________

Total Points Earned: __________ Multiplied by 100 = __________ Divided by Total Possible Points = __________ %

PASS ❑ **FAIL** ❑ **COMMENTS:**

Student's signature ____________________ Date __________

Partner's signature ____________________ Date __________

Instructor's signature ____________________ Date __________

PSY PROCEDURE 8-3 Releasing Medical Records

Name: ____________________ **Date:** __________ **Time:** __________ **Grade:** __________

EQUIPMENT/SUPPLIES: Simulated patient medical record (paper or electronic)

STANDARDS: Given the needed equipment and a place to work, the student will perform this skill with ______ % accuracy in a total of _____ minutes. *(Your instructor will tell you what the percentage and time limits will be before you begin.)*

KEY: 4 = Satisfactory 0 = Unsatisfactory NA = This step is not counted

PROCEDURE STEPS	SELF	PARTNER	INSTRUCTOR
1. Verify the patient's name and another piece of identifying information in order to pull the correct medical record	❑	❑	❑
2. Determine if a release of medical record must be signed before the records can be released	❑	❑	❑
3. Choose the correct document(s) to be released and provide a copy of the documentation if it not sent electronically	❑	❑	❑
4. Determine whether or not a fee should be assessed for copies of the medical record	❑	❑	❑
5. AFF Explain how you would handle copying the requested medical documentation when using a copier	❑	❑	❑

____

____

____

____

CALCULATION

Total Possible Points: __________

Total Points Earned: __________ Multiplied by 100 = __________ Divided by Total Possible Points = __________ %

PASS ❑ **FAIL** ❑ **COMMENTS:**

Student's signature ____________________ Date __________

Partner's signature ____________________ Date __________

Instructor's signature ____________________ Date __________

CHAPTER

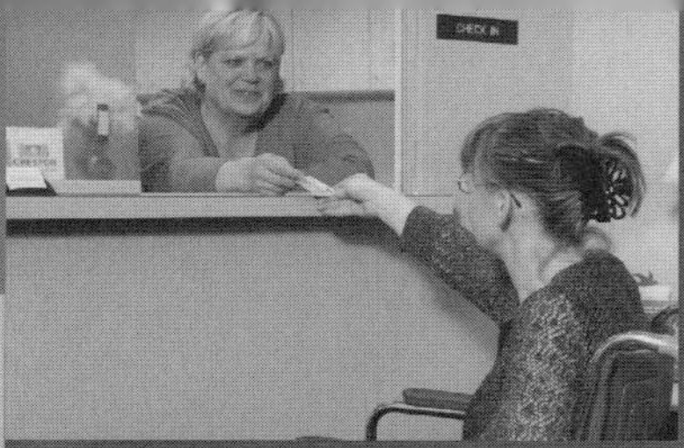

9 Electronic Applications in the Medical Office

Learning Outcomes

COG Cognitive Domain

1. Spell and define the key words
2. Identify the basic computer components
3. Explain the purpose of routine maintenance of administrative and clinical equipment
4. Explain the basics of connecting to the Internet
5. Discuss the safety concerns for online searching
6. Describe how to use a search engine
7. List sites that can be used by professionals and sites geared for patients
8. Describe the benefits of an intranet and explain how it differs from the Internet
9. Describe the various types of clinical software that might be used in a physician's office
10. Describe the various types of administrative software that might be used in a physician's office
11. Discuss applications of electronic technology in professional communication
12. Describe the considerations for purchasing a computer
13. Describe various training options
14. Discuss the adoption of electronic health records
15. Describe the steps in making the transition from paper to electronic records
16. Discuss the ethics related to computer access
17. Differentiate between electronic medical records (EMR) and a practice management system.

AFF Affective Domain

1. Apply ethical behaviors, including honest/integrity in the performance of medical assisting practice

PSY Psychomotor Domain

1. Perform routine maintenance of administrative or clinical equipment (Procedure 9-1)
2. Use the Internet to access information related to the medical office (Procedure 9-2)
3. Input patient data utilizing a practice management system (Procedure 9-3)

ABHES Competencies

1. Apply electronic technology
2. Receive, organize, prioritize, and transmit information expediently
3. Locate information and resources for patients and employers
4. Apply computer application skills using variety of different electronic programs including both practice management software and EMR software

Name: ______________________ Date: ____________ Grade: ____________

COG MULTIPLE CHOICE

1. Another name for a central processing unit is a:
- **a.** silicon chip.
- **b.** USB port.
- **c.** modem.
- **d.** microprocessor.
- **e.** handheld computer.

2. The purpose of a zip drive in a computer is to:
- **a.** scan information.
- **b.** delete information.
- **c.** store information.
- **d.** research information.
- **e.** translate information.

3. The acronym *DSL* stands for:
- **a.** data storage location.
- **b.** digital subscriber line.
- **c.** digital storage link.
- **d.** data saved/lost.
- **e.** digital software link.

4. In a physician's practice, the HIPAA officer:
- **a.** checks for security threats or gaps in electronic information.
- **b.** purchases new technological equipment.
- **c.** maintains computer equipment and fixes problems.
- **d.** trains staff in how to use computer equipment.
- **e.** monitors staff who may be misusing computer equipment.

Scenario for questions 5 and 6: A parent approaches you and asks how he can keep his 9-year-old daughter safe on the Internet.

5. Which of these actions would you recommend to the parent?
- **a.** Don't allow the daughter on the Internet after 7 PM.
- **b.** Stand behind the daughter the entire time she is using the Internet.
- **c.** Don't permit the daughter to use the Internet until she is 10 years old.
- **d.** Add a filter to the daughter's computer to only allow safe sites as decided by the parent.
- **e.** Ask other parents for advice.

6. Which of these Web sites might be helpful to the parent?
- **a.** www.skyscape.com
- **b.** www.pdacortec.com
- **c.** www.ezclaim.com
- **d.** www.cyberpatrol.com
- **e.** www.nextgen.com

7. To protect your computer from a virus, you should:
- **a.** make sure that your computer is correctly shut down every time you use it.
- **b.** avoid opening any attachments from unknown Web sites.
- **c.** only download material from government Web sites.
- **d.** consult a computer technician before you use new software.
- **e.** only open one Web site at a time.

8. What is the advantage of encrypting an e-mail?
- **a.** It makes the e-mail arrive at its intended destination faster.
- **b.** It marks the e-mail as *urgent*.
- **c.** It scrambles the e-mail so that it cannot be read until it reaches the recipient.
- **d.** It translates the e-mail into another language.
- **e.** It informs the sender when the e-mail has been read by the recipient.

9. Which of these is an example of an inappropriate e-mail?
- **a.** "There will be a staff meeting on Wednesday at 9 AM."
- **b.** "Please return Mrs. Jay's call: Her number is 608-223-3444."
- **c.** "If anyone has seen a lost pair of sunglasses, please return them to reception."
- **d.** "Mr. Orkley thinks he is having a stroke. Please advise."
- **e.** "Mrs. Jones called to confirm her appointment."

10. Which of the following is a peripheral?
- **a.** Zip drive
- **b.** Monitor
- **c.** Keyboard
- **d.** Internet
- **e.** Modem

11. Which of these would you most likely find on an intranet?
- **a.** Advice about health insurance
- **b.** Minutes from staff meetings
- **c.** Information about Medicare
- **d.** Descriptions of alternative treatments
- **e.** National guidelines on medical ethics

12. What is the difference between clinical and administrative software packages?
a. Clinical software helps provide good medical care, whereas administrative software keeps the office efficient.
b. Administrative software is designed to be used by medical assistants, whereas clinical software is used by physicians.
c. Clinical software is cheaper than administrative software because it offers fewer technical features.
d. Administrative software lasts longer than clinical software because it is of higher quality.
e. Clinical software does not allow users to access it without a password, whereas anyone can use administrative software.

13. Which of these should you remember to do when paging a physician?
a. Follow up the page with a phone call to make sure the physician got the message.
b. Keep track of what time the message is sent and repage if there is no response.
c. Document the fact that you sent a page to the physician.
d. Contact the person who left the message to let him or her know you have paged the physician.
e. E-mail the physician with a copy of the paged message.

14. You can use the Meeting Maker software program to:
a. contact patients about appointment changes.
b. coordinate internal meetings and calendars.
c. print patient reminders for annual checkups.
d. create slideshow presentations for meetings.
e. page office staff when a meeting is about to start.

15. Which of these is an important consideration when purchasing a new computer for the office?
a. Whether the computer's programs are HIPAA compliant
b. Whether the computer will be delivered to the office
c. The number of people who will be using the computer
d. The amount of space the computer will take up in the office
e. Which is the best-selling computer on the market?

16. When assigning computer log-in passwords to staff, a physician should:
a. make sure that everyone has the code for the hospital computers.
b. give staff two log-in passwords: one for professional use and one for personal use.
c. issue all new employees their own password.
d. make sure that everyone has access to his or her e-mails, in case he or she is out of the office.
e. use a standard log-in password for all the office computers.

17. It is a good idea to lock the hard drive when you are moving a computer to:
a. prevent the zip drive from falling out.
b. make sure that no information is erased.
c. stop viruses from attacking the computer.
d. protect the CPU and disk drives.
e. avoid damaging the keyboard.

18. A modem is a:
a. communication device that connects a computer to other computers, including the Internet.
b. piece of software that enables the user to perform advanced administrative functions.
c. name for the Internet.
d. method of storing data on the computer.
e. type of networking technology for local area networks.

19. Which of the following is true of an abstract found during a literary search?
a. Abstracts are only found on government Web sites.
b. Only physicians can access an abstract during a literary search.
c. An abstract is a summary of a journal article.
d. Most medical offices cannot afford to download an abstract.
e. Abstracts can only be printed at a hospital library.

20. If a computer is exposed to static electricity, there is the potential risk of:
a. electrical fire.
b. memory loss.
c. dust accumulation.
d. slow Internet connection.
e. viruses.

21. You have been asked to train new employees on how to use an administrative application. However, you do not have a lot of time or extra funding to spend on training. Circle the best option for training the new employees.
a. Have them read the user manual.
b. Have them call the help desk.
c. Have them ask another colleague.
d. Have them take a tutorial on the program.
e. Hire experts from the software company.

22. When shopping for prescription management software, what is the minimum that a physician should be able to do with the program? Circle the correct answer.
a. Find a patient name in a database, write the prescription, and download it to the pharmacy.
b. Find a patient name in a database, check the prescription for contraindication, and download it to the pharmacy.
c. Find a patient name in a database, write the prescription, and print it out for the patient.
d. Find a medication in a database, write the prescription, and download the data to a handheld computer.
e. Find a patient name in a database, write the prescription, download it to the pharmacy, and check that the medication is covered by insurance.

COG MATCHING

Grade: _____

Match the following key terms to their definitions.

Key Terms	Definitions
23. _____ cookies	a. a system that allows the computer to be connected to a cable or DSL system
24. _____ downloading	b. a private network of computers that share data
25. _____ encryption	c. a global system used to connect one computer to another
26. _____ Ethernet	d. tiny files left on your computer's hard drive by a Web site without your permission
27. _____ Internet	e. a dangerous invader that enters your computer through a source and can destroy your files, software programs, and possibly even the hard drive
28. _____ intranet	f. transferring information from an outside location to your computer's hard drive
29. _____ literary search	g. the process of scrambling e-mail messages so that they cannot be read until they reach the recipient
30. _____ search engine	h. the process of navigating Web sites
31. _____ surfing	i. a program that allows you to find information on the Web related to specific terms
32. _____ virus	j. a search that involves finding journal articles that present new facts or data about a given topic
33. _____ virtual	k. simulated by your computer

COG SHORT ANSWER

Grade: _____

34. List three benefits of having appointment scheduling software in the office.

_____

_____

_____

_____

35. You receive an e-mail from a patient saying that his medication is working out well and is not causing any side effects. He will be in for his appointment next Tuesday. How do you document this information in the patient's medical record?

____

____

____

____

36. What are three benefits of using electronic medical records instead of paper charts?

____

____

____

____

37. Mr. Jones requires special treatment that uses a laser machine. He makes an appointment for Thursday morning and takes time off work to attend. When he arrives at the facility, he is told that the machine is only available on Mondays and that the new receptionist was unaware of this fact when she made his appointment. How could an administrative software program have helped to prevent this situation?

____

____

____

____

COG PSY PATIENT EDUCATION

Grade: __________

38. A patient has told you of his decision to start buying prescription medication on the Internet. What warnings/information should you give to him?

____

____

____

____

COG PSY ACTIVE LEARNING

Grade: __________

39. Perform research using the Internet to find information about a disease and possible treatments. Try using different key words to see which ones produce the most useful results. Make a list of the Web sites you have used and observe whether each one has the logo of a verification program such as the HON (Health on the Net) seal.

40. Use the PowerPoint program on the computer to turn your Internet research about a common disease into a presentation. Use the program to make handouts of your presentation for quick office reference. You can use the tutorial feature on the software if you are unsure how to perform certain functions.

41. Visit the Medicare Web site at www.medicare.gov. Find the part of the Web site that addresses FAQs, or frequently asked questions. Choose five of these questions that might be relevant to your patients and print the questions and answers. Then use presentation software to highlight these five questions in a presentation that you will give to your class.

COG IDENTIFICATION

Grade: ___________

42. Your office has started converting many of your paper files into digital online files to save time. Recently, you have realized that accessing these records through your Internet service provider (ISP) is taking a very long time. Circle the solutions to this problem.

a. Upgrade your office's ISP to cable.Q2.
b. Switch your Web browser.
c. Switch your search engine.
d. Upgrade your printer.
e. Eliminate viruses with a virus scan.
f. Upgrade your monitor.
g. Upgrade your office's ISP to DSL.

43. A patient has asked you for information on how she can lower her cholesterol. You have decided to surf the Internet to find the latest information. Place a check in the "Yes" column for those key words that would lead to a faster, more efficient search. Place a check in the "No" column for those key words that would lead to a slower, less efficient search.

Key Words	Yes	No
a. Cholesterol		
b. Lowering cholesterol		
c. Cholesterol diet		
d. How do people lower their cholesterol?		
e. Cholesterol reduction		

44. A diabetic patient has been researching information on the disease. He has asked you to review a list of Web sites he has been reading. Place a check in the "Patient" box for sites that are more useful for patients. Place a check in the "Professional" box for sites that are more useful to physicians and medical assistants.

Web sites	Patient	Professional
a. www.mywebmd.com		
b. www.lancet.org		
c. www.jama.com		
d. www.healthfinder.gov		
e. www.tifaq.com		

COG PSY PATIENT EDUCATION

Grade: ______

45. A patient has expressed an interest in learning more about her food allergies on the Internet. You decide to give her advice on what to look out for when surfing. Place a check in the "Yes" column indicating that the statement is good advice. Place a check in the "No" column indicating that the statement is bad advice.

Key Words	Yes	No
a. Almost all testimonials can be trusted.		
b. Don't trust sites that claim to have secret formulas, medical miracles, or breakthroughs.		
c. Some treatments found online are best to not tell your physician about.		
d. No matter how professional the Web site, you cannot learn lifesaving skills on the Internet.		

TRUE OR FALSE?

Grade: ______

46. Determine whether the following statements are true or false. If false, explain why.

a. The advanced search feature of a search engine should return more results.

______

b. Internal job postings are often found on the Internet.

______

c. The most popular program used to write presentations is PowerPoint.

______

d. A computer system is divided into three areas: hardware, peripherals, and software.

______

AFF PSY WHAT WOULD YOU DO?

Grade: ______

47. You perform most of the administrative tasks in a physician's office and have been asked for your input concerning a new office computer. The physician asks you which administrative features you would find helpful in a new computer. List three administrative software programs that you would find useful and explain what functions they perform.

______

______

______

______

48. A patient tells you that her medicine has not been working properly and that she is thinking of researching alternative treatments on the Internet. What is the best advice you can give her?

___

___

___

___

49. One of your coworkers has a habit of getting up from her computer and leaving confidential patient information visible on the screen. She says that she sits too far away from patients for them to read anything on the screen, but you have seen several patients near the computer while your coworker is away from her desk. What do you say to her?

___

___

___

___

50. It is your first week working at a physician's office. You notice that the computer is dusty and in the morning sunlight. Disks are in a neat pile next to the uncovered computer. What steps would you take to maintain this computer?

___

___

___

___

AFF CASE STUDY FOR CRITICAL THINKING

Grade: ___

You are teaching a new employee to use the computer system in the office where you work. Ginger is excited and enthusiastic about her new job. At every possible opportunity, Ginger checks her Facebook and Twitter pages. You know that this is against the office policy regarding accepted use of office computers.

51. Circle all appropriate actions from the list below.
- **a.** Beg the office manager to get someone else to train Ginger.
- **b.** Show her the policy in the office *Policies and Procedures Manual.*
- **c.** Tell her if she continues this practice she will get fired.
- **d.** Tell her that the IT department can and will track her use of the office computer.
- **e.** Suggest that she wait until she gets off work for personal computer use.
- **f.** Suggest that people should talk to each other the way they used to, face to face.

52. Circle the accurate statements from the list below. Businesses control personal use of their computers because:
- **a.** it reduces wear and tear on the computers.
- **b.** it is inefficient for employees to be doing personal things while at work.
- **c.** it is dishonest to use someone else's computer.
- **d.** it is unprofessional and unethical.
- **e.** you should never disobey the office rules, no matter what.
- **f.** they are not paying you to be on Facebook and Twitter.
- **g.** it is illegal.

53. You are teaching Ginger how to care for her computer. Why is it important to perform routine maintenance on the office computer? Circle all appropriate answers from the list below.

a. It enhances the performance and prolongs the life of the equipment.
b. It is a rule and you *always* follow the rules, no matter what.
c. It shows that you are a clean person.
d. It looks bad for the patients to see dust.
e. It is in the office *Policy and Procedure Manual*.

PSY PROCEDURE 9-1 Care for and Maintain Computer Hardware

Name: ______________________ **Date:** __________ **Time:** __________ **Grade:** __________

EQUIPMENT/SUPPLIES: Computer CPU, monitor, keyboard, mouse, printer, duster, simulated warranties

STANDARDS: Given the needed equipment and a place to work, the student will perform this skill with _____ % accuracy in a total of _____ minutes. *(Your instructor will tell you what the percentage and time limits will be before you begin.)*

KEY: 4 = Satisfactory 0 = Unsatisfactory NA = This step is not counted

PROCEDURE STEPS	SELF	PARTNER	INSTRUCTOR
1. Place the monitor, keyboard, and printer in a cool, dry area out of direct sunlight.	❑	❑	❑
2. Place the computer desk on an antistatic floor mat or carpet.	❑	❑	❑
3. Clean the monitor screen with antistatic wipes.	❑	❑	❑
4. Use dust covers for the keyboard and the monitor when they are not in use.	❑	❑	❑
5. Lock the hard drive when moving the computer.	❑	❑	❑
6. Keep keyboard and mouse free of debris and liquids; dust and/or vacuum the keyboard.	❑	❑	❑
7. Create a file for maintenance and warranty contracts for the computer system.	❑	❑	❑
8. Handle data storage disks with special care.	❑	❑	❑
9. AFF If you were the office manager, explain how you would respond to an employee who continued to spill soft drinks on her keyboard.	❑	❑	❑

____

____

____

____

CALCULATION

Total Possible Points: __________

Total Points Earned: __________ Multiplied by 100 = __________ Divided by Total Possible Points = __________ %

PASS ❑ **FAIL** ❑ **COMMENTS:**

Student's signature ____________________ Date __________

Partner's signature ____________________ Date __________

Instructor's signature ____________________ Date __________

PSY PROCEDURE 9-2 Searching on the Internet

Name: ______________________ **Date:** ________ **Time:** ________ **Grade:** ________

EQUIPMENT/SUPPLIES: Computer with Web browser software, modem, active Internet connection account

STANDARDS: Given the needed equipment and a place to work, the student will perform this skill with _____ % accuracy in a total of _____ minutes. *(Your instructor will tell you what the percentage and time limits will be before you begin.)*

KEY: 4 = Satisfactory 0 = Unsatisfactory NA = This step is not counted

PROCEDURE STEPS	SELF	PARTNER	INSTRUCTOR
1. Connect computer to the Internet.	❑	❑	❑
2. Locate a search engine.	❑	❑	❑
3. Select two or three key words and type them at the appropriate place on the Web page.	❑	❑	❑
4. View the number of search results. If no sites are found, check spelling and retype or choose new key words.	❑	❑	❑
5. If the search produces a long list, do an advanced search and refine key words.	❑	❑	❑
6. Select an appropriate site and open its home page.	❑	❑	❑
7. If satisfied with the site's information, either download the material or bookmark the page. If unsatisfied with its information, either visit a site listed on the results page or return to the search engine.	❑	❑	❑
8. AFF You sit down to use your office computer to search for information with a patient when a coworker's Facebook page pops up. You are embarrassed at the unprofessionalism this displays in front of the patient. Explain how you would respond in this situation.	❑	❑	❑

____

____

____

____

CALCULATION

Total Possible Points: __________

Total Points Earned: __________ Multiplied by 100 = __________ Divided by Total Possible Points = __________ %

PASS ❑ **FAIL** ❑ **COMMENTS:**

Student's signature ____________________ Date __________

Partner's signature ____________________ Date __________

Instructor's signature ____________________ Date __________

PSY PROCEDURE 9-3 Entering Patient Demographics into a Practice Management System

Name: ______________________ **Date:** __________ **Time:** __________ **Grade:** __________

EQUIPMENT/SUPPLIES: Computer, completed patient demographics form, and a practice management system such as Caretracker

STANDARDS: Given the needed equipment and a place to work, the student will perform this skill with _____ % accuracy in a total of _____ minutes. *(Your instructor will tell you what the percentage and time limits will be before you begin.)*

KEY: 4 = Satisfactory 0 = Unsatisfactory NA = This step is not counted

PROCEDURE STEPS	SELF	PARTNER	INSTRUCTOR
1. Open the practice management application and verify that the patient is not already in the system.	❑	❑	❑
2. Open the patient module and enter all of the patient's personal information on the demographics tab and save.	❑	❑	❑
3. Enter the insurance/subscriber information for the primary insurance and save.	❑	❑	❑
4. Verify correct information has been entered from the patient information form.	❑	❑	❑
5. AFF While entering the patient's demographic information you are interrupted by the physician and walk away from your computer. What choices could you have made to protect the patient's private information?	❑	❑	❑

____

____

____

____

CALCULATION

Total Possible Points: __________

Total Points Earned: __________ Multiplied by 100 = __________ Divided by Total Possible Points = __________ %

PASS ❑ **FAIL** ❑ **COMMENTS:**

Student's signature ____________________ Date __________

Partner's signature ____________________ Date __________

Instructor's signature ____________________ Date __________

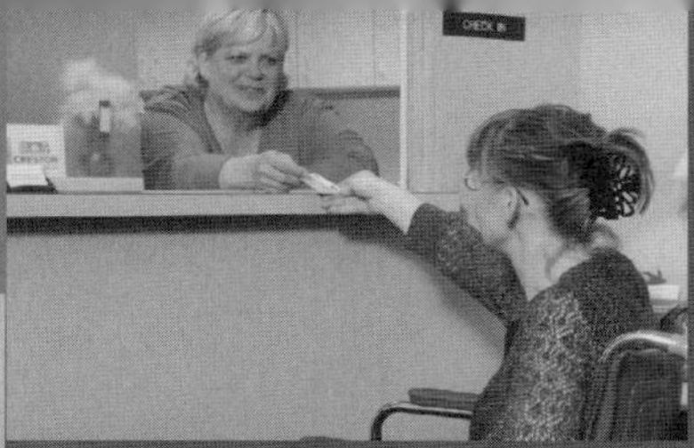

CHAPTER

10 Managing the Medical Office

Learning Outcomes

COG Cognitive Domain

1. Spell and define the key terms
2. Describe what is meant by organizational structure
3. List seven responsibilities of the medical office manager
4. Explain the five staffing issues that a medical office manager will be responsible for handling
5. List the types of policies and procedures that should be included in a medical office's policy and procedures manual
6. List five types of promotional materials that a medical office may distribute
7. Discuss financial concerns that the medical office manager must be capable of addressing
8. Describe the duties regarding office maintenance, inventory, and service contracts
9. Discuss the need for continuing education
10. Describe liability, professional, personal injury, and third-party insurance
11. List three services provided by most medical malpractice companies
12. List six guidelines for completing incident reports
13. List four regulatory agencies that require medical offices to have quality improvement programs
14. Describe the accreditation process of The Joint Commission
15. Describe the steps to developing a quality improvement program
16. Identify safety techniques that can be used to prevent accidents and maintain a safe work environment
17. Describe the purpose of Safety Data Sheets (SDS) in a health care setting
18. Discuss fire safety issues in an ambulatory health care environment
19. Explain the evacuation plan for a physician's office
20. Discuss requirements for disposing of hazardous material
21. Identify principles of body mechanics and ergonomics
22. List and discuss legal and illegal applicant interview questions
23. Discuss all levels of governmental legislation and regulation as they apply to medical assisting practice
24. Apply local, state, and federal health care legislation and regulation appropriate to the medical assisting practice setting
25. Describe the process in compliance reporting: unsafe activities, errors in patient care, conflicts of interest, and incident reports

PSY Psychomotor Domain

1. Create a policy and procedures manual (Procedure 10-1)
2. Perform an inventory with documentation (Procedure 10-2)
3. Report relevant information concisely and accurately (Procedures 10-3 and 10-4)
4. Evaluate the work environment to identify unsafe working conditions (Procedure 10-3)
5. Complete an incident report related to an error in patient care (Procedure 10-4)
6. Apply local, state, and federal health care legislation and regulation appropriate to the medical assisting practice setting (Procedure 10-3)

AFF Affective Domain

1. Recognize the effects of stress on all persons involved in emergency situations
2. Demonstrate self-awareness in responding to emergency situations
3. Apply active listening skills
4. Use appropriate body language and other nonverbal skills in communicating with patients, family, and staff
5. Recognize the importance of local, state, and federal legislation and regulation in the practice setting

ABHES Competencies

1. Perform routine maintenance of administrative and clinical equipment
2. Maintain inventory, equipment, and supplies
3. Maintain medical facility
4. Serve as liaison between physician and others
5. Interview effectively
6. Comprehend the current employment outlook for the medical assistant
7. Understand the importance of maintaining liability coverage once employed in the industry
8. Perform risk management procedures
9. Comply with federal, state, and local health laws and regulations

Name: ______________________ Date: __________ Grade: __________

COG MULTIPLE CHOICE

Scenario for questions 1 and 2: It's your first day on the job as the medical office manager, so there's a lot you don't know yet about this office.

1. You want to know who's responsible for what in the office. Where is the best place to find that information?
a. Payroll records
b. The work schedule
c. The chain-of-command chart
d. The recent employee evaluations
e. The bulletin board

2. You know the office is running low on paper and syringes. You're most likely to find out how to order supplies in:
a. the QI plan.
b. the service contracts folder.
c. the operating budget.
d. the policy and procedures manual.
e. the communication notebook.

3. An SDS is required to contain:
a. general information about safety.
b. a written hazard communication plan.
c. information regarding hazardous chemicals found in a facility.
d. the appropriate amount of bleach that can be stored in a medical office.
e. a complete list of the hazardous materials in a facility.

4. The office keeps running out of tongue depressors. Which action should you take first?
a. Establish a recycling program.
b. Determine whether someone is stealing supplies.
c. Review the system for keeping track of supplies.
d. Tell the physicians not to use so many tongue depressors.
e. Borrow some tongue depressors from the nearest medical office.

5. Which item should be in any job description?
a. Age requirements
b. Salary or hourly pay
c. Physical requirements
d. The preferred gender of the applicant
e. Medical and dental benefits

6. Which task should you be expected to perform as medical office manager?
a. Clean the waiting room.
b. Assign someone to make coffee.
c. Develop promotional pamphlets.
d. Assist with simple medical procedures.
e. Sign prescription refills.

7. Which of the following is a medical office manager's responsibility?
a. Completing all incident reports
b. Teaching CPR
c. Evaluating the physicians
d. Hiring and firing employees
e. Teaching employees about malpractice insurance

8. Which statement is true of an incident report about a patient?
a. It should be mailed to the attorney of your choice.
b. It should be written by a physician.
c. It should be written within 24 hours of the incident.
d. It should be written from the patient's point of view.
e. It should be kept in the medical office.

9. Which action should be taken if an employee is stuck by a patient's needle?
a. The patient should be informed.
b. The physician should take disciplinary action against the employee.
c. The employee should write an incident report.
d. The employee should be kept away from patients.
e. The employee should sign a form admitting liability.

10. Which of the following categories is part of a capital budget?
a. Payroll
b. Medical supplies
c. Building maintenance
d. Heating and air conditioning
e. Electricity

11. Which item should be part of any medical office budget?
a. Merit bonuses
b. Billing service
c. Continuing education
d. Magazine subscriptions
e. Children's play facility

12. Which agency licenses and monitors health care organizations and enforces regulations?
a. CMS
b. State health department
c. The Joint Commission
d. OSHA
e. HCFA

13. General liability and medical malpractice insurance is for:
a. all medical professionals.
b. all physicians.
c. physicians who perform risky procedures.
d. medical professionals with high-risk profiles.
e. physicians and nurses.

14. The first step in creating a quality improvement plan is to:
a. form a task force.
b. identify the problem.
c. establish a monitoring plan.
d. assign an expected threshold.
e. explore the problem.

15. Which of the following items should be included in an emergency kit?
a. Alcohol wipes
b. Syringe
c. Penicillin
d. Oscilloscope
e. Sample containers

16. If you fill out an incident report, you should:
a. keep a copy of the report.
b. have a supervisor review it.
c. give your title but not your name.
d. fill out only the sections that apply.
e. summarize what happened in the report.

17. Which of the following is used to estimate expenditures and revenues?
a. Budget
b. Tracking file
c. Expected threshold
d. Financial statement
e. Previous expenditures

18. Risk management is a(n):
a. process begun only after a sentinel event.
b. process intended to identify potential problems.
c. external process that deals with OSHA violations.
d. internal process that deals with recurring problems.
e. process undertaken by managers to reduce annual expenditure.

19. Which of the following is true of an expected threshold for a quality improvement program?
a. It is the expected percentage reduction in risk.
b. It is a way to measure the success of the program.
c. It should be set higher for more dangerous problems.
d. It should be set lower than you think you can achieve.
e. It should only be used for particularly severe problems.

20. General liability and medical malpractice insurance is needed:
a. only by employees in offices that use new medical procedures.
b. by physicians sued for malpractice, but not by nurses or office personnel.
c. to protect medical professionals from financial loss due to lawsuits or settlements.
d. because visitors who are hurt in the waiting room can sue unless an incident report is completed.

COG MATCHING

Grade: ________

Match the following key terms to their definitions.

Key Terms	Definitions
21. ______ bioterrorism	**a.** numerical goal for a given problem
22. ______ body mechanics	**b.** statement of work-related responsibilities
23. ______ budget	**c.** series of steps required to perform a given task
24. ______ compliance officer	**d.** written account of untoward patient, visitor, or staff event
25. ______ epidemic	**e.** description of the goals of the practice and whom it serves
26. ______ ergonomics	**f.** statement regarding the organization's rules on a given topic
27. ______ expected threshold	**g.** purposeful infliction of a dangerous agent into a populated area with intent to harm
28. ______ incident report	**h.** financial planning tool used to estimate anticipated expenditures and revenues
29. ______ job description	

Key Terms	Definitions
30. ______ mission statement	**i.** staff member who ensures compliance with the rules and regulations of the office
31. ______ organizational chart	**j.** implementation of practices that will help ensure high-quality patient care and service
32. ______ pandemic	**k.** flow sheet that allows staff to identify team members and see where they fit into the team
33. ______ policy	**l.** group of employees with different roles brought together to solve a problem
34. ______ procedure	**m.** using the correct muscles and posture to complete a task safely and efficiently
35. ______ quality improvement	**n.** the study of the fit between a worker and his or her physical work environment
36. ______ task force	**o.** a disease affecting many people in a specific geographic area
	p. a disease infecting numerous people in many areas of the world at the same time

SHORT ANSWER

Grade: ______

37. List three responsibilities of the office manager regarding service contractors.

______

______

______

______

38. List five types of promotional materials that a medical office might use.

______

______

______

______

39. List six items that should be included in employee fire safety training.

______

______

______

______

______

______

40. List the four basic principles of proper body mechanics.

______

______

______

______

41. List five techniques used to reduce fatigue as you work.

____

____

____

____

COG IDENTIFICATION

Grade: _______

42. Below is a list of the steps for creating a quality improvement plan. Put the steps in logical order. Then explain the reason for each step.

Steps

Assign an expected threshold.
Document the entire process.
Establish a monitoring plan.
Explore the problem and propose solutions.
Form a task force.
Identify the problem.
Implement the solution.
Obtain feedback.

Step	Reason
1.	
2.	
3.	
4.	
5.	
6.	
7.	
8.	

COG YES OR NO?

Grade: ______

Answer "Yes," "No," or "Yes But" to the following questions about evaluating employees. If you answer "No" or "Yes But," be able to explain why.

	Yes	No	Yes But ...
43. Are employee evaluations your responsibility as a medical office manager?			
44. Should new employees be evaluated annually?			
45. Should you coach new employees about how to do their jobs well?			
46. Can annual performance appraisals be done orally?			
47. Should you communicate with employees about performance problems when one of the physicians asks you to?			
48. Should you inform a good employee yearly that she or he is doing a good job?			

COG IDENTIFICATION

Grade: ______

49. Medical offices usually have an operating budget and a capital budget. Separate the following items into the two categories by checking the column for operating budget or capital budget.

Budget Item	Operating Budget	Capital Budget
a. Payroll		
b. Medical equipment		
c. Office supplies		
d. Internet service		
e. Medical supplies		
f. Building maintenance		
g. Telephone service		
h. Electricity		
i. Expensive furniture		
j. Patient materials		
k. Continuing education		

COG PSY ACTIVE LEARNING

Grade: ________

50. When you complete your program of study, you would like to find a job as a medical office manager. Write the job description for your ideal job. Be sure to include all the essential elements, including a position summary, hours, location, and duties.

51. Your office manager has assigned you to a task force that will write a plan for fire prevention in your office. Your role in the group is to establish the headings for the plan. List five items that should be included.

____

____

____

____

____

____

____

____

52. Working together with a partner, search the local classified ads for an open job as a medical office manager. Then prepare to role-play the interview process with your partner, taking turns acting as the interviewer and the interviewee. Make a list of questions that you would ask as both the interviewer and the interviewee. Switch places so you both get to experience the job interview process from each perspective.

____

____

____

____

COG IDENTIFICATION

Grade: ________

53. Circle all the following tasks that are the responsibility of the medical office manager.

a. Scheduling staff

b. Ordering supplies

c. Writing the budget

d. Keeping up to date on legal issues

e. Assisting with medical procedures

f. Cleaning the office and waiting room

g. Revising policy and procedures manuals

h. Presenting continuing education seminars

i. Developing HIPAA and OSHA regulations

j. Developing promotional pamphlets or newsletters

54. Inventory control is the responsibility of the office manager. On the checklist below, put an **M** beside the inventory tasks the manager should do and an **A** beside the things an assistant or other office staff member can do.

_____________ Receive supplies

_____________ Initial the packing slip

_____________ Develop a system to keep track of supplies

_____________ Determine the procedures for ordering supplies

_____________ Transfer supplies from packing boxes to supply shelves

_____________ Check the packing slip against the actual supply contents

_____________ Keep receipts or packing slips in a bills-pending file for payment

_____________ Develop a process to check that deliveries of supplies are complete and accurate

COG YES OR NO?

Grade: _____________

55. Indicate by a check mark in the "Yes" or "No" column whether an item should be included in a medical office's policy and procedures manual.

Policy	Yes	No
a. A chain-of-command chart		
b. A list of employee benefits		
c. Infection control guidelines		
d. The office operating budget		
e. Annual employee evaluations		
f. Procedures for bill collections		
g. Copies of completed incident reports		
h. A description of the goals of the practice		
i. Responsibilities and procedures for ordering supplies		
j. A list of responsibilities for the last employee to leave the office each day		

COG LISTING

Grade: ___________

56. List six of the elements that should be included in any job description.

a. ______________________________

b. ______________________________

c. ______________________________

d. ______________________________

e. ______________________________

f. ______________________________

57. In addition to writing job descriptions and managing employee evaluations, list the three other staffing issues that are the responsibility of the medical office manager?

a. ______________________________

b. ______________________________

c. ______________________________

58. List three services provided by most medical malpractice companies.

a. ______________________________

b. ______________________________

c. ______________________________

COG FALSE THEN TRUE

Grade: ___________

59. Each of the following statements about incident reports is false or incomplete. Rewrite each statement to make it true and complete.

a. You should write up an incident report as the event was reported to you.

____

b. The witness should summarize and explain the event.

____

c. You should remain anonymous when you fill out a report.

____

d. The form should be completed within 48 hours of the event.

____

e. If a particular section of the report does not apply, it should be left blank.

____

f. Keep a copy of the incident report for your own personal record.

____

g. If the incident happened to a patient, put a copy of the report in the patient's chart.

____

h. The report should be reviewed by a supervisor to make sure the office is not liable.

____

i. Incident reports are written when negative events happen to patients or visitors.

____

COG MATCHING

Grade: ___________

60. Below is a list of four regulatory agencies that require medical offices to have quality improvement programs. Draw a line between the two columns to match the regulatory agency with its description.

Agencies	Descriptions
1. CMS	**a.** federal agency that regulates and runs Medicare and Medicaid
2. OSHA	**b.** nonfederal agency to license and monitor health care organizations and enforce regulations
3. The Joint Commission	**c.** federal agency that enforces regulations to protect the health and welfare of patients and employees
4. State health department	**d.** agency that sets voluntary health care standards and evaluates a health care organization's implementation of those standards

COG WHICH IS WHICH?

Grade: ___________

61. Explain how quality improvement programs and risk management work together in a medical office.

____

____

____

____

COG TRUE OR FALSE?

Grade: ___________

62. Determine whether the following statements are true or false. If false, explain why.

a. Health care organizations are required to follow the regulations of the Joint Commission.

____

b. Accreditation by The Joint Commission is valid for 5 years.

____

c. If The Joint Commission's initial site review identifies unsatisfactory areas, the health care organization may later prove that corrections have been made by passing a focus survey.

____

d. The health care organization should prepare for the Joint Commission survey by assessing its compliance with OSHA standards.

____

AFF WHAT WOULD YOU DO?

Grade: __________

63. As you enter the office on the first day of your new job as the medical office manager, you notice a thick layer of dust on the plastic plants in the waiting room and see that the magazines are old and tattered. The staff greets you with enthusiasm, saying you are just what they need to deal with the patients' complaints about spending too much time waiting to be seen. Someone has left an incident report file on your desk. You look through it right away and learn that a needlestick has been reported almost every Wednesday evening for a month. What would you do first, and why?

____

____

____

64. You have a patient who lost her home and several pets to a recent tornado in your city. You know she is at risk for the development of a major psychiatric disorder. What are five ways to help this patient who has been exposed to trauma from natural or manmade disasters?

____

____

____

____

65. Mrs. Hadley, who is blind and walks with a cane, slipped on the wet floor near a leaky water cooler and fell, cutting her forearm. One of the nurses examined and treated her wound and apologized. Mrs. Hadley said it was no problem and left the office. The nurse told you she wasn't going to file an incident report because the wound was minor and Mrs. Hadley had accepted her apology. As the medical office manager, what should you do?

____

____

____

____

AFF CASE STUDY FOR CRITICAL THINKING

Grade: ____________

You have been asked by your physician employer to inspect the office for possible safety hazards. He wants a report of any negative findings by the end of the week.

66. Circle the most appropriate first step.

a. Ask if you can assign a task force to help you.

b. Design a form for checking off items as you inspect them.

c. Tell him you are too busy with patients to take on such a large task.

d. Call the local fire department to perform the inspection.

e. Call the local OSHA representative to perform the inspection.

67. From the following list of actions, circle all that are appropriate.

a. Check closets for the storage of flammable liquids.

b. Check areas where oxygen is in use.

c. Check to be sure all cylinders and tanks that contain flammable gases or liquids are uncapped and ready for use.

d. Check to see that equipment and carts are on the right side of each hallway.

e. Check the CMA schedule to be sure there is enough coverage to keep everyone safe.

PSY PROCEDURE 10-1 Create a Procedures Manual

Name: ________________ **Date:** ________ **Time:** ________ **Grade:** ________

EQUIPMENT/SUPPLIES: Word processor, three-ring binder, paper, choose any procedure approved by your instructor

STANDARDS: Given the needed equipment and a place to work, the student will perform this skill with _____ % accuracy in a total of _____ minutes. *(Your instructor will tell you what the percentage and time limits will be before you begin.)*

KEY: 4 = Satisfactory 0 = Unsatisfactory NA = This step is not counted

PROCEDURE STEPS	SELF	PARTNER	INSTRUCTOR
1. Check the latest information from key governmental agencies, local, and state health departments, and health care organizations, such as OSHA and the CDC to make sure that the policies and procedures being written comply with federal and state legislation and regulations.	❑	❑	❑
2. Gather product information; consult government agencies, if needed. Secure educational pamphlets.	❑	❑	❑
3. Title the procedure properly.	❑	❑	❑
4. Number the procedure appropriately.	❑	❑	❑
5. Define the overall purpose of the procedure in a sentence or two explaining the intent of the procedure.	❑	❑	❑
6. List all necessary equipment and forms. Include everything needed to complete the task.	❑	❑	❑
7. List each step with its rationale.	❑	❑	❑
8. Provide spaces for signatures.	❑	❑	❑
9. Record the date the procedure was written.	❑	❑	❑
10. AFF Describe how you would explain to employees why they were asked to work in a group to create a procedure manual.	❑	❑	❑

____

____

____

____

CALCULATION

Total Possible Points: ________

Total Points Earned: ________ Multiplied by 100 = ________ Divided by Total Possible Points = ________ %

PROCEDURE 10-1 Create a Procedures Manual (continued)

Pass ❑ **Fail** ❑ **Comments:**

Student's signature ____________________ Date __________

Partner's signature ____________________ Date __________

Instructor's signature ____________________ Date __________

PSY PROCEDURE 10-2 Perform an Office Inventory

Name: ______________________ **Date:** __________ **Time:** __________ **Grade:** __________

EQUIPMENT: Inventory form, reorder form

STANDARDS: Given the needed equipment and a place to work, the student will perform this skill with _____ % accuracy in a total of _____ minutes. *(Your instructor will tell you what the percentage and time limits will be before you begin.)*

KEY: 4 = Satisfactory 0 = Unsatisfactory NA = This step is not counted

PROCEDURE STEPS	SELF	PARTNER	INSTRUCTOR
1. Using forms supplied by your instructor, count and record the amounts of specified supplies.	❑	❑	❑
2. Record amount of each item.	❑	❑	❑
3. Compare amount on hand with amount needed.	❑	❑	❑
4. Complete reorder form based on these numbers.	❑	❑	❑
5. Submit reorder forms to office manager.	❑	❑	❑
6. Document your actions per the ordering procedure.	❑	❑	❑
7. AFF Explain how you would respond to an employee who continually takes a vacation day when the office plans to take inventory.	❑	❑	❑

____

____

____

____

CALCULATION

Total Possible Points: __________

Total Points Earned: __________ Multiplied by 100 = __________ Divided by Total Possible Points = __________ %

PASS ❑ **FAIL** ❑ **COMMENTS:**

Student's signature ____________________ Date __________

Partner's signature ____________________ Date __________

Instructor's signature ____________________ Date __________

PSY PROCEDURE 10-3 Perform Medical Office Safety Checklist

Name: ____________________ **Date:** __________ **Time:** __________ **Grade:** __________

EQUIPMENT: Office Safety Checklist, pen

STANDARDS: Given the needed equipment and a place to work, the student will perform this skill with _____ % accuracy in a total of _____ minutes. *(Your instructor will tell you what the percentage and time limits will be before you begin.)*

KEY: 4 = Satisfactory 0 = Unsatisfactory NA =This step is not counted

PROCEDURE STEPS	SELF	PARTNER	INSTRUCTOR
1. After obtaining a floor plan of the medical office, perform a general visual inspection of every room/area for potential hazards.	❑	❑	❑
2. Inspect office equipment for potential hazards	❑	❑	❑
3. Examine all fire extinguishers and determine that they are in their appropriate places, fully charged, and operating properly.	❑	❑	❑
4. Verify that the following items are properly displayed: Evacuation routes in every room; and an OSHA poster (publication 3165) in a prominent location in the office. Also, verify that lighted exit signs are working.	❑	❑	❑
5. Verify that the SDS are accessible to all employees in a prominent location in the office.	❑	❑	❑
6. AFF Advise the physician of any hazardous situations that you may find that need corrective action.	❑	❑	❑

____

____

____

____

CALCULATION

Total Possible Points: __________

Total Points Earned: __________ Multiplied by 100 = __________ Divided by Total Possible Points = __________ %

PASS ❑ **FAIL** ❑ **COMMENTS:**

Student's signature ____________________ Date __________

Partner's signature ____________________ Date __________

Instructor's signature ____________________ Date __________

Great Falls Medical Center Physician Offices
WORKPLACE SAFETY CHECKLIST

Name of person conducting the inspection:	Inspection Date:

GENERAL VISUAL INSPECTION:

Reception Area	Yes	No	Comments
1. Is this area clean and uncluttered?			
2. Is there a posted office diagram showing evacuation routes in the event of an emergency?			
3. Are the exits unobstructed?			
4. Are the emergency exit lights working properly?			
5. Is there anything stacked up that could fall?			
6. Are all electrical cables in good condition (not frayed or damaged) and neatly tied up?			
7. Is electrical equipment working properly with adequate ventilation?			
8. Is there adequate clearance for electrical equipment from combustible material?			
Exam Room 1	**Yes**	**No**	**Comments**
1. Is this area clean and uncluttered?			
2. Is there a posted office diagram showing evacuation routes in the event of an emergency?			
3. Are the exits unobstructed?			
4. Are the emergency exit lights working properly?			
5. Is there anything stacked up that could fall?			
6. Are all electrical cables in good condition (not frayed or damaged) and neatly tied up?			
7. Is electrical equipment working properly with adequate ventilation?			
8. Is there adequate clearance for electrical equipment from combustible material?			
Exam Room 2	**Yes**	**No**	**Comments**
1. Is this area clean and uncluttered?			
2. Is there a posted office diagram showing evacuation routes in the event of an emergency?			

3. Are the exits unobstructed?			
4. Are the emergency exit lights working properly?			
5. Is there anything stacked up that could fall?			
6. Are all electrical cables in good condition (not frayed or damaged) and neatly tied up?			
7. Is electrical equipment working properly with adequate ventilation?			
8. Is there adequate clearance for electrical equipment from combustible material?			

Lunch Room/Break Area	**Yes**	**No**	**Comments**
1. Is this area clean and uncluttered?			
2. Is there a posted office diagram showing evacuation routes in the event of an emergency?			

Lunch Room/Break Area continued:	**Yes**	**No**	**Comments**
3. Are the exits unobstructed?			
4. Are the emergency exit lights working properly?			
5. Is there anything stacked up that could fall?			
6. Are all electrical cables in good condition (not frayed or damaged) and neatly tied up?			
7. Is electrical equipment working properly with adequate ventilation?			
8. Is there adequate clearance for electrical equipment from combustible material?			
9. Is the OSHA poster "Job Safety and Health" prominently displayed?			

Fire Emergencies	**Yes**	**No**	
1. Are fire extinguishers visible and current throughout the office?			
2. Have all fire extinguishers been checked within the last 6 months?			

CLINICAL AREA INSPECTIONS:

All Exam Rooms:	**YES**	**NO**	**Comments**
1. Are medical records inaccessible and PHI protected while in the exam rooms?			
2. Are there any syringes or needles accessible in the exam rooms?			
3. Are medications accessible in the exam rooms?			
4. Are there Sharps containers in each exam room for disposal of needles and biohazard material?			

Lab Area:			
5. Is food kept in the lab refrigerator?			
6. Is there food or drink consumed in the lab area?			
7. Do specimen containers have biohazard labels?			
8. Are chemicals stored in an unlabeled container?			
9. Is there a biohazard container in the lab?			
Personal Protective Equipment Inspection:	**YES**	**NO**	
10. Are employees provided with and using proper PPE for procedures in which there is a potential for contamination with bloodborne pathogens?			
11. Are the Safety Data Sheets current and accessible to all employees			

EMPLOYEE TRAINING:

Required Training Inservices	**YES**	**NO**	**Last Training Date:**
1. Training for proper selection and use of PPE			
2. Bloodborne Pathogens Training			
3. Emergency Preparedness Training			
4. Fire Safety Training including use of fire extinguishers			
5. HIPAA Privacy Training			

PSY PROCEDURE 10-4 Complete an Incident Report

Name: ______________________ **Date:** __________ **Time:** __________ **Grade:** __________

EQUIPMENT: Incident Form, pen

STANDARDS: Given the needed equipment and a place to work the student will perform this skill with _____ % accuracy in a total of _____ minutes. *(Your instructor will tell you what the percentage and time limits will be before you begin.)*

KEY: 4 = Satisfactory 0 = Unsatisfactory NA = This step is not counted

PROCEDURE STEPS	SELF	PARTNER	INSTRUCTOR
1. Recognize the error in patient care or accident occurring in the office	❑	❑	❑
2. Complete the incident report as per office policies and procedures	❑	❑	❑
3. Sign and date the incident report form and file with the office or practice manager.	❑	❑	❑
4. AFF Explain what steps can be taken to ensure that this accident does not occur in the future.	❑	❑	❑

____

____

____

____

CALCULATION

Total Possible Points: __________

Total Points Earned: __________ Multiplied by 100 = __________ Divided by Total Possible Points = __________ %

PASS ❑ **FAIL** ❑ **COMMENTS:**

Student's signature ____________________ Date __________

Partner's signature ____________________ Date __________

Instructor's signature ____________________ Date __________

WORK PRODUCT 1

Grade: ___________

USE METHODS OF QUALITY CONTROL

Louise Baggins, a 55-year-old patient, was visiting the physician for a physical exam. While waiting for her appointment, she asked you to direct her to the restroom. On her way into the restroom, she slipped and fell on a magazine that had fallen on the floor in the reception area. You did not see her fall, but she yelled out in pain after she fell. She was able to get up on her own but injured her wrist. Her wrist was immediately red, swollen, and painful to touch. Dr. Mikuski looked at her wrist and suggested she go to the hospital emergency room to have x-rays. You called an ambulance to transfer Mrs. Baggins to the hospital.

Fill in the incident report below to document this event.

Great Falls Medical Center Physician Offices

Employee Incident/Injury Report Form

Please complete this form as soon as possible when an accident, injury, or illness occurs in the workplace.

Employee Name:	**Title:**
Location:	Date and Time of Injury/Illness:
Person or Employee the Injury/Illness Reported to:	Title of Person or Employee Injury or Illness Reported to:

Describe the details of your accident, injury, or illness. Be as specific as possible:

____

____

____

____

Explain what you were doing at the time of your accident, injury, or illness:

____

____

____

____

For injuries, list the part or parts of your body that were injured. Be specific (i.e., right index finger, left ankle, etc…):

____

If there was a delay in reporting the injury or illness, explain the reason for this delay:

____

____

____

Names and Titles of Any Witnesses to your Injury or Illness:

____

____

____

____

Employee Signature: **Date:**

WORK PRODUCT 2

Grade: __________

USE METHODS OF QUALITY CONTROL

After Mrs. Baggins fell in the reception area (see Work Product 1), your supervisor asks you to review any other injuries in the reception area in the past 6 months. There are seven incident reports involving patient falls, and all of those occurred in some part of the reception area. Three patients slipped by the doorway on rainy days. Two more tripped on the corner of the doormat. The last two patients fell in the main lobby—one tripped over a children's toy, and the other slipped on a magazine, just like Mrs. Baggins did.

You are named to represent the medical assistants on a task force addressing these complaints. Assign an expected threshold using measurable, realistic goals. Explore the problem and propose solutions. Establish a QI monitoring plan explaining how data will be collected. Document the entire process and print the information to attach to this sheet. Using the blank memorandum below, write a memo to the staff with instructions to implement the solutions.

Memo

To:

From:

Date:

Re:

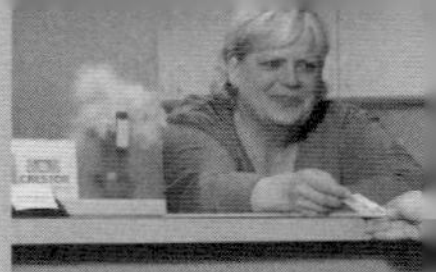

UNIT THREE MANAGING THE FINANCES IN THE PRACTICE

CHAPTER 11 Diagnostic Coding

Learning Outcomes

Cognitive Domain

1. Spell and define the key terms
2. Describe the relationship between coding and reimbursement
3. Name and describe the coding system used to describe diseases, injuries, and other reasons for encounters with a medical provider
4. Explain the format of the ICD-9-CM
5. Give four examples of ways E codes are used
6. Describe how to use the most current diagnostic coding classification system
7. Describe the ICD-10-CM version and its differences from ICD-9

Psychomotor Domain

1. Perform diagnostic coding (Procedure 11-1)
2. Utilize medical necessity guidelines (Procedure 11-1)

Affective Domain

1. Work with physician to achieve the maximum reimbursement
2. Utilize tactful communication skills with medical providers to ensure accurate code selection.

ABHES Competencies

1. Apply third-party guidelines
2. Perform diagnostic and procedural coding
3. Comply with federal, state, and local health laws and regulations

Name: ______________________ Date: __________ Grade: __________

COG MULTIPLE CHOICE

1. Which most accurately states the purpose of coding?
a. Coding assists patients in accessing insurance databases.
b. Coding determines the reimbursement of medical fees.
c. Coding is used to track a physician's payments.
d. Coding is used to index patients' claims forms.
e. Coding identifies patients in a database.

2. A patient signs an advance beneficiary notice (ABN) to:
a. consent to medically necessary procedures.
b. assign payment to Medicare.
c. accept responsibility for payment.
d. assign responsibility for payment to a beneficiary.
e. consent to a medically unnecessary procedure.

3. The content of the ICD-9-CM and ICD-10-CM is a(n):
a. classification of diseases and list of procedures.
b. statistical grouping of trends in diseases.
c. clinical modification of codes used by hospitals.
d. index of diseases.
e. international document for monitoring coding.

4. Which is true of Volume 3 of the ICD-9-CM and ICD-10-PCS?
a. It is organized by location on the patient's body.
b. It is used to code mostly outpatient procedures.
c. It is an alphabetical listing of diseases.
d. It is used by hospitals to report procedures and services.
e. It is an index of Volumes 1 and 2.

5. Physicians' services are reported:
a. on the UB-04.
b. on the CMS-1500.
c. on the uniform bill.
d. on the advance beneficiary notice.
e. on bills from health institutions.

6. Which of these would not be considered outpatient coding?
a. Hospital same-day surgery
b. Hour-long testing in a hospital CAT scan
c. Treatment in the emergency room
d. Observation status in a hospital
e. Meals and testing during a hospital stay

7. In ICD-10-CM and Volume 1 of the ICD-9-CM, chapters are grouped:
a. by alphabetic ordering of diseases and injuries.
b. alphabetically by eponym.
c. by location in the body.
d. by etiology and anatomic system.
e. by surgical specialty.

8. The fourth and fifth digits in an ICD-9-CM code indicate the:
a. anatomical location where a procedure was performed.
b. number of times a test was executed.
c. higher definitions of a code.
d. code for the patient's general disease.
e. traumatic origins of a disease (i.e., injury, deliberate violence).

9. An ICD-9-CM V-code or a code from Chapter 20 in ICD-10-CM might indicate a(n):
a. immunization.
b. poisoning.
c. accident.
d. diagnosis.
e. treatment.

10. ICD-9-CM V-codes or Chapter 20 in ICD-10-CM are used:
a. for outpatient coding.
b. when reimbursement is not needed.
c. when a patient is not sick.
d. to indicate testing for HIV.
e. for infectious diseases.

11. What is the purpose of ICD-9-CM E-codes?
a. They code for immunizations and other preventive procedures.
b. They are used to code medical testing before a diagnosis.
c. They assist insurance companies in making reimbursements.
d. They indicate why a patient has an injury or poisoning.
e. They indicate if a procedure was inpatient or outpatient.

12. How is Volume 2 of the ICD-9-CM different from Volume 1?
- **a.** Volume 2 contains diagnostic terms that are not used in Volume 1.
- **b.** Volume 2 is organized into 17 chapters rather than 3 sections.
- **c.** Volume 2 does not contain E-codes, but Volume 1 does.
- **d.** Volume 2 contains hospital coding to cross-reference with Volume 1.
- **e.** Volume 2 provides information about the fourth and fifth digits of a code.

13. After finding a code in Volume 2 in ICD-9-CM, you should:
- **a.** record the code on the CMS-1500.
- **b.** consult Volume 3 for subordinate terms.
- **c.** cross-reference the code with Volume 1.
- **d.** indicate if the code is inpatient or outpatient.
- **e.** record the code on the UB-04.

14. Volume 3 of the ICD-9-CM is organized:
- **a.** by disease.
- **b.** by anatomy.
- **c.** into 17 chapters.
- **d.** into three sections.
- **e.** by surgical specialty.

15. One example of an eponym is:
- **a.** Crohn disease.
- **b.** bacterial meningitis.
- **c.** influenza virus.
- **d.** pruritus.
- **e.** pneumonia.

16. What is the first step to locating a diagnostic code?
- **a.** Determine where the diagnosis occurs in the body.
- **b.** Choose the main term within the diagnostic statement.
- **c.** Begin looking up the diagnosis in the tabular index .
- **d.** Consult the CMS-1500 for reimbursement codes.
- **e.** Use Volume 3 of the ICD-9-CM to find the disease.

17. Which code is listed first on a CMS-1500?
- **a.** A reasonable second opinion
- **b.** Relevant laboratory work
- **c.** Diagnostic tests
- **d.** The symptoms of an illness
- **e.** The primary diagnosis

18. How do you code for late effects?
- **a.** Code for the treatment of the disease that causes late effects.
- **b.** Code for the disease that is causing the current condition.
- **c.** First code for the current condition, and then list the cause.
- **d.** Only code for the current condition.
- **e.** Only code for the cause of the current condition.

19. You should not code for a brain tumor:
- **a.** when the patient comes in for an MRI.
- **b.** after the tumor is confirmed on an MRI.
- **c.** when the diagnosed patient comes in for treatment.
- **d.** any time after the patient has been diagnosed.
- **e.** when the patient seeks specialist care.

COG MATCHING

Grade: ________

Match the following key terms to their definitions.

Key Terms

20. ______ advance beneficiary notice
21. ______ audits
22. ______ conventions
23. ______ cross-reference
24. ______ E-codes
25. ______ eponym
26. ______ etiology
27. ______ inpatient
28. ______ International Classification of Diseases, Clinical Modification
29. ______ late effects
30. ______ main terms
31. ______ medical necessity

Definitions

- **a.** ICD-9-CM codes indicating the external causes of injuries and poisoning
- **b.** conditions that result from another condition
- **c.** general notes, symbols, typeface, format, and punctuation that direct and guide a coder to the most accurate diagnosis code
- **d.** the condition or chief complaint that brings a person to a medical facility for treatment
- **e.** a procedure or service that would have been performed by any reasonable physician under the same or similar circumstances
- **f.** a document that informs covered patients that Medicare may not cover a certain service and the patient will be responsible for the bill
- **g.** a word based on or derived from a person's name
- **h.** ICD-9-CM codes assigned to patients who receive service but have no illness, injury, or disorder

Key Terms	Definitions
32. ______ outpatient	**i.** the billable tasks performed by a physician
33. ______ primary diagnosis	**j.** refers to a medical setting in which patients are admitted for diagnostic, radiographic, or treatment purposes
34. ______ service	**k.** an investigation performed by government, managed health care companies, and health care organizations to determine compliance and to detect fraud
35. ______ specificity	**l.** a system for transforming verbal descriptions of disease, injuries, conditions, and procedures to numeric codes
36. ______ V-codes	**m.** refers to the cause of disease
	n. refers to a medical setting in which patients receive care but are not admitted
	o. verification against another source
	p. relating to a definite result
	q. words in a multiple-word diagnosis that a coder should locate in the alphabetic listing

COG SHORT ANSWER

Grade: ___________

37. Why is the ICD-10-PCS not used at a hospital's emergency department?

____

____

____

____

38. What is the title of the new edition of the ICD manuals?

____

____

____

____

39. You are reading a patient's chart and notice that it is marked with an E-code. However, the patient has experienced no physical injuries. Why might an E-code be used in this situation?

____

____

____

____

40. You ask a veteran medical assistant for advice on coding, especially how to go about finding a diagnosis with more than one word. Her response is, "Find the condition, not the location." What does she mean by this?

____

____

____

____

41. What is listed first in the diagnosis section of the CMS-1500? What does it represent?

42. If a construction worker falls from a ladder and suffers an ankle fracture, what supplemental code is used for ICD-9-CM? What supplemental code is used for ICD10-CM?

43. When would you use a supplemental ICD-9-CM V-code for laboratory examination?

44. What should you do after finding a seemingly appropriate code in the alphabetic listing of ICD-10-CM?

45. If you do not know the medical terminology for a diagnosis for a common problem, what would be a good first plan of action?

46. What is the purpose of additional digits often appended to categories?

COG PSY ACTIVE LEARNING

Grade: ___________

47. A reasonable and capable physician believes that a patient needs a chest x-ray to rule out pneumonia. Does the procedure meet the grounds for medical necessity? Why? Why not?

48. A patient comes in complaining of chest pain, and tests are ordered to rule out myocardial infarction. When you enter the codes for this patient encounter, you code that the patient has "acute myocardial infarction." Why would it be better to code this encounter "chest pain "?

49. George Cregan has been seen by the physician for controlled non–insulin-dependent type 2 diabetes mellitus for about 10 years. While being seen for a routine check of his blood sugar, he complains of numbness and tingling in his left lower leg and foot. An x-ray of both legs is performed because poor circulation in the extremities can be a complication of diabetes. The x-ray confirms the diagnosis of peripheral neuropathy. Which diagnosis code should be listed with the office visit? Which code indicates the reason for the x-ray? Which code should be placed on the CMA-1500 first as the primary diagnosis or reason for the visit?

Determine the main term for the following multiple-word diagnoses.

Diagnosis	Main Term
50. Chronic fatigue syndrome	
51. Severe acute respiratory syndrome	
52. Hemorrhagic encephalitis	
53. Acute fulminating multiple sclerosis	
54. Fractured left tibia	
55. Breast cyst	

COG IDENTIFICATION

Grade: ___________

56. Review the list of circumstances below and place a check mark to indicate whether a patient would be forced, given the circumstance, to sign an ABN. All of the patients below are covered by Medicare.

Circumstance	ABN	No ABN
a. The patient wishes to receive a service or procedure that is not covered by Medicare.		
b. The patient is undergoing a regularly scheduled checkup.		
c. The patient demands to be tested for an illness that the physician considers an impossibility.		
d. The patient has a badly sprained ankle and wishes to be treated.		
e. The patient is undergoing x-ray imaging per order of a physician.		

57. When it comes to coding, it makes a difference if the patient is seen in an inpatient or outpatient facility. Review the list of places below. Place an *I* next to those places that are considered "Inpatient" and an O next to those places that are considered "Outpatient."

a. ___________ Hospital clinic

b. ___________ Health care provider's office

c. ___________ Hospital for less than 24 hours

d. ___________ Hospital for 24 hours or more

e. ___________ Hospital emergency room

58. Circle the main terms where you will find obstetric conditions.

delivery	fetus	pregnancy	labor
baby	obstetrics	puerperal	gestational

COG TRUE OR FALSE?

Grade: ___________

True or False? Determine whether the following statements are true or false. If false, explain why.

59. Only the first three digits of a code are necessary.

____

60. One should never code directly from the alphabetic index.

____

61. The main term describes a condition, not an aspect of anatomy.

____

62. In the outpatient setting, coders list conditions after the patient's testing is complete.

____

AFF WHAT WOULD YOU DO?

Grade: ___________

63. A patient calls complaining of pain and swelling in the right hand since awakening this morning. The patient comes in, sees the doctor, and returns to the front desk with an encounter form that states his diagnosis is "gout." In order to make this diagnosis, the physician would need to know the patient's uric acid level. You know that the patient just had blood drawn for the test. It is a test that must be sent to an outside lab. Do you still code today's visit as "gout"? What would you do?

____

____

____

____

64. A patient is concerned that her insurance provider will not cover her visit because the diagnosis is for a very minor ailment. She requests that you mark her CMA-1500 with a more severe disorder that demands similar treatment. How would you deal with this situation? What would you tell the patient? How might you involve the physician?

____

____

____

____

65. A patient entered the office complaining of abdominal pain that radiates into the right lower quadrant. After examination, the physician decided to order laboratory tests in order to rule out the possibility of appendicitis. . Which code should be placed on the CMA-1500 first as the primary diagnosis or reason for the visit? Why?

____

____

____

____

AFF CASE STUDY FOR CRITICAL THINKING

Grade: ___________

Your physician employer works with you closely to choose the most appropriate codes. He tells you that he would like for you to code patients who have B_{12} injections with "pernicious anemia." You ask if these patients should have a lab work to substantiate that diagnosis, and he says, "don't worry about that."

66. What would you say to him?

____

____

____

____

67. What would be the possible consequences of such an action?

---

68. Which of these is an unethical act? Explain why.

a. Coding multiple conditions on the same CMS-1500

---

b. Coding an unsupported diagnosis in order to make a service appear medically necessary

---

---

c. Using a supplemental ICD-9-CM V-code or a code from Chapter 20 in ICD-10-CM to better explain the reason for a patient's visit

---

---

d. Using diagnosis coding search software to more easily access the codes contained in the ICD-9-CM or ICD-10-CM.

PSY PROCEDURE 11-1 Locating A Diagnostic Code

Name: ______________________ **Date:** __________ **Time:** __________ **Grade:** __________

EQUIPMENT: Diagnosis, current volume of ICD-9-CM, Volumes 1 and 2 or ICD-10-CM codebook medical dictionary.

STANDARDS: Given the needed equipment and a place to work, the student will perform this skill with _____ % accuracy in a total of _____ minutes. *(Your instructor will tell you what the percentage and time limits will be before you begin.)*

KEY: 4 = Satisfactory 0 = Unsatisfactory NA = This step is not counted

PROCEDURE STEPS	SELF	PARTNER	INSTRUCTOR
1. Using the diagnosis "chronic rheumatoid arthritis," choose the main term within the diagnostic statement. If necessary, look up the word(s) in your dictionary.	❑	❑	❑
2. Locate the main term in the alphabetic index.	❑	❑	❑
3. Refer to all notes and conventions under the main term.	❑	❑	❑
4. Find the appropriate indented subordinate term.	❑	❑	❑
5. Follow any relevant instructions, such as "see also."	❑	❑	❑
6. Confirm the selected code by cross-referencing to the tabular index. Make sure you have added any fourth or fifth digits necessary.	❑	❑	❑
7. Assign the code.	❑	❑	❑
8. AFF Your office manager instructs you to assign a diagnosis code to a claim for a patient that you know does not have the diagnosis. Explain how you would respond.	❑	❑	❑

____

____

____

____

CALCULATION

Total Possible Points: __________

Total Points Earned: __________ Multiplied by 100 = __________ Divided by Total Possible Points = __________ %

PASS ❑ **FAIL** ❑ **COMMENTS:**

Student's signature ____________________ Date __________

Partner's signature ____________________ Date __________

Instructor's signature ____________________ Date __________

WORK PRODUCT 1

Grade: ____________

Underline the main term in these diagnoses with more than one word. Using a current diagnoses coding book, then code the diagnoses:

1. Sick sinus syndrome
2. Congestive heart failure with malignant hypertension
3. Bilateral stenosis of carotid artery
4. Aspiration pneumonia
5. Massive blood transfusion thrombocytopenia
6. Acute rheumatic endocarditis
7. Acute viral conjunctivitis with hemorrhage
8. *Escherichia coli* intestinal infection
9. Postgastrectomy diarrhea
10. Congenital syphilitic osteomyelitis

WORK PRODUCT 2

Grade: ____________

Determine the diseases associated with the following ICD-9-CM codes:

1. 555.9

   ____

2. 676.54

   ____

3. 314.01

   ____

4. 726.71

   ____

5. 722.93

   ____

WORK PRODUCT 3

Grade: ____________

Determine the supplemental *External Causes of Injury (or Morbidity)* for the following:

Description	ICD-9-CM Code	ICD-10-CM Code
Injured when hot air balloon crashed		
Skin frozen, contact with dry ice		
Bicyclist injured by train in a traffic accident		
Injured by fireworks		
Hand slashed by circular saw		

WORK PRODUCT 4

Grade: __________

Code Sequencing

Kayla Moore, age 38 years, is seen in the clinic today. She has a few chronic conditions but is seen today for fluttering in her chest. Because she is here, and it is time for her regular diabetes checkup, the doctor orders a test to check on her blood sugar. Because Ms. Moore is a breast cancer survivor, in addition she was given a mammogram. Her physician also prescribed a tetanus booster as well, because she has been renovating an old stable and has suffered several small skin punctures over the past few weeks. Her encounter form indicates the following charges:

- An EKG to monitor a previously diagnosed arrhythmia
- Fasting blood sugar for known diabetes
- Mammogram
- Tetanus booster
- List the diagnoses in the proper order to be placed on line #21 of the CMS-1500 form.

21.

1. __________ 3. __________

2. __________ 4. __________

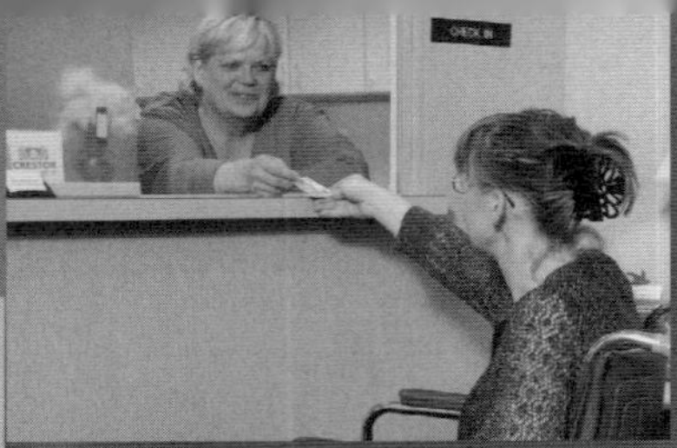

CHAPTER

12 Outpatient Procedural Coding

Learning Outcomes

COG Cognitive Domain

1. Spell and define the key terms
2. Explain the Healthcare Common Procedure Coding System (HCPCS), levels I and II
3. Explain the format of level I, Current Procedural Terminology (CPT-4), and its use
4. Describe the relationship between coding and reimbursement
5. Describe how to use the most current procedure coding system
6. Discuss the effects of upcoding and downcoding
7. Describe how to use the most current HCPCS coding
8. Describe the concept of RBRVS
9. Define both medical terms and abbreviations related to all body systems
10. Define medical necessity as it applies to procedural coding.

PSY Psychomotor Domain

1. Perform procedural coding (Procedure 12-1)

AFF Affective Domain

1. Work with physician to achieve the maximum reimbursement
2. Interact professionally with third-party representatives
3. Display tactful behavior when communicating with medical providers regarding third-party requirements
4. Utilize tactful communication skills with medical providers to ensure accurate code selection
5. Apply ethical behaviors, including honesty/integrity in performance of medical assisting practice

ABHES Competencies

1. Apply third-party guidelines
2. Perform diagnostic and procedural coding
3. Comply with federal, state, and local health laws and regulations

AFF WHAT WOULD YOU DO?

Grade: ___________

62. Read the scenario below. Then, highlight or underline the medical decision-making section.
Anikka was seen today for a follow-up on her broken wrist. The cast was removed 2 weeks ago, and she said she is still unable to achieve full range of movement in her wrist without pain. On exam, her wrist appeared swollen, and she mentioned tenderness. X-ray revealed slight fracture in carpals. Dr. Levy splinted the wrist and referred her to an orthopedic surgeon for possible surgery. I spoke with Anikka, instructing her to avoid exerting her wrist and to keep it splinted until she has seen the surgeon. Dr. Levy suggested aspirin for pain.

63. Now, read the same scenario again. Circle the history section.
Anikka was seen today for a follow-up on her broken wrist. The cast was removed 2 weeks ago, and she said she is still unable to achieve full range of movement in her wrist without pain. On exam, her wrist appeared swollen, and she mentioned tenderness. X-ray revealed slight fracture in carpals. Dr. Levy splinted the wrist and referred her to an orthopedic surgeon for possible surgery. I spoke with Anikka, instructing her to avoid exerting her wrist and to keep it splinted until she has seen the surgeon. Dr. Levy suggested aspirin for pain.

64. Read the scenario below.
Mr. Ekko presents today for removal of stitches from calf wound. Upon inspection, wound seems to have healed well, but scar tissue is still slightly inflamed. I prescribed antibacterial cream for him to apply twice a day, and instructed him to still keep the area bandaged. I told him to let us know if the swelling has not gone down within a week and to come in if it gets any worse.

Circle the correct level of medical decision making involved.

Straightforward | Low complexity

Moderate complexity | High complexity

COG IDENTIFICATION

Grade: ___________

Fill in the medical terminology chart below about the CPT subcategory on repair, revision, or reconstruction.

Suffix	Meaning
65. -pexy	
	66. surgical repair
67. -rrhaphy	

AFF CASE STUDY FOR CRITICAL THINKING

Grade: ___________

68. A patient will be undergoing surgery to remove her gallbladder. Her insurance company labels this sort of operation as an outpatient surgery. She lives alone with no assistance after surgery. She wants to stay in the hospital overnight. The patient asks if you can do anything in the coding of the procedure to make her insurance company pay for a night in the hospital. What do you say to her? Can you do anything to code this information on the claim form for more reimbursement?

____

____

____

____

PSY PROCEDURE 12-1 Locating a CPT Code

Name: ______________________ **Date:** __________ **Time:** __________ **Grade:** __________

EQUIPMENT: CPT-4 codebook, patient chart, scenario (Work Product 1)

STANDARDS: Given the needed equipment and a place to work the student will perform this skill with _____ % accuracy in a total of _____ minutes. *(Your instructor will tell you what the percentage and time limits will be before you begin.)*

KEY: 4 = Satisfactory 0 = Unsatisfactory NA = This step is not counted

PROCEDURE STEPS	SELF	PARTNER	INSTRUCTOR
1. Identify the exact procedure performed.	❑	❑	❑
2. Obtain the documentation of the procedure in the patient's chart.	❑	❑	❑
3. Choose the proper codebook.	❑	❑	❑
4. Using the alphabetic index, locate the procedure.	❑	❑	❑
5. Locate the code or range of codes given in the tabular section.	❑	❑	❑
6. Read the descriptors to find the one that most closely describes the procedure.	❑	❑	❑
7. Check the section guidelines for any special circumstances.	❑	❑	❑
8. Review the documentation to be sure it justifies the code.	❑	❑	❑
9. Determine if any modifiers are needed.	❑	❑	❑
10. Select the code and place it in the appropriate field of the CMS-1500 form.	❑	❑	❑
8. AFF Your physician is helping you find a code in the CPT-4 codebook. He chooses a code based on what the surgery entailed, but the operative report does not support what he says he did. Explain how you would advise the physician to correct the problem and proceed.	❑	❑	❑

____

____

____

____

PSY PROCEDURE 12-1 Locating a CPT Code (continued)

CALCULATION

Total Possible Points: ____________

Total Points Earned: ____________ Multiplied by 100 = ____________ Divided by Total Possible Points = ____________ %

PASS **FAIL** **COMMENTS:**

❑ ❑

Student's signature ______________________ Date ____________

Partner's signature ______________________ Date ____________

Instructor's signature ______________________ Date ____________

WORK PRODUCT 1

Grade: ____________

Perform Procedural Coding

Kayla Moore, age 38 years, has just completed a general physical. Her examination consisted of the following:

- An EKG to monitor a previously diagnosed arrhythmia
- Urine collection to test for diabetes
- Blood sampling to test cholesterol levels

Because Ms. Moore is a breast cancer survivor, in addition to the routine examination, she was given a mammogram. Her physician prescribed a tetanus booster as well, because she has been renovating an old stable and has suffered several small skin punctures over the past few weeks.

Complete the CMS-1500 form with the proper procedural coding for the patient's visit. Use the same personal patient information you used for Work Product 1 in Chapter 11 to fill in all essential details when completing the CMS-1500.

HEALTH INSURANCE CLAIM FORM

APPROVED BY NATIONAL UNIFORM CLAIM COMMITTEE (NUCC) 02/12

PICA — PICA

CARRIER

1. MEDICARE (Medicare#) MEDICAID (Medicaid#) TRICARE (ID#/DoD#) CHAMPVA (Member ID#) GROUP HEALTH PLAN (ID#) FECA BLK LUNG (ID#) OTHER (ID#)

1a. INSURED'S I.D. NUMBER (For Program in Item 1)

2. PATIENT'S NAME (Last Name, First Name, Middle Initial)

3. PATIENT'S BIRTH DATE MM DD YY SEX M F

4. INSURED'S NAME (Last Name, First Name, Middle Initial)

5. PATIENT'S ADDRESS (No., Street)

6. PATIENT RELATIONSHIP TO INSURED Self Spouse Child Other

7. INSURED'S ADDRESS (No., Street)

CITY STATE

8. RESERVED FOR NUCC USE

CITY STATE

ZIP CODE TELEPHONE (Include Area Code) ( )

ZIP CODE TELEPHONE (Include Area Code) ( )

9. OTHER INSURED'S NAME (Last Name, First Name, Middle Initial)

10. IS PATIENT'S CONDITION RELATED TO:

11. INSURED'S POLICY GROUP OR FECA NUMBER

a. OTHER INSURED'S POLICY OR GROUP NUMBER

a. EMPLOYMENT? (Current or Previous) YES NO

a. INSURED'S DATE OF BIRTH MM DD YY SEX M F

b. RESERVED FOR NUCC USE

b. AUTO ACCIDENT? YES NO PLACE (State)

b. OTHER CLAIM ID (Designated by NUCC)

c. RESERVED FOR NUCC USE

c. OTHER ACCIDENT? YES NO

c. INSURANCE PLAN NAME OR PROGRAM NAME

d. INSURANCE PLAN NAME OR PROGRAM NAME

10d. CLAIM CODES (Designated by NUCC)

d. IS THERE ANOTHER HEALTH BENEFIT PLAN? YES NO *If yes*, complete items 9, 9a, and 9d.

READ BACK OF FORM BEFORE COMPLETING & SIGNING THIS FORM.

12. PATIENT'S OR AUTHORIZED PERSON'S SIGNATURE I authorize the release of any medical or other information necessary to process this claim. I also request payment of government benefits either to myself or to the party who accepts assignment below.

SIGNED ____________ DATE ____________

13. INSURED'S OR AUTHORIZED PERSON'S SIGNATURE I authorize payment of medical benefits to the undersigned physician or supplier for services described below.

SIGNED ____________

PATIENT AND INSURED INFORMATION

14. DATE OF CURRENT ILLNESS, INJURY, or PREGNANCY (LMP) MM DD YY QUAL.

15. OTHER DATE QUAL. MM DD YY

16. DATES PATIENT UNABLE TO WORK IN CURRENT OCCUPATION FROM MM DD YY TO MM DD YY

17. NAME OF REFERRING PROVIDER OR OTHER SOURCE

17a.

17b. NPI

18. HOSPITALIZATION DATES RELATED TO CURRENT SERVICES FROM MM DD YY TO MM DD YY

19. ADDITIONAL CLAIM INFORMATION (Designated by NUCC)

20. OUTSIDE LAB? YES NO $ CHARGES

21. DIAGNOSIS OR NATURE OF ILLNESS OR INJURY Relate A-L to service line below (24E) ICD Ind.

A. B. C. D.

E. F. G. H.

I. J. K. L.

22. RESUBMISSION CODE ORIGINAL REF. NO.

23. PRIOR AUTHORIZATION NUMBER

24. A. DATE(S) OF SERVICE From MM DD YY To MM DD YY	B. PLACE OF SERVICE	C. EMG	D. PROCEDURES, SERVICES, OR SUPPLIES (Explain Unusual Circumstances) CPT/HCPCS MODIFIER	E. DIAGNOSIS POINTER	F. $ CHARGES	G. DAYS OR UNITS	H. EPSDT Family Plan	I. ID. QUAL.	J. RENDERING PROVIDER ID. #
1								NPI	
2								NPI	
3								NPI	
4								NPI	
5								NPI	
6								NPI	

25. FEDERAL TAX I.D. NUMBER SSN EIN

26. PATIENT'S ACCOUNT NO.

27. ACCEPT ASSIGNMENT? (For govt. claims, see back) YES NO

28. TOTAL CHARGE $

29. AMOUNT PAID $

30. Rsvd for NUCC Use

31. SIGNATURE OF PHYSICIAN OR SUPPLIER INCLUDING DEGREES OR CREDENTIALS (I certify that the statements on the reverse apply to this bill and are made a part thereof.)

SIGNED DATE

32. SERVICE FACILITY LOCATION INFORMATION

a. NPI b.

33. BILLING PROVIDER INFO & PH # ( )

a. NPI b.

PHYSICIAN OR SUPPLIER INFORMATION

NUCC Instruction Manual available at: www.nucc.org **_PLEASE PRINT OR TYPE_** APPROVED OMB-0938-1197 FORM 1500 (02-12)

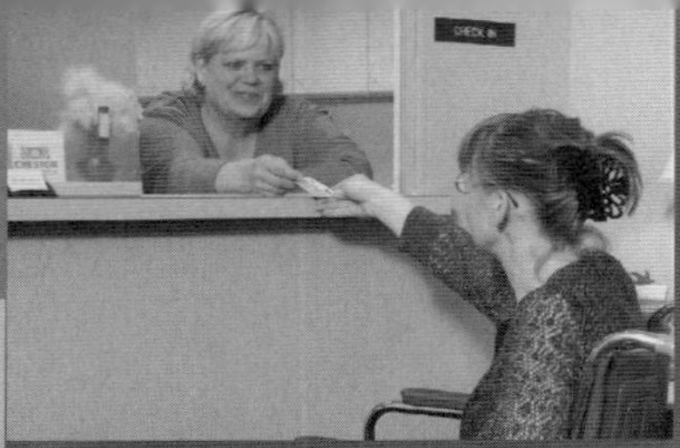

CHAPTER 13 Health Insurance and Reimbursement

Learning Outcomes

COG Cognitive Domain

1. Spell and define the key terms
2. Identify types of:
   a. third-party plans
   b. information required to file a third-party claim
   c. the steps for filing a third-party claim
3. Discuss workers' compensation as it applies to patients
4. Describe procedures for implementing both managed care and insurance plans
5. Discuss utilization review principles
6. Outline managed care requirements for patient referral
7. Compare processes for filing insurance claims both manually and electronically
8. Describe guidelines for third-party claims
9. Discuss types of physician fee schedules
10. Describe the concept of resource-based relative value scale (RBRVS)
11. Define diagnosis-related groups (DRGs)
12. Name two legal issues affecting claims submissions
13. Describe processes for verification of eligibility for services, precertification, and preauthorization
14. Define a patient-centered medical home (PCMH)
15. Differentiate between fraud and abuse

PSY Psychomotor Domain

1. Complete an insurance claim form (Procedure 13-1)
2. Apply both managed care policies and procedures
3. Apply third-party guidelines
4. Interpret information on an insurance card (Procedure 13-2)
5. Obtain precertification or preauthorization, including documentation (Procedure 13-2)
6. Verify eligibility for services including documentation (Procedure 13-2)
7. Utilize medical necessity guidelines (Procedure 13-2)

AFF Affective Domain

1. Interact professionally with third-party representatives
2. Display tactful behavior when communicating with medical providers regarding third-party requirements
3. Communicate in language the patient can understand regarding managed care and insurance plans
4. Show sensitivity when communicating with patients regarding third-party requirements
5. Apply ethical behaviors, including honesty/integrity in performance of medical assisting practice

ABHES Competencies

1. Prepare and submit insurance claims
2. Serve as liaison between physician and others
3. Comply with federal, state, and local health laws and regulations

PSY PROCEDURE 13-1 Completing a CMS-1500 Claim Form

Name: ______________________________ **Date:** __________ **Time:** __________ **Grade:** __________

EQUIPMENT: Case scenario (see work product), completed encounter form, blank CMS-1500 Claim Form, pen

STANDARDS: Given the needed equipment and a place to work, the student will perform this skill with _____ % accuracy in a total of _____ minutes. *(Your instructor will tell you what the percentage and time limits will be before you begin.)*

KEY: 4 = Satisfactory 0 = Unsatisfactory NA = This step is not counted

PROCEDURE STEPS	SELF	PARTNER	INSTRUCTOR
1. Using the information provided in the case scenario, complete the demographic information in lines 1 through 11d.	❑	❑	❑
2. Insert "SOF" (signature on file) on lines 12 and 13. Check to be sure there is a current signature on file in the chart and that it is specifically for the third-party payer being filed.	❑	❑	❑
3. If the services being filed are for a hospital stay, insert information in lines 16, 18, and 32.	❑	❑	❑
4. If the services are related to an injury, insert the date of the accident in line 14.	❑	❑	❑
5. Insert dates of service.	❑	❑	❑
6. Using the encounter form, place the CPT code listed for each service and procedure checked off in column D of lines 21–24 on the form.	❑	❑	❑
7. Place the diagnostic codes indicated on the encounter form in lines 21 (A–L) . List the reason for the encounter on line 21.A and any other diagnoses listed on the encounter form that relate to the services or procedures.	❑	❑	❑
7. Reference the codes placed in lines 21 (A–L) to each line listing a different CPT code by placing the corresponding one digit in line 24, column e.	❑	❑	❑
8. AFF You notice that Mr. Dishman has no signature on file, but the box on line 12 of his claim form says he does. Explain how you would respond.	❑	❑	❑

____

____

____

____

PSY PROCEDURE 13-1 Completing a CMS-1500 Claim Form (continued)

CALCULATION

Total Possible Points: ________

Total Points Earned: ________ Multiplied by 100 = ________ Divided by Total Possible Points = ________ %

PASS ❑ **FAIL** ❑ **COMMENTS:**

Student's signature ________________ Date ________

Partner's signature ________________ Date ________

Instructor's signature ________________ Date ________

PSY PROCEDURE 13-2 Obtain Preauthorization for Services

Name: ______________________ **Date:** __________ **Time:** __________ **Grade:** __________

EQUIPMENT: Case scenario (see work product 2), patient's demographic information including insurance card information, a physician's order for treatment, preauthorization form, pen

STANDARDS: Given the needed equipment and a place to work, the student will perform this skill with _____ % accuracy in a total of _____ minutes. *(Your instructor will tell you what the percentage and time limits will be before you begin.)*

KEY: 4 = Satisfactory 0 = Unsatisfactory NA = This step is not counted

PROCEDURE STEPS	SELF	PARTNER	INSTRUCTOR
1. Using the information provided in the case scenario, verify the physician's order with the patient's demographic/insurance information.	❑	❑	❑
2. Complete the preauthorization form (preauth form) as provided by the insurance company or the practice's form with details involving the requested services including the date the preauthorization is being requested.	❑	❑	❑
3. Contact the insurance company's preauthorization department by calling the number listed on the back of the patient's insurance card to verify the patient's eligibility for the services and document on the preauth form	❑	❑	❑
4. Determine whether or not the patient's insurance benefits require preauthorization or precertification from the insurance company for the requested service	❑	❑	❑
5. Note the name or identification of the insurance preauthorization representative on the preauth form.	❑	❑	❑
6. Provide details noted on the completed preauthorization form for the requested services and/or treatment to the insurance preauthorization representative	❑	❑	❑
7. Accurately document the preauthorization number given for the service or treatment on the preauth form. This information must be given to the provider performing the authorized services.	❑	❑	❑
8. Sign the preauthorization form as the person who got the authorization, and file it in the patient's medical record.	❑	❑	❑
9. AFF Describe how you would handle advising a patient that his or her insurance benefits did not cover the ordered service or treatment.	❑	❑	❑

____

____

____

____

PSY PROCEDURE 13-2 Obtain Preauthorization for Services (continued)

CALCULATION

Total Possible Points: __________

Total Points Earned: __________ Multiplied by 100 = __________ Divided by Total Possible Points = __________ %

PASS ❑ **FAIL** ❑ **COMMENTS:**

Student's signature ____________________ Date __________

Partner's signature ____________________ Date __________

Instructor's signature ____________________ Date __________

WORK PRODUCT 1

Grade: __________

COMPLETE INSURANCE CLAIM FORMS

Jackson Dishman is a 58-year-old man who is seen in the office for acute abdominal pain. Complete the CMS-1500 form using the information provided below:

297-01-2222
Jackson W. Dishman   Group #68735
123 Smith Avenue
Winston-Salem NC 27103   Date of Birth: 06-01-49

He is charged for an office visit, which carries the CPT code 99213 and costs $150.00. The doctor has the CMA do a radiologic examination, abdomen; complete acute abdomen series (the CPT code 74022); and the charge for the x-rays is $250.00. The x-rays are normal. He pays nothing today. The physician sends Mr. Dishman home with a diagnosis of acute right lower abdominal pain (IDC-10-CM code is R10.31). He is to return in 2 days unless the pain becomes unbearable.

HEALTH INSURANCE CLAIM FORM

APPROVED BY NATIONAL UNIFORM CLAIM COMMITTEE (NUCC) 02/12

PICA | PICA

CARRIER

1. MEDICARE (Medicare#) | MEDICAID (Medicaid#) | TRICARE (ID#/DoD#) | CHAMPVA (Member ID#) | GROUP HEALTH PLAN (ID#) | FECA BLK LUNG (ID#) | OTHER (ID#)

1a. INSURED'S I.D. NUMBER (For Program in Item 1)

2. PATIENT'S NAME (Last Name, First Name, Middle Initial)

3. PATIENT'S BIRTH DATE MM DD YY SEX M F

4. INSURED'S NAME (Last Name, First Name, Middle Initial)

5. PATIENT'S ADDRESS (No., Street)

6. PATIENT RELATIONSHIP TO INSURED Self Spouse Child Other

7. INSURED'S ADDRESS (No., Street)

CITY STATE

8. RESERVED FOR NUCC USE

CITY STATE

ZIP CODE TELEPHONE (Include Area Code) ( )

ZIP CODE TELEPHONE (Include Area Code) ( )

9. OTHER INSURED'S NAME (Last Name, First Name, Middle Initial)

10. IS PATIENT'S CONDITION RELATED TO:

11. INSURED'S POLICY GROUP OR FECA NUMBER

a. OTHER INSURED'S POLICY OR GROUP NUMBER

a. EMPLOYMENT? (Current or Previous) YES NO

a. INSURED'S DATE OF BIRTH MM DD YY SEX M F

b. RESERVED FOR NUCC USE

b. AUTO ACCIDENT? YES NO PLACE (State)

b. OTHER CLAIM ID (Designated by NUCC)

c. RESERVED FOR NUCC USE

c. OTHER ACCIDENT? YES NO

c. INSURANCE PLAN NAME OR PROGRAM NAME

d. INSURANCE PLAN NAME OR PROGRAM NAME

10d. CLAIM CODES (Designated by NUCC)

d. IS THERE ANOTHER HEALTH BENEFIT PLAN? YES NO *If yes*, complete items 9, 9a, and 9d.

READ BACK OF FORM BEFORE COMPLETING & SIGNING THIS FORM.

12. PATIENT'S OR AUTHORIZED PERSON'S SIGNATURE I authorize the release of any medical or other information necessary to process this claim. I also request payment of government benefits either to myself or to the party who accepts assignment below.

SIGNED ______ DATE ______

13. INSURED'S OR AUTHORIZED PERSON'S SIGNATURE I authorize payment of medical benefits to the undersigned physician or supplier for services described below.

SIGNED ______

PATIENT AND INSURED INFORMATION

14. DATE OF CURRENT ILLNESS, INJURY, or PREGNANCY (LMP) MM DD YY QUAL.

15. OTHER DATE QUAL. MM DD YY

16. DATES PATIENT UNABLE TO WORK IN CURRENT OCCUPATION FROM MM DD YY TO MM DD YY

17. NAME OF REFERRING PROVIDER OR OTHER SOURCE 17a. 17b. NPI

18. HOSPITALIZATION DATES RELATED TO CURRENT SERVICES FROM MM DD YY TO MM DD YY

19. ADDITIONAL CLAIM INFORMATION (Designated by NUCC)

20. OUTSIDE LAB? YES NO $ CHARGES

21. DIAGNOSIS OR NATURE OF ILLNESS OR INJURY Relate A-L to service line below (24E) ICD Ind.

A. B. C. D.
E. F. G. H.
I. J. K. L.

22. RESUBMISSION CODE ORIGINAL REF. NO.

23. PRIOR AUTHORIZATION NUMBER

24. A. DATE(S) OF SERVICE From MM DD YY To MM DD YY	B. PLACE OF SERVICE	C. EMG	D. PROCEDURES, SERVICES, OR SUPPLIES (Explain Unusual Circumstances) CPT/HCPCS MODIFIER	E. DIAGNOSIS POINTER	F. $ CHARGES	G. DAYS OR UNITS	H. EPSDT Family Plan	I. ID. QUAL.	J. RENDERING PROVIDER ID. #
1								NPI	
2								NPI	
3								NPI	
4								NPI	
5								NPI	
6								NPI	

25. FEDERAL TAX I.D. NUMBER SSN EIN

26. PATIENT'S ACCOUNT NO.

27. ACCEPT ASSIGNMENT? (For govt. claims, see back) YES NO

28. TOTAL CHARGE $

29. AMOUNT PAID $

30. Rsvd for NUCC Use

31. SIGNATURE OF PHYSICIAN OR SUPPLIER INCLUDING DEGREES OR CREDENTIALS (I certify that the statements on the reverse apply to this bill and are made a part thereof.)

SIGNED DATE

32. SERVICE FACILITY LOCATION INFORMATION

a. NPI b.

33. BILLING PROVIDER INFO & PH # ( )

a. NPI b.

PHYSICIAN OR SUPPLIER INFORMATION

NUCC Instruction Manual available at: www.nucc.org **_PLEASE PRINT OR TYPE_** APPROVED OMB-0938-1197 FORM 1500 (02-12)

WORK PRODUCT 2

Grade: ________

COMPLETE PREAUTHORIZATION FOR SERVICES

Charlene Adams is a 31-year-old woman who has been having right shoulder pain for the last 3 months that is causing her to wake several times during the night because of the severe pain. Dr. Kyle Dunn has requested an MRI of her right shoulder with contrast, and her insurance requires preauthorization. Complete a preauthorization form using the information provided below:

880-43-9770
Charlene Adams
Southeast Insurance Company Member ID #19923VT
167 Maple Ave.
Winston-Salem NC 27103 Date of Birth: 03/22/1984

The diagnosis is right shoulder pain, ICD-10-CM M25.511, and preauthorization is necessary for CPT 73222. The patient recently finished 10 physical therapy sessions for her right shoulder without relief. Ms. Adams is also an insulin-dependent diabetic.

Great Falls Medical Center Physician Offices

Insurance Preauthorization/Precertification Form

Please complete this form as accurately and with as many details as possible when preauthorizing or precertifying services or treatments with insurance companies. The completed form is filed in the patient's medical record for future reference.

Employee Name and Title:	**Date of Completion:**
Ordering Physician:	
Patient's Name:	
Patient's DOB:	Insurance ID:
Insurance Company:	
Description of service or treatment requested with CPT Code(s):	
Diagnoses codes supporting medical necessity for the service or treatment requested:	
Comorbid conditions and diseases (Diagnoses Codes):	
Other information to support medical necessity (i.e., physical therapy, medication regimen, etc.)	
Name or ID number of Insurance Representative:	
AUTHORIZATION NUMBER:	AUTHORIZED FROM: TO:
Employee Signature:	Date Authorization Obtained:

48. List four items that should be readily available in case your office is audited.

49. What is a returned check fee?

50. Why might you run a trial daily report before you run a final daily report?

51. The office you are working in has recently updated its bookkeeping system from pegboard to computer. Now, the physician wants to utilize all the capabilities the new system offers. One particular function that interests her is the computer accounting reports. List the different types of reports and briefly describe their uses.

COG PSY ACTIVE LEARNING

Grade: ____________

52. During a staff meeting, the issue of ordering supplies comes up. The office has been buying small quantities of all supplies, causing some items to quickly run out, while others are stockpiled in disuse. The physician wants to figure out a way to spend the budget more efficiently and asks you to be in charge of the next order. What steps can you take to determine which items you will order in the office's next purchase? How can you further improve the office's expenditure?

53. Your office currently is using a checking account at a local bank. However, the physician you work for is thinking about changing over to a money market account, because he has heard the interest is much better in a money market account. He knows about an offer through another bank that will waive the minimum balance of $500 for 3 months. What important information should you look into before you give him your opinion? Discuss the differences between a checking account and a money market account, and include the advantages and disadvantages to switching accounts.

____

____

____

____

COG IDENTIFICATION

Grade: ___________

54. There are several advantages of a computerized system over a manual system. Read the selection below, and circle the functions that are computerized accounting functions only.

a. Entries are recorded in a patient's file.

b. Quickly create invoices and receipts.

c. Calculation of each transaction is made, as well as a total at the end of the day.

d. Performs bookkeeping, making appointments, and generating office reports.

e. Daily activities are recorded.

f. Bill reminders are placed to keep track of expenses.

55. A medical office is just starting up, and one of the first things the bookkeeper needs to do is find a bank. Fill in the chart below with descriptions of checking, savings, and money market accounts.

Checking Account	Savings Account	Money Market Account

56. The office you are working in has an accounting cycle that begins in June. Describe what the accounting cycle is, and what kind of year your office follows.

____

____

____

____

57. The office manager ordered a new endorsement stamp from the bank. In the meantime, you need to deposit a check for Rinku Banjere, MD, into account number 123-4567-890. Endorse the check below for deposit.

ENDORSE HERE ______________________________________ ______________________________________ ______________________________________ DO NOT SIGN/WRITE/STAMP BELOW THIS LINE FOR FINANCIAL INSTITUTION USE ONLY*

PSY WHAT WOULD YOU DO?

Grade: __________

58. A patient's check has been returned for insufficient funds. The patient asks you to send it back through the bank. What would you do?

____

____

____

____

59. Explain the process of ordering supplies and paying invoices.

____

____

____

____

COG TRUE OR FALSE?

Grade: __________

Determine whether the following statements are true or false. If false, explain why.

60. Once you have entered a patient transaction on the daysheet, you give the ledger to the patient as a receipt.

____

61. As long as your bookkeeping records are accurate and the figures balance, you do not need to save receipts.

____

62. You should always compare the prices and quality of office supplies when you are placing an order.

____

63. Audits are performed in the office yearly by the IRS.

____

64. Packing slips are used by the manufacturer and can be destroyed upon opening a package of supplies.

____

COG PATIENT EDUCATION

Grade: __________

65. Your patient is a young woman who does not understand what happens to the difference between what a physician charges and what her insurance company will pay. In her case, the physician's charge is $100, but insurance only allows for $80. The insurance company will pay for 75% of the cost. How much will the patient pay? Explain to her how this works, and how the charge is determined.

____

____

____

____

AFF CASE STUDY FOR CRITICAL THINKING

Grade: __________

You have been working at a small, one-physician practice for about 2 weeks. You share the front office with the office manager, who has been working there for 20 years. She goes on vacation and in the course of covering some of her duties, you discover suspicious entries in the accounts payable records. You wonder if she is paying her own bills out of the office account.

66. What should you do? Choose all appropriate actions from the list below.

a. Nothing, she is your boss and you are new here.

b. Ask your coworkers for advice.

c. Question her about what you found when she returns.

d. Tell the physician immediately.

e. Tell the physician's wife of your suspicions.

f. Keep it to yourself; it is none of your business.

g. Post the situation on Facebook and ask for advice.

h. Investigate further while she is away by going over all of the check entries.

PSY PROCEDURE 14-1 Post Charges on a Daysheet

Name: ______________________ **Date:** __________ **Time:** __________ **Grade:** __________

EQUIPMENT/SUPPLIES: Pen, pegboard, calculator, daysheet, encounter forms, ledger cards, previous day's balance, list of patients and charges, fee schedule

STANDARDS: Given the needed equipment and a place to work, the student will perform this skill with _____ % accuracy in a total of _____ minutes. *(Your instructor will tell you what the percentage and time limits will be before you begin.)*

KEY: 4 = Satisfactory 0 = Unsatisfactory NA = This step is not counted

PROCEDURE STEPS	SELF	PARTNER	INSTRUCTOR
1. Place a new daysheet on the pegboard and record the totals from the previous daysheet.	❑	❑	❑
2. Align the patient's ledger card with the first available line on the daysheet.	❑	❑	❑
3. Place the receipt to align with the appropriate line on the ledger card.	❑	❑	❑
4. Record the number of the receipt in the appropriate column.	❑	❑	❑
5. Write the patient's name on the receipt.	❑	❑	❑
6. Record any existing balance the patient owes in the previous balance column of the daysheet.	❑	❑	❑
7. Record a brief description of the charge in the description line.	❑	❑	❑
8. Record the total charges in the charge column. Press hard so that the marks go through to the ledger card and the daysheet.	❑	❑	❑
9. Add the total charges to the previous balance and record in the current balance column.	❑	❑	❑
10. Return the ledger card to appropriate storage.	❑	❑	❑

PSY PROCEDURE 14-1 Post Charges on a Daysheet (continued)

CALCULATION

Total Possible Points: __________

Total Points Earned: __________ Multiplied by 100 = __________ Divided by Total Possible Points = __________ %

PASS ❑ **FAIL** ❑ **COMMENTS:**

Student's signature ____________________ Date __________

Partner's signature ____________________ Date __________

Instructor's signature ____________________ Date __________

PSY PROCEDURE 14-2 Post Payments on a Daysheet

Name: ______________________________ **Date:** __________ **Time:** __________ **Grade:** __________

EQUIPMENT/SUPPLIES: Pen, pegboard, calculator, daysheet, encounter forms, ledger cards, previous day's balance, list of patients and charges, fee schedule

COMPUTER AND MEDICAL OFFICE SOFTWARE: Follow the software requirements for posting credits to patient accounts.

STANDARDS: Given the needed equipment and a place to work, the student will perform this skill with _____ % accuracy in a total of _____ minutes. *(Your instructor will tell you what the percentage and time limits will be before you begin.)*

KEY: 4 = Satisfactory 0 = Unsatisfactory NA = This step is not counted

PROCEDURE STEPS	SELF	PARTNER	INSTRUCTOR
1. Place a new daysheet on the pegboard and record the totals from the previous daysheet.	❑	❑	❑
2. Align the patient's ledger card with the first available line on the daysheet.	❑	❑	❑
3. Place receipt to align with the appropriate line on the ledger card.	❑	❑	❑
4. Record the number of the receipt in the appropriate column.	❑	❑	❑
5. Write the patient's name on the receipt.	❑	❑	❑
6. Record any existing balance the patient owes in the previous balance column of the daysheet.	❑	❑	❑
7. Record the source and type of the payment in the description line.	❑	❑	❑
8. Record appropriate adjustments in adjustment column.	❑	❑	❑
9. Record the total payment in the payment column. Press hard so that marks go through to the ledger card and the daysheet.	❑	❑	❑
10. Subtract the payment and adjustments from the outstanding/previous balance, and record the current balance.	❑	❑	❑
11. Return the ledger card to appropriate storage.	❑	❑	❑

____

____

____

____

PSY PROCEDURE 14-2 Post Payments on a Daysheet (continued)

CALCULATION

Total Possible Points: __________

Total Points Earned: __________ Multiplied by 100 = __________ Divided by Total Possible Points = __________ %

PASS ❑ **FAIL** ❑ **COMMENTS:**

Student's signature ____________________ Date __________

Partner's signature ____________________ Date __________

Instructor's signature __________________ Date __________

PSY PROCEDURE 14-3 Process a Credit Balance

Name: ______________________ **Date:** __________ **Time:** __________ **Grade:** __________

EQUIPMENT/SUPPLIES: Pen, pegboard, calculator, daysheet, ledger card

STANDARDS: Given the needed equipment and a place to work, the student will perform this skill with _____ % accuracy in a total of _____ minutes. *(Your instructor will tell you what the percentage and time limits will be before you begin.)*

KEY: 4 = Satisfactory 0 = Unsatisfactory NA = This step is not counted

PROCEDURE STEPS	SELF	PARTNER	INSTRUCTOR
1. Determine the reason for the credit balance.	❑	❑	❑
2. Place brackets around the balance indicating that it is a negative number.	❑	❑	❑
3. Write a refund check and follow the steps in Procedure 14-4.	❑	❑	❑

CALCULATION

Total Possible Points: __________

Total Points Earned: __________ Multiplied by 100 = __________ Divided by Total Possible Points = __________ %

PASS ❑ **FAIL** ❑ **COMMENTS:**

Student's signature ____________________ Date __________

Partner's signature ____________________ Date __________

Instructor's signature ____________________ Date __________

PSY PROCEDURE 14-4 Process Refunds

Name: ______________________________ **Date:** __________ **Time:** __________ **Grade:** __________

EQUIPMENT/SUPPLIES: Pen, pegboard, calculator, daysheet, ledger card, checkbook, check register, word processor letterhead, envelope, postage, copy machine, patient's chart, refund file

STANDARDS: Given the needed equipment and a place to work, the student will perform this skill with _____ % accuracy in a total of _____ minutes. *(Your instructor will tell you what the percentage and time limits will be before you begin.)*

KEY: 4 = Satisfactory 0 = Unsatisfactory NA = This step is not counted

PROCEDURE STEPS	SELF	PARTNER	INSTRUCTOR
1. Determine who gets the refund, the patient or the insurance company.	❏	❏	❏
2. Pull patient's ledger card and place on current daysheet aligned with the first available line.	❏	❏	❏
3. Post the amount of the refund in the adjustment column in brackets indicating it is a debit, not a credit, adjustment.	❏	❏	❏
4. Add the adjustment to the outstanding/previous balance, and record in the current balance column.	❏	❏	❏
5. Write "Refund to Patient" or "Refund to _______" (name of insurance company) in the description column.	❏	❏	❏
6. Write a check for the credit amount made out to the appropriate party.	❏	❏	❏
7. Record the amount and name of payee in the check register.	❏	❏	❏
8. Mail check with letter of explanation to patient or insurance company.	❏	❏	❏
9. Place copy of check and copy of letter in the patient's record or in refund file.	❏	❏	❏
10. Return the patient's ledger card to its storage area.	❏	❏	❏

PSY PROCEDURE 14-4 **Process Refunds** (continued)

CALCULATION

Total Possible Points: __________

Total Points Earned: __________ Multiplied by 100 = __________ Divided by Total Possible Points = __________ %

PASS **FAIL** **COMMENTS:**

❑ ❑

Student's signature ____________________ Date __________

Partner's signature ____________________ Date __________

Instructor's signature __________________ Date __________

PSY PROCEDURE 14-5 Post Adjustments to a Daysheet

Name: ______________________ **Date:** __________ **Time:** __________ **Grade:** __________

EQUIPMENT/SUPPLIES: Pen, pegboard, calculator, daysheet, encounter forms, ledger cards, previous day's balance, list of patients and charges, fee schedule

COMPUTER AND MEDICAL OFFICE SOFTWARE: Follow the software requirements for posting credits to patient accounts.

STANDARDS: Given the needed equipment and a place to work, the student will perform this skill with _____ % accuracy in a total of _____ minutes. *(Your instructor will tell you what the percentage and time limits will be before you begin.)*

KEY: 4 = Satisfactory 0 = Unsatisfactory NA = This step is not counted

PROCEDURE STEPS	SELF	PARTNER	INSTRUCTOR
1. Pull patient's ledger card and place on current daysheet aligned with the first available line.	❑	❑	❑
2. Post the amount to be written off in the adjustment column as a credit adjustment.	❑	❑	❑
3. Subtract the adjustment from the outstanding/previous balance, and record in the current balance column.	❑	❑	❑
4. Return the ledger card to appropriate storage.	❑	❑	❑

____

____

____

____

CALCULATION

Total Possible Points: __________

Total Points Earned: __________ Multiplied by 100 = __________ Divided by Total Possible Points = __________ %

PASS ❑ **FAIL** ❑ **COMMENTS:**

Student's signature ______________________ Date __________

Partner's signature ______________________ Date __________

Instructor's signature ______________________ Date __________

PSY PROCEDURE 14-6 Post Collection Agency Payments

Name: ______________________ **Date:** __________ **Time:** __________ **Grade:** __________

EQUIPMENT/SUPPLIES: Pen, pegboard, calculator, daysheet, patient's ledger card

STANDARDS: Given the needed equipment and a place to work, the student will perform this skill with ____ % accuracy in a total of _____ minutes. *(Your instructor will tell you what the percentage and time limits will be before you begin.)*

KEY: 4 = Satisfactory 0 = Unsatisfactory NA = This step is not counted

PROCEDURE STEPS	SELF	PARTNER	INSTRUCTOR
1. Review check stub or report from the collection agency explaining the amounts to be applied to the accounts.	❑	❑	❑
2. Pull the patients' ledger cards.	❑	❑	❑
3. Post the amount to be applied in the payment column for each patient.	❑	❑	❑
4. Adjust off the amount representing the percentage of the payment charged by the collection agency.	❑	❑	❑

____

____

____

____

CALCULATION

Total Possible Points: __________

Total Points Earned: __________ Multiplied by 100 = __________ Divided by Total Possible Points = __________ %

PASS **FAIL** **COMMENTS:**

❑ ❑

Student's signature ______________________ Date __________

Partner's signature ______________________ Date __________

Instructor's signature ______________________ Date __________

PSY PROCEDURE 14-7 Process NSF Checks

Name: ______________________ **Date:** __________ **Time:** __________ **Grade:** __________

EQUIPMENT/SUPPLIES: Pen, pegboard, calculator, daysheet, patient's ledger card

STANDARDS: Given the needed equipment and a place to work, the student will perform this skill with _____ % accuracy in a total of _____ minutes. *(Your instructor will tell you what the percentage and time limits will be before you begin.)*

KEY: 4 = Satisfactory 0 = Unsatisfactory NA = This step is not counted

PROCEDURE STEPS	SELF	PARTNER	INSTRUCTOR
1. Pull patient's ledger card and place on current daysheet aligned with the first available line.	❑	❑	❑
2. Write the amount of the check in the payment column in brackets indicating it is a debit, not a credit, adjustment.	❑	❑	❑
3. Add it to the outstanding/previous balance, and record in the current balance column.	❑	❑	❑
4. Write "Check Returned For Nonsufficient Funds" in the description column.	❑	❑	❑
5. Post a returned check charge with an appropriate explanation in the charge column.	❑	❑	❑
6. Write "Bank Fee for Returned Check" in the description column.	❑	❑	❑
7. Call the patient to advise him of the returned check and the fee.	❑	❑	❑
8. Construct a proper letter of explanation and a copy of the ledger card and mail to patient.	❑	❑	❑
9. Place a copy of the letter and the check in the patient's file.	❑	❑	❑
10. Make arrangements for the patient to pay cash.	❑	❑	❑
11. Flag the patient's account as a credit risk for future transactions.	❑	❑	❑
12. Return the patient's ledger card to its storage area.	❑	❑	❑
13. AFF You see a patient whose check was returned for nonsufficient funds out at a soccer game. He whispers to you to keep quiet about the bad check. Explain how you would respond.	❑	❑	❑

____

____

____

____

PSY PROCEDURE 14-7 **Process NSF Checks** (continued)

CALCULATION

Total Possible Points: __________

Total Points Earned: __________ Multiplied by 100 = __________ Divided by Total Possible Points = __________ %

PASS ❑ **FAIL** ❑ **COMMENTS:**

Student's signature ____________________ Date __________

Partner's signature ____________________ Date __________

Instructor's signature ____________________ Date __________

PSY PROCEDURE 14-8 Balance a Daysheet

Name: ______________________ **Date:** __________ **Time:** __________ **Grade:** __________

EQUIPMENT/SUPPLIES: Daysheet with totals brought forward, simulated exercise, calculator, pen

STANDARDS: Given the needed equipment and a place to work, the student will perform this skill with _____ % accuracy in a total of _____ minutes. *(Your instructor will tell you what the percentage and time limits will be before you begin.)*

KEY: 4 = Satisfactory 0 = Unsatisfactory NA = This step is not counted

PROCEDURE STEPS	SELF	PARTNER	INSTRUCTOR
1. Be sure the totals from the previous daysheet are recorded in the column for previous totals.	❑	❑	❑
2. Total the charge column and place that number in the proper blank.	❑	❑	❑
3. Total the payment column and place that number in the proper blank.	❑	❑	❑
4. Total the adjustment column and place that number in the proper blank.	❑	❑	❑
5. Total the current balance column and place that number in the proper blank.	❑	❑	❑
6. Total the previous balance column and place that number in the proper blank.	❑	❑	❑
7. Take the grand total of the previous balances, add the grand total of the charges, and subtract the grand total of the payments and adjustments. This number must equal the grand total of the current balance.	❑	❑	❑
8. If the numbers do not match, calculate your totals again, and continue looking for errors until the numbers match. This will prove that the daysheet is balanced, and there are no errors.	❑	❑	❑
9. Record the totals of the columns in the proper space on the next daysheet. You will be prepared for balancing the new daysheet.	❑	❑	❑

PSY PROCEDURE 14-8 Balance a Daysheet (continued)

CALCULATION

Total Possible Points: __________

Total Points Earned: __________ Multiplied by 100 = __________ Divided by Total Possible Points = __________ %

PASS ❑ **FAIL** ❑ **COMMENTS:**

Student's signature ____________________ Date __________

Partner's signature ____________________ Date __________

Instructor's signature ____________________ Date __________

PSY PROCEDURE 14-9 Complete a Bank Deposit Slip and Make a Deposit

Name: ______________________ **Date:** __________ **Time:** __________ **Grade:** __________

EQUIPMENT/SUPPLIES: Calculator with tape, currency, coins, checks for deposit, deposit slip, endorsement stamp, deposit envelope

STANDARDS: Given the needed equipment and a place to work, the student will perform this skill with _____ % accuracy in a total of _____ minutes. *(Your instructor will tell you what the percentage and time limits will be before you begin.)*

KEY: 4 = Satisfactory 0 = Unsatisfactory NA = This step is not counted

PROCEDURE STEPS	SELF	PARTNER	INSTRUCTOR
1. Separate cash from checks.	❑	❑	❑
2. Arrange bills face up and sort with the largest denomination on top.	❑	❑	❑
3. Record the total in the cash block on the deposit slip	❑	❑	❑
4. Endorse the back of each check with "For Deposit Only."	❑	❑	❑
5. Record the amount of each check beside an identifying number on the deposit slip.	❑	❑	❑
6. Total and record the amounts of checks in the total of checks line on the deposit slip.	❑	❑	❑
7. Total and record the amount of cash and the amount of checks.	❑	❑	❑
8. Record the total amount of the deposit in the office checkbook register.	❑	❑	❑
9. Make a copy of both sides of the deposit slip for office records.	❑	❑	❑
10. Place the cash, checks, and the completed deposit slip in an envelope or bank bag for transporting to the bank for deposit.	❑	❑	❑

____

____

____

____

PSY PROCEDURE 14-9 Complete a Bank Deposit Slip and Make a Deposit (continued)

CALCULATION

Total Possible Points: __________

Total Points Earned: __________ Multiplied by 100 = __________ Divided by Total Possible Points = __________ %

PASS ❑ **FAIL** ❑ **COMMENTS:**

Student's signature ____________________ Date __________

Partner's signature ____________________ Date __________

Instructor's signature ____________________ Date __________

PSY PROCEDURE 14-10 Reconcile a Bank Statement

Name: ______________________ **Date:** __________ **Time:** __________ **Grade:** __________

EQUIPMENT/SUPPLIES: Simulated bank statement, reconciliation worksheet, calculator, pen

STANDARDS: Given the needed equipment and a place to work, the student will perform this skill with _____ % accuracy in a total of _____ minutes. *(Your instructor will tell you what the percentage and time limits will be before you begin.)*

KEY: 4 = Satisfactory 0 = Unsatisfactory NA = This step is not counted

PROCEDURE STEPS	SELF	PARTNER	INSTRUCTOR
1. Compare the opening balance on the new statement with the closing balance on the previous statement.	❑	❑	❑
2. List the bank balance in the appropriate space on the reconciliation worksheet.	❑	❑	❑
3. Compare the check entries on the statement with the entries in the check register.	❑	❑	❑
4. List the amounts of checks without check marks (outstanding checks).	❑	❑	❑
5. Total outstanding checks.	❑	❑	❑
6. Subtract from the checkbook balance items such as withdrawals, automatic payments, or service charges that appeared on the statement but not in the checkbook.	❑	❑	❑
7. Add to the bank statement balance any deposits not shown on the bank statement.	❑	❑	❑
8. Make sure balance in the checkbook and the bank statement agree.	❑	❑	❑

____

____

____

____

CALCULATION

Total Possible Points: __________

Total Points Earned: __________ Multiplied by 100 = __________ Divided by Total Possible Points = __________ %

PASS ❑ **FAIL** ❑ **COMMENTS:**

Student's signature ____________________ Date __________

Partner's signature ____________________ Date __________

Instructor's signature ____________________ Date __________

PSY PROCEDURE 14-11 Maintain a Petty Cash Account

Name: ________________________ **Date:** __________ **Time:** __________ **Grade:** __________

EQUIPMENT/SUPPLIES: Cash box, play money, checkbook, simulated receipts, and/or vouchers representing expenditures

STANDARDS: Given the needed equipment and a place to work, the student will perform this skill with _____ % accuracy in a total of _____ minutes. *(Your instructor will tell you what the percentage and time limits will be before you begin.)*

KEY: 4 = Satisfactory 0 = Unsatisfactory NA =This step is not counted

PROCEDURE STEPS	SELF	PARTNER	INSTRUCTOR
1. Count the money remaining in the box.	❑	❑	❑
2. Total the amounts of all vouchers in the petty cash box and determine the amount of expenditures.	❑	❑	❑
3. Subtract the amount of receipts from the original amount in petty cash, to equal the amount of cash remaining in the box.	❑	❑	❑
4. Balance the cash against the receipts.	❑	❑	❑
5. Write a check only for the amount that was used.	❑	❑	❑
6. Record totals on the memo line of the check stub.	❑	❑	❑
7. Sort and record all vouchers to the appropriate accounts.	❑	❑	❑
8. File the list of vouchers and attached receipts.	❑	❑	❑
9. Place cash in petty cash fund.	❑	❑	❑
10. AFF A coworker asks to borrow money from petty cash for bus fair home. She promises to pay it back tomorrow. Explain how you would respond.	❑	❑	❑

____

____

____

____

PSY PROCEDURE 14-11 Maintain a Petty Cash Account (continued)

CALCULATION

Total Possible Points: __________

Total Points Earned: __________ Multiplied by 100 = __________ Divided by Total Possible Points = __________ %

PASS ❑ **FAIL** ❑ **COMMENTS:**

Student's signature ____________________ Date __________

Partner's signature ____________________ Date __________

Instructor's signature ____________________ Date __________

PSY PROCEDURE 14-12 Order Supplies

Name: ______________________ **Date:** __________ **Time:** __________ **Grade:** __________

EQUIPMENT/SUPPLIES: 5 × 7 index cards, file box with divider cards, computer with Internet (optional), medical supply catalogues

STANDARDS: Given the needed equipment and a place to work, the student will perform this skill with _____ % accuracy in a total of _____ minutes. *(Your instructor will tell you what the percentage and time limits will be before you begin.)*

KEY: 4 = Satisfactory 0 = Unsatisfactory NA = This step is not counted

PROCEDURE STEPS	SELF	PARTNER	INSTRUCTOR
1. Create a list of supplies to be ordered that is based on inventory done by employees.	❑	❑	❑
2. Create an index card for each supply on the list including the name of the supply in the top left corner, the name and contact information of vendor(s), and product identification number.	❑	❑	❑
3. File the index cards in the file box with divider cards alphabetically or by product type.	❑	❑	❑
4. Record the current price of the item and how the item is supplied.	❑	❑	❑
5. Record the reorder point.	❑	❑	❑

____

____

____

____

CALCULATION

Total Possible Points: __________

Total Points Earned: __________ Multiplied by 100 = __________ Divided by Total Possible Points = __________ %

PASS **FAIL** **COMMENTS:**

❑ ❑

Student's signature ____________________ Date __________

Partner's signature ____________________ Date __________

Instructor's signature ____________________ Date __________

PSY PROCEDURE 14-13 Write a Check

Name: ______________________ **Date:** __________ **Time:** __________ **Grade:** __________

EQUIPMENT/SUPPLIES: Simulated page of checks from checkbook, scenario giving amount of check, check register

STANDARDS: Given the needed equipment and a place to work, the student will perform this skill with _____ % accuracy in a total of _____ minutes. *(Your instructor will tell you what the percentage and time limits will be before you begin.)*

KEY: 4 = Satisfactory 0 = Unsatisfactory NA = This step is not counted

PROCEDURE STEPS	SELF	PARTNER	INSTRUCTOR
1. Fill out the check register with the following information: **a.** check number **b.** date **c.** payee information **d.** amount **e.** previous balance **f.** new balance	❑	❑	❑
2. Enter date on check.	❑	❑	❑
3. Enter payee on check.	❑	❑	❑
4. Enter the amount of check using numerals.	❑	❑	❑
5. Write out the amount of the check beginning as far left as possible and make a straight line to fill in space between dollars and cents.	❑	❑	❑
6. Record cents as a fraction with 100 as the denominator.	❑	❑	❑
7. Obtain appropriate signature(s).	❑	❑	❑
8. Proofread for accuracy.	❑	❑	❑

CALCULATION

Total Possible Points: __________

Total Points Earned: __________ Multiplied by 100 = __________ Divided by Total Possible Points = __________ %

PASS ❑ **FAIL** ❑ **COMMENTS:**

Student's signature ____________________ Date __________

Partner's signature ____________________ Date __________

Instructor's signature ____________________ Date __________

WORK PRODUCT 1

Grade: ____________

PERFORM AN INVENTORY OF SUPPLIES

When you are working in a medical office, you may need to keep an inventory of all supplies. The inventory will help you decide when to order new supplies. It will also help you calculate how much money you will need to spend on supplies. Supplies are those items that are consumed quickly and need to be reordered on a regular basis.

If you are currently working in a medical office, use the form below to take an inventory of the supplies in the office. If you do not have access to a medical office, complete an inventory of the supplies in your kitchen or bathroom at home.

Third Street
Physician's Office, Inc.
123 Main Street
Baltimore, MD 21201
410-895-6214

Supply Inventory

Item Description	Item Number or Code	Number Needed in Stock	Number Currently in Stock	Date Ordered	Number Ordered	Unit Price	Total	Actual Delivery Date

WORK PRODUCT 2

Grade: ____________

PERFORM AN INVENTORY OF EQUIPMENT

When you are working in a medical office, you may need to keep an inventory of all equipment. The inventory will help you decide when to order new equipment. It will also help you calculate how much money you will need to spend on new equipment. Equipment includes items that can be used over and over and generally last many years.

If you are currently working in a medical office, use the form below to take an inventory of the equipment in the office. If you do not have access to a medical office, complete an inventory of the equipment in your kitchen or bathroom at home.

Third Street
Physician's Office, Inc.
123 Main Street
Baltimore, MD 21201
410-895-6214

Equipment Inventory

Item Description	Item Number or Code	Purchase Date	Condition	Comments	Expected New Purchase Date	Cost if Purchased This Year

WORK PRODUCT 3

Grade: ___________

PROCESS A CREDIT BALANCE

Mr. Juan Rodriguez has switched to a different insurance company. His copay with his old carrier was $35 per visit. His new copay is $20 per visit. However, there was a billing oversight, and Mr. Rodriguez paid his old copay. Process Mr. Rodriguez's credit balance on the daysheet.

			CREDITS				
Date	Description	Charges	Payments	Adjust ments	Current Balance	Previous Balance	NAME

Totals This Page					
Totals Previous Page					
Month-To-Date Totals					

WORK PRODUCT 4

Grade: ________

PROCESS A REFUND

Mr. Rodriguez has a credit balance of $15 on his account. You need to mail him a refund check. Post this transaction on the daysheet.

			CREDITS				
Date	**Description**	**Charges**	**Payments**	**Adjust ments**	**Current Balance**	**Previous Balance**	**NAME**

Totals This Page					
Totals Previous Page					
Month-To-Date Totals					

WORK PRODUCT 5

Grade: ___________

POST ADJUSTMENTS

Mr. Rodriguez visits your office for an x-ray of his knee. Your office normally charges $225 for a knee x-ray. However, your physician is a participating provider for Mr. Rodriguez's insurance carrier. His insurance pays your office only $175 for a knee x-ray. Post the proper adjustment on the daysheet.

			CREDITS				
Date	Description	Charges	Payments	Adjust ments	Current Balance	Previous Balance	NAME

Totals This Page					
Totals Previous Page					
Month-To-Date Totals					

WORK PRODUCT 6

Grade: ____________

POST NSF CHECKS

You have just received a check that was returned for nonsufficient funds. The check was written by Martha Montgomery for $750. Post the proper information on the daysheet.

			CREDITS				
Date	**Description**	**Charges**	**Payments**	**Adjust ments**	**Current Balance**	**Previous Balance**	**NAME**

Totals This Page					
Totals Previous Page					
Month-To-Date Totals					

WORK PRODUCT 7

Grade: ____________

POST COLLECTION AGENCY PAYMENTS

You receive a check for $787.50 and the following statement from your collection agency.
Jones & Jones Collections
Account:d. Larsen, MD

Debtor	Amount Collected	Fee	Balance
Martha Montgomery	$750.00	$187.50	$562.50
Johan Johansen	$300.00	$75.00	$225.00
		Total	$787.50

Post the payments to the daysheet.

			CREDITS				
Date	Description	Charges	Payments	Adjust ments	Current Balance	Previous Balance	NAME

Totals This Page					
Totals Previous Page					
Month-To-Date Totals					

WORK PRODUCT 8

Grade: ____________

POSTING PAYMENTS FROM MEDICARE

On a blank daysheet provided, post the following Medicare payments. You will need to calculate the adjustments by subtracting the amount allowed from the amount charged. The patient's previous balance will be the amount charged back on the date of service.

Keep in mind that on an actual Medicare EOB, the CPT-4 codes would be used instead of OV, x-ray, etc.

MEDICARE EXPLANATION OF BENEFITS

Name	Charges	Date of Service	Amount Allowed	Amount Paid to Provider	Patient's Responsibility
Smith, John	OV 40.00	3-2-xx	18.00	14.40	3.60
Jones, Anne Total:	OV 100.00 Lab 50.00 150.00	3-2-xx	65.00 50.00 115.00	52.00 40.00 92.00	13.00 10.00 23.00
Stevens, Sally Total:	OV 150.00 X-ray 200.00 350.00	3-2-xx	120.00 160.00 280.00	96.00 128.00 224.00	24.00 32.00 56.00
Reynolds, Susan	Consult 300.00	3-2-xx	250.00	200.00	50.00

CREDITS

Date	Description	Charges	Payments	Adjustments	Current Balance	Previous Balance	NAME

Totals This Page					
Totals Previous Page					
Month-To-Date Totals					

WORK PRODUCT 9

Grade: __________

PUTTING IT ALL TOGETHER

On a blank daysheet provided, complete 1–8.

Post the following transactions on the daysheet provided. Use today's date.

1. Stanley Gleber came in and paid $25.00 in cash on his account. His previous balance is $100.00.
2. Lisa Moore sent a check in the mail for $100.00 to be paid on her account, which carries a balance of $500.00.
3. Elaine Newman came in and handed you a check she received from Blue Cross Blue Shield for $700.00 to be paid on her account, which has a balance of $900.00. The explanation attached to the check indicates it is for surgery she had on 03/01/09. Your physician does NOT participate with Blue Cross Blue Shield. Post the payment with an appropriate description. Will there be an adjustment?
4. Madeline Bell saw the doctor and brings out an encounter form with a charge for an office visit at $50.00 and lab at $150.00. Post her charges. She does not pay today. Her previous balance was zero.
5. Post the collection agency payment for John Simms. His account with a balance of $250.00 was turned over to Equifax on 03/01/12. They collected the entire amount. You receive a check from Equifax. They charge 30% of what they collect, so the check is for 200.00. His balance was not written off when turned over to Equifax, so his previous balance should be 250.00.
6. Hazel Wilbourne paid her charges of $200.00 in full at her last visit. Now you receive a check from Aetna for that visit. The check is for $130.00. Your physician participates with this insurance company, which means he agrees to accept what they pay. In other words, you will not bill the patient for the difference. Post the check to Ms. Wilbourne's account.
7. Ms. Wilbourne now has a credit balance. You will need to send her a check from the office account as a refund. Post the appropriate entry for this transaction. In accounting, a credit balance is put in angle brackets: <200.00>.
8. Calculate and record each column total. Make sure the columns balance by starting with your previous balance, adding the charges, subtracting the payments and adjustments, and this should give you the total of your current balance column. Remember, brackets in accounting mean that you do the opposite when adding your columns, so instead of adding a credit balance when totaling, you will subtract it.

Date	Description	Charges	CREDITS Payments	CREDITS Adjustments	Current Balance	Previous Balance	NAME

Totals This Page					
Totals Previous Page					
Month-To-Date Totals					

WORK PRODUCT 10

Grade: ________

PREPARE A BANK DEPOSIT

Prepare a bank deposit for the following:

- Check for $750 from Martin Montgomery.
- Check for $35 from Rita Gonzalez.
- $125 cash

Use fictitious demographic information for the account holder on the deposit slip.

Newtown Bank, N.A.

DEPOSIT

Name and account number will be verifi ed when presented.

Name	Date
Address	
Signature	Sign here only if cash is received from deposit

ITEMS DEPOSITED	DOLLARS	CENTS
Currency	.	
Coin	.	
Checks 1	.	
2	.	
3	.	
4	.	
Sub Total	.	
Less Cash	.	
Total Deposit	$.	

Store Number (Commercial Accounts Only) *

Account Number (For CAP Accounts, use 10-digit number.) *

36. What are some of the negative aspects of extending credit to patients? Consider costs, patient attitudes, and legal requirements in your answer.

____

____

____

____

COG ACTIVE LEARNING

Grade: __________

37. Use the Internet to research the three major credit bureaus and find out how to check a new patient's credit history. Specifically, find out what's available to help you decide how to handle payment from people without traditional credit histories. This group includes college students, young adults, recent immigrants, traditional housewives, and people who choose not to use credit cards.

38. Many people feel uncomfortable asking other people for money. However, you need to feel comfortable discussing finance and account information with patients. Working with a partner, role-play a scenario in which a patient has an overdue account that the medical assistant must address. Take turns playing the parts of the medical assistant and the patient to understand both perspectives.

39. In recent years, the government has called into question the practice of professional courtesy extended to other health care professionals. Perform research online or talk to health care professionals to find out more about the issues surrounding professional courtesy. Then, write a viewpoint paper arguing for or against the practice of professional courtesy.

COG FALSE THEN TRUE

Grade: __________

40. All the statements below are false or inaccurate. Rewrite each statement so that it accurately reflects the consumer protection laws regarding credit collection.

a. You cannot contact a patient directly about an unpaid bill.

____

b. You should not try to contact a debtor before 9:00 am or after 5:00 pm.

____

c. You have every right to call debtors at work.

____

d. You should keep calling a patient about a debt after turning the case over to a collection agency, in order to increase your chances of recovering the money.

____

e. It's okay to use abusive language to intimidate a debtor, as long as you don't give false or misleading information.

____

f. If a patient dies and the estate can't meet all of his or her debts, the probate court will pay the medical bills first.

____

COG SHORT ANSWER

Grade: _______

41. List three situations in which calling a patient to collect an overdue payment may be least helpful.

____

____

____

____

42. What should be in a mailing that asks a patient to settle an overdue account?

____

____

____

____

43. What is a good way to use a patient's visit as an opportunity to try to collect payment on an overdue bill?

____

____

____

____

44. What should you say and not say if you call a patient to collect on a bill and you are asked to leave a message?

____

____

____

____

COG TRUE OR FALSE?

Grade: _______

45. Determine whether the following statements are true or false. If false, explain why.

a. A physician's fee schedule takes into consideration the costs of operating the office, such as rent, utilities, malpractice insurance, and salaries.

____

b. If a patient has insurance, you must charge him the insurance carrier's allowed fee for a procedure.

____

c. To maintain good relations with patients, you should be vague and polite when you ask them to pay their bills.

___

d. You should monitor the activity on a patient's credit account in order to keep the collection ratio low.

___

PSY AFF WHAT WOULD YOU DO?

Grade: ___

46. You have several patients who have long-standing debts. They don't come into the office anymore, and they don't respond to your telephone calls or letters. You outsourced your overdue billing to a collections agency, but these longtime patients have told you that they have been very upset by the "nastiness" of the collections people who contacted them. You spoke with a collections agency representative who assured you his employees were doing nothing illegal or inappropriate. You have considered changing collection agencies, but this one's rates are better, and they did collect the debts. What would you do?

___

___

___

___

47. Mrs. Sanchez is seeing Dr. Roland for the first time and has asked you to explain the physician's fees. How would you explain to Mrs. Sanchez how Dr. Roland establishes the fees he charges his patients?

___

___

___

___

AFF CASE STUDY FOR CRITICAL THINKING

Grade: ___

Mr. Green has been a patient with your practice for more than 20 years and has always paid his copayment or bill before he left the office. Recently, however, he has not been paying anything at all, and his outstanding bill is 60 days past due. You have called his home and left several phone messages, but you still haven't heard from him.

48. What should you do? Circle all appropriate actions from the following list.

a. Send him a letter demanding that he pay his balance immediately.

b. Flag his account for the credit manager to speak with him about his bill when he comes in for a visit.

c. Send a letter asking him to please call the office. State in the letter that you are worried about him.

d. Flag his record to warn anyone making an appointment for him that he is not to be seen until he pays on his bill.

e. Terminate the physician–patient contract in writing.

49. A coworker tells you that the patient is very rich. She says that he is just getting old and can't keep up with his bills any longer. Circle all appropriate actions in the list below.

a. Tell the coworker to mind her own business.

b. Do not consider this gossip in your dealings with the patient.

c. Contact the patient's next of kin and tell them that he needs help.

d. Send the patient a letter telling him you know he has the funds to pay his bill.

e. Do nothing until you reach the patient.

f. Do not mention this new information when you do speak with him.

PSY PROCEDURE 15-1 Evaluate and Manage a Patient's Account

Name: ______________________ **Date:** __________ **Time:** __________ **Grade:** __________

EQUIPMENT: Simulation including scenario; sample patient ledger card with transactions; yellow, blue, and red stickers (yellow for accounts 30 days past due; blue for accounts 60 days past due; red for accounts 90 days past due). See Work Product 1.

STANDARDS: Given the needed equipment and a place to work, the student will perform this skill with _____ % accuracy in a total of _____ minutes. *(Your instructor will tell you what the percentage and time limits will be before you begin.)*

KEY: 4 = Satisfactory 0 = Unsatisfactory NA = This step is not counted

PROCEDURE STEPS	SELF	PARTNER	INSTRUCTOR
1. Review the patient's account history to determine the "age" of the account. If payment has not been made between 30 and 59 days from today's date, the account is 40 days past due, and so on.	❑	❑	❑
2. Flag the account for appropriate action. Place a yellow flag (sticker) on accounts that are 30 days old. Place a blue flag on accounts that are 60 days old. Place a red flag on accounts that are 90 days old.	❑	❑	❑
3. Set aside accounts that have had no payment in 91 days or longer.	❑	❑	❑
4. Set aside accounts that have had no payment in 91 days or longer.	❑	❑	❑
5. Sort the copies by category: 30, 60, 90 days.	❑	❑	❑
6. Write or stamp the copies with the appropriate message.	❑	❑	❑
7. Mail the statements to the patients.	❑	❑	❑
8. Follow through with the collection process by continually reviewing past due accounts.	❑	❑	❑
9. AFF When you call a patient with a seriously past due account, he informs you that he has not paid because his wife passed away and he cannot hardly get through the day. Explain how you would respond.	❑	❑	❑

____

____

____

____

PSY PROCEDURE 15-1 Evaluate and Manage a Patient's Account (continued)

CALCULATION

Total Possible Points: __________

Total Points Earned: __________ Multiplied by 100 = __________ Divided by Total Possible Points = __________ %

PASS **FAIL** **COMMENTS:**

❑ ❑

Student's signature ____________________ Date __________

Partner's signature ____________________ Date __________

Instructor's signature ____________________ Date __________

PSY PROCEDURE 15-2 Composing a Collection Letter

Name: ______________________ **Date:** __________ **Time:** __________ **Grade:** __________

EQUIPMENT: Ledger cards generated in Procedure 15-1, word processor, and stationery with letterhead

STANDARDS: Given the needed equipment and a place to work, the student will perform this skill with _____ % accuracy in a total of _____ minutes. *(Your instructor will tell you what the percentage and time limits will be before you begin.)*

KEY: 4 = Satisfactory 0 = Unsatisfactory NA = This step is not counted

PROCEDURE STEPS	SELF	PARTNER	INSTRUCTOR
1. Review the patients' accounts and sort the accounts by age.	❑	❑	❑
2. Design a rough draft of a form letter that can be used for collections.	❑	❑	❑
3. In the first paragraph, tell the patient why you are writing.	❑	❑	❑
4. Inform the patient of the action you expect. For example: "To avoid further action, please pay $50.00 on this account by Friday, May 1, 20 _____	❑	❑	❑
5. Proofread the rough draft for errors, clarity, accuracy, and retype.	❑	❑	❑
6. Take the collection letter to a supervisor or physician for approval.	❑	❑	❑
7. Fill in the appropriate amounts and dates on each letter. Ask for at least half of the account balance within a 2-week period.	❑	❑	❑
8. Print, sign, and mail the letter.	❑	❑	❑
9. AFF You are helping a coworker get her collections letters in the mail. You notice several errors in the letters. Explain how you would respond.	❑	❑	❑

____

____

____

____

CALCULATION

Total Possible Points: __________

Total Points Earned: __________ Multiplied by 100 = __________ Divided by Total Possible Points = __________ %

PASS ❑ **FAIL** ❑ **COMMENTS:**

Student's signature ____________________ Date __________

Partner's signature ____________________ Date __________

Instructor's signature ____________________ Date __________

WORK PRODUCT 1

Grade: ________

PERFORM ACCOUNTS RECEIVABLE PROCEDURES

Your office's billing cycle posts bills on the first of every month. Review the list of outstanding payments and organize in the Aging of Accounts Receivable Report below.

- Oliver Santino visited the office on April 27 for a physical and blood work. The bill was $250.
- Warren Gates visited the office on May 8. His bill was $55.
- Tamara Jones visited the office on June 18 for a physical examination. The cost for the physical was $125, with an additional $55 for lab work.
- Amir Shell visited the office on June 25 for a physical exam and chest x-rays. The bill was $315.
- Nora Stevenson visited the office on July 9 to have a wound sutured. The bill was $100.

Below is an aging schedule as of August 30, 2012. Fill in the information for these patients. You may enter an account number of 000-00-0000 for all patients.

Aging of Accounts Receivable Report: August 30, 2012

Patient Name	Account Number	Due Date	Amount
Accounts 30 Days Past Due:			
________	________	________	________
________	________	________	________
________	________	________	________
________	________	________	________
________	________	________	________
Accounts 60 Days Past Due:			
________	________	________	________
________	________	________	________
________	________	________	________
________	________	________	________
________	________	________	________
Accounts 90 Days Past Due:			
________	________	________	________
________	________	________	________
________	________	________	________
________	________	________	________
________	________	________	________
Accounts 120 Days or More Past Due:			
________	________	________	________
________	________	________	________
________	________	________	________
________	________	________	________
________	________	________	________
Total Overdue Accounts Receivable			________

WORK PRODUCT 2

Grade: __________

PERFORM BILLING AND COLLECTION PROCEDURES

Caroline Cusick has an outstanding balance of $415 due to the medical office Pediatric Associates, 1415 San Juan Way, Santa Cruz, CA 95060. Write a collection letter to the patient to tell her about her overdue account. Her contact information is as follows: Caroline Cusick, 24 Beach Street, Santa Cruz, CA 95060. Print the letter and attach to this sheet.

PART

3

The Clinical Medical Assistant

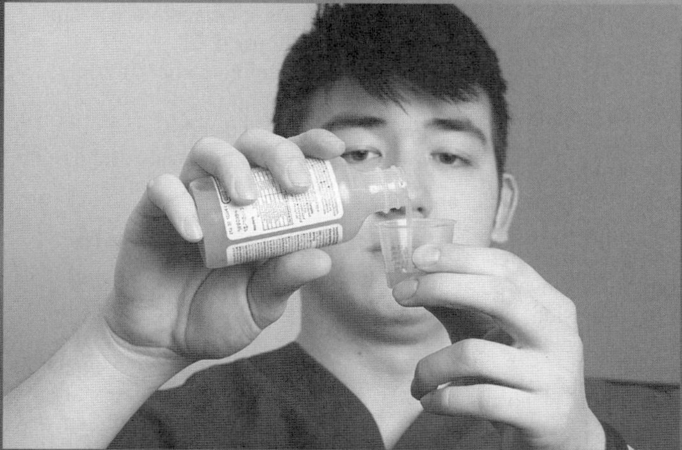

UNIT FOUR FUNDAMENTALS OF CLINICAL MEDICAL ASSISTING

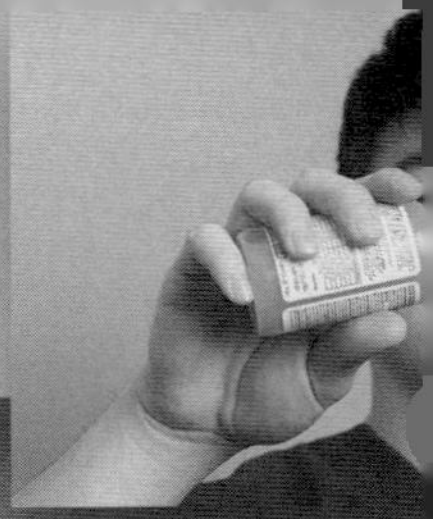

CHAPTER 16 Nutrition and Wellness

Learning Outcomes

COG Cognitive Domain

1. Spell and define the key terms
2. Identify body systems
3. List major organs in each body system
4. Identify the anatomical location of major organs in each body system
5. Describe the normal function of the digestive system
6. Analyze health care results as reported in graphs, and/or tables (BMI)
7. Describe dietary nutrients including carbohydrates, fat, protein, minerals, electrolytes, vitamins, fiber, and water.
8. Discuss the body's basal metabolic rate and its importance in weight management
9. Explain how to use the food pyramid and MyPlate guides to promote healthy food choices
10. Read and explain the information on food labels
11. Identify the special dietary needs for weight control, cardiovascular disease, and hypertension.
12. Define the function of dietary supplements
13. List the components of physical fitness
14. Discuss suggestions for a healthy lifestyle
15. Explain the importance of disease prevention
16. List and describe the effects of the substances most commonly abused
17. Recognize the dangers of substance abuse

PSY Psychomotor Domain

1. Teach a patient how to read food labels (Procedure 16-1)
2. Document patient care accurately in the medical record
3. Develop a meal plan utilizing basic principles of nutrition (Procedure 16-2)
4. Instruct a patient according to patient's special dietary needs (Procedure 16-2)
5. Coach patients appropriately considering:
   a. cultural diversity
   b. developmental life stage
   c. communication barriers

AFF Affective Domain

1. Incorporate critical thinking skills when performing patient assessment
2. Incorporate critical thinking skills when performing patient care
3. Show awareness of a patient's concerns regarding dietary changes
4. Protect the integrity of the medical record
5. Demonstrate:
   a. empathy
   b. active listening
   c. nonverbal communication
6. Demonstrate the principles of self-boundaries
7. Demonstrate respect for individual diversity including
   a. gender
   b. race
   c. religion
   d. age
   e. economic status
   f. appearance
8. Explain to a patient the rationale for performance of a procedure

ABHES Competencies

1. Comprehend and explain to the patient the importance of diet and nutrition
2. Effectively convey and educate patients regarding the proper diet and nutrition guidelines
3. Identify categories of patients that require special diets or diet modifications
4. Document accurately

10. Your 17-year-old patient comes in to the physician's office because he has a bad cough. This is the second time this winter that he has seen the physician for respiratory problems. When you review the patient's chart, you see that he had asthma when he was younger. You ask the patient if he smokes and he says that he does occasionally with his friends but also indicates that he is "not a smoker" because he's not addicted to nicotine. He also notes that he would prefer that his parents not know that he smokes, even occasionally. What should you say to this patient about his breathing issues? Would it be appropriate to tell his parents? Why or why not?

____

____

____

____

PSY PROCEDURE 16-1 Teach a Patient How to Read Food Labels

Name: ______________________ **Date:** __________ **Time:** __________ **Grade:** __________

EQUIPMENT/SUPPLIES: Two boxes of the same item, one low calorie or "lite," the other regular; measuring cup; two bowls

STANDARDS: Given the needed equipment and a place to work, the student will perform this skill with _____ % accuracy in a total of _____ minutes. *(Your instructor will tell you what the percentage and time limits will be before you begin.)*

KEY: 4 = Satisfactory 0 = Unsatisfactory NA = This step is not counted

PROCEDURE STEPS	SELF	PARTNER	INSTRUCTOR
1. Identify the patient.	❑	❑	❑
2. Introduce yourself and explain the procedure including the rationale.	❑	❑	❑
3. Have the patient look at the labels comparing the two.	❑	❑	❑
4. Ask the patient to pour out a normal serving.	❑	❑	❑
5. Measure the exact serving size printed on the label.	❑	❑	❑
6. Compare the two. Discuss the difference, if any.	❑	❑	❑
7. Explain to the patient the sections of the label: serving size and servings per package.	❑	❑	❑
8. Explain column for amount in serving.	❑	❑	❑
9. Explain column for percent daily value (formerly RDA).	❑	❑	❑
10. Explain calories and calories from fat.	❑	❑	❑
11. Have the patient calculate the percentage of fat calories and compare with the label.	❑	❑	❑
12. Read down the label and discuss each nutrient, pointing out the amounts and percentages.	❑	❑	❑
13. Have the patient compare the two labels and tell you how many total carbohydrates are in each label, sugars, protein, etc.	❑	❑	❑
14. AFF Explain how to respond to a patient who has religious or personal beliefs against eating specific food groups, such as meats.	❑	❑	❑

____

____

____

____

PSY PROCEDURE 16-1 Teach a Patient How to Read Food Labels (continued)

15. Ask the patient if she has any questions.	❑	❑	❑
16. Log into the Electronic Medical Record (EMR) using your username and secure password OR obtain the paper medical record from a secure location and assure it is kept away from public access.	❑	❑	❑
17. Chart the verbal and written instructions given to the patient. When finished, log out of the EMR and/or replace the paper medical record in an appropriate and secure location.	❑	❑	❑

CALCULATION

Total Possible Points: __________

Total Points Earned: __________ Multiplied by 100 = __________ Divided by Total Possible Points = __________ %

PASS ❑ **FAIL** ❑ **COMMENTS:**

Student's signature ____________________ Date __________

Partner's signature ____________________ Date __________

Instructor's signature ____________________ Date __________

PSY PROCEDURE 16-2 Develop a Meal Plan Utilizing Basic Principles of Nutrition; Instruct a Patient according to Patient's Special Dietary Needs

Name: ______________________ **Date:** __________ **Time:** __________ **Grade:** __________

EQUIPMENT/SUPPLIES: Reference materials related to dietary choices that include nutritional components (i.e., calories and nutrient amounts such as protein, fat, and carbohydrates), a physician order, and the patient medical record.

STANDARDS: Given the needed equipment and a place to work, the student will perform this skill with _____ % accuracy in a total of _____ minutes. *(Your instructor will tell you what the percentage and time limits will be before you begin.)*

KEY: 4 = Satisfactory 0 = Unsatisfactory NA = This step is not counted

PROCEDURE STEPS	SELF	PARTNER	INSTRUCTOR
1. Review the physician order to determine the specific nutritional information necessary for patient instruction.	❏	❏	❏
2. Identify the patient.	❏	❏	❏
3. Introduce yourself and explain the procedure including the rationale.	❏	❏	❏
4. Develop a meal plan based on a regular (i.e., no special dietary needs) 2,000 calorie diet and include information on basic nutrition (nutrients, serving sizes, and calories). Printable materials may be used during instruction from the choosemyplate.gov website if approved by the physician.	❏	❏	❏
5. Observe the patient during instruction for non-verbal signs such as confusion, interest or disinterest, emotions, etc.	❏	❏	❏
6. Explain how to respond to a patient who verbalizes concern about the ability to purchase fresh fruits and vegetables due to lack of monetary resources and reliance on public transportation to shop for groceries.	❏	❏	❏
7. Instruct a patient according to one of the following special dietary needs as ordered by the physician: **a.** low sodium **b.** low fat **c.** low carbohydrate **d.** high protein **e.** restricted calorie (i.e., 500, 1,800, etc.) **f.** lactose free **g.** gluten free **h.** high fiber	❏	❏	❏
8. Ask the patient questions during instruction and allow the opportunity for them to ask questions during instruction and at the end.	❏	❏	❏

PSY PROCEDURE 16-2 Develop a Meal Plan Utilizing Basic Principles of Nutrition; Instruct a Patient according to Patient's Special Dietary Needs (continued)

9. Explain how to respond to a patient who has a religious or personal belief against specific food groups such as a vegetarian.	❑	❑	❑
10. Log into the Electronic Medical Record (EMR) using your username and secure password OR obtain the paper medical record from a secure location and assure it is kept away from public access.	❑	❑	❑
11. Chart the verbal and written instructions given to the patient. When finished, log out of the EMR and/or replace the paper medical record in an appropriate and secure location.	❑	❑	❑

____

____

____

____

CALCULATION

Total Possible Points: __________

Total Points Earned: __________ Multiplied by 100 = __________ Divided by Total Possible Points = __________ %

PASS ❑ **FAIL** ❑ **COMMENTS:**

Student's signature ____________________ Date __________

Partner's signature ____________________ Date __________

Instructor's signature ____________________ Date __________

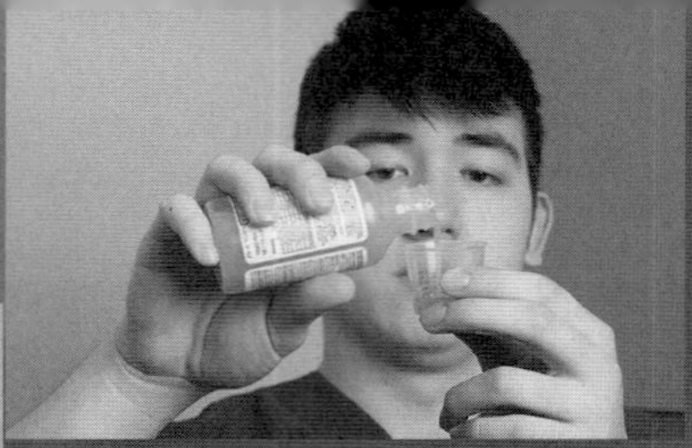

CHAPTER 17 Medical Asepsis and Infection Control

Learning Outcomes

COG Cognitive Domain

1. Spell and define key terms
2. Describe the infection cycle, including the infectious agent, reservoir, susceptible host, means of transmission, portals of entry, and portals of exit
3. List major types of infectious agents
4. Identify different methods of controlling the growth of microorganisms
5. Define the following as practiced within an ambulatory care setting: (a) medical asepsis; (b) surgical asepsis
6. List the various ways microbes are transmitted
7. Define the principles of standard precautions
8. Compare the effectiveness in reducing or destroying microorganisms using the various levels of infection control
9. Identify personal safety precautions as established by the Occupational Safety and Health Administration (OSHA)
10. Define personal protective equipment (PPE) for: (a) all body fluids, secretions, and excretions; (b) blood; (c) nonintact skin; (d) mucous membranes
11. Identify Center for Disease Control (CDC) regulations that impact health care practices
12. List the required components of an exposure control plan
13. Explain the facts pertaining to the transmission and prevention of the hepatitis B virus and the human immunodeficiency virus in the medical office

PSY Psychomotor Domain

1. Perform a medical aseptic hand-washing procedure (Procedure 17-1)
2. Select appropriate PPE and remove contaminated gloves (Procedure 17-2)
3. Clean and decontaminate biohazardous spills (Procedure 17-3)
4. Participate in bloodborne pathogen training (Procedure 17-4)

AFF Affective Domain

1. Incorporate critical thinking skills when performing patient care
2. Recognize the implications for failure to comply with the Center for Disease Control (CDC) regulations in health care settings.

ABHES Competencies

1. Apply principles of aseptic techniques and infection control
2. Use standard precautions
3. Dispose of biohazardous materials

38. Name four factors that affect the disinfection process.

____

____

____

____

39. You accidentally stick yourself with a bloody needle. After washing the site, describe what you should do next.

____

____

____

____

COG TRUE OR FALSE?

Grade: __________

40. Indicate whether the statements are true or false by placing the letter T (true) or F (false) on the line preceding the statement.

a. __________ Adhering to "clean technique," or medical asepsis, ensures that an object or area is free from all microorganisms.

b. __________ Sterilization is the highest level of infection control.

c. __________ Low-level disinfection destroys bacteria, but not viruses.

d. __________ There are three levels of disinfection: minor, moderate, and severe.

e. __________ Handwashing is a form of surgical or sterile asepsis.

COG AFF CASE STUDIES FOR CRITICAL THINKING

Grade: __________

1. Mei Lin is a clinical medical assistant who works in an outpatient clinic. Today she arrives at work with a minor cold. Over the course of an hour, she sees four patients. She draws a blood sample from one patient and retrieves a urine sample from another patient. During the hour, she sneezes three times. She is preparing to leave for her lunch break. How many times should she have washed her hands during this time period?

____

____

____

____

2. Your patient is a 24-year-old female who has been diagnosed with bacterial pneumonia. The physician has ordered antibiotic therapy and bedrest. When leaving the office, she tells you that she is concerned about the fact that she has a 7-month-old baby at home. What information could you give her to clearly explain what steps she can take to avoid transmitting her illness to her child?

3. An established patient in your office is a 38-year-old female with AIDS. One of your coworkers, Steve, is afraid of interacting with this patient and has made disparaging remarks about her in the back office. You worry that Steve's attitude will affect patient care and you decide to talk to him privately. What points will you make? Should you also talk with your supervisor about Steve? Why, or why not?

4. The test results for 15-year-old Ashley Lewis come in and show that she is positive for hepatitis C. Her mother phones and asks you for the results. Is it appropriate for you to give her mother the test results? Why, or why not? How would you handle this call?

5. A middle-aged male comes into the medical office with a low-grade fever and productive cough that has lasted several weeks. The physician orders a chest x-ray to aid in diagnosis. After the patient leaves to get his chest x-ray, you begin to clean the room for the next patient. What level of disinfection will you use? What product(s) will you use? Provide detailed information about your actions, including dilution instructions, if appropriate.

6. You work in a pediatrician's office and have been working extra hours to save for a new, more reliable vehicle. Between work and school, you are tired and rundown. This morning, you woke up with a sore throat and headache. The last thing you want to do is call in sick because you need the money and you want your supervisor to think you are reliable. What should you do? Explain your answer.

PSY **PROCEDURE 17-1 Perform Medical Aseptic Handwashing Procedure**

Name: ______________________ **Date:** __________ **Time:** __________ **Grade:** __________

EQUIPMENT/SUPPLIES: Liquid soap, disposable paper towels, a waste can

STANDARDS: Given the needed equipment and a place to work, the student will perform this skill with _____ % accuracy in a total of _____ minutes. *(Your instructor will tell you what the percentage and time limits will be before you begin.)*

KEY: 4 = Satisfactory 0 = Unsatisfactory NA =This step is not counted

PROCEDURE STEPS	SELF	PARTNER	INSTRUCTOR
1. Remove all rings and wristwatch.	❑	❑	❑
2. Stand close to the sink without touching it.	❑	❑	❑
3. Turn on the faucet and adjust the temperature of the water to warm.	❑	❑	❑
4. Wet hands and wrists, apply soap, and work into a lather.	❑	❑	❑
5. Rub palms together and rub soap between your fingers at least 10 times.	❑	❑	❑
6. Scrub one palm with fingertips, work soap under nails, and then reverse hands.	❑	❑	❑
7. Rinse hands and wrists under warm running water.	❑	❑	❑
8. Hold hands lower than elbows and avoid touching the inside of the sink.	❑	❑	❑
9. Clean under the nails by scraping the fingernails of one hand against the soapy palm of the other hand for 10 seconds. Repeat with other hand.	❑	❑	❑
10. Reapply liquid soap and rewash hands and wrists.	❑	❑	❑
11. Rinse hands again while holding hands lower than the wrists and elbows.	❑	❑	❑
12. Use a dry paper towel to dry your hands and wrists gently.	❑	❑	❑
13. Use a dry paper towel to turn off the faucets and discard the paper towel.	❑	❑	❑

PSY PROCEDURE 17-1 Perform Medical Aseptic Handwashing Procedure (continued)

CALCULATION

Total Possible Points: __________

Total Points Earned: __________ Multiplied by 100 = __________ Divided by Total Possible Points = __________ %

PASS **FAIL** **COMMENTS:**

❑ ❑

Student's signature ____________________ Date __________

Partner's signature ____________________ Date __________

Instructor's signature ____________________ Date __________

PSY PROCEDURE 17-2 Select Appropriate Personal Protective Equipment and Remove Contaminated Gloves

Name: ______________________ **Date:** __________ **Time:** __________ **Grade:** __________

EQUIPMENT/SUPPLIES: PPE (Clean examination gloves; goggles or disposable masks with eye/splash guard; disposable masks; disposable gown); biohazard waste container

STANDARDS: Given the needed equipment and a place to work, the student will perform this skill with _____ % accuracy in a total of _____ minutes. *(Your instructor will tell you what the percentage and time limits will be before you begin.)*

KEY: 4 = Satisfactory 0 = Unsatisfactory NA = This step is not counted

PROCEDURE STEPS	SELF	PARTNER	INSTRUCTOR
1. Given a potentially biohazardous situation, choose the correct PPE: **a.** Cleaning up spilled urine **b.** Irrigating a wound **c.** Giving an injection **d.** Disinfecting examination tables	❑	❑	❑
2. Apply appropriately chosen PPE. If a gown, mask, and goggles are necessary, apply the gown and mask/goggles first. Choose the appropriate size gloves for your hands and put them on last.	❑	❑	❑
3. Make sure clothing is protected if a gown is worn and no skin is showing.	❑	❑	❑
4. After the procedure is finished, appropriately remove PPE by removing the gloves first, next the gown, and last the goggles and mask or face shield.	❑	❑	❑
5. To remove gloves, grasp the glove of your nondominant hand at the palm and pull the glove away.	❑	❑	❑
6. Slide your hand out of the glove, rolling the glove into the palm of the gloved dominant hand.	❑	❑	❑
7. Holding the soiled glove in the palm of your gloved hand, slip your ungloved fingers under the cuff of the glove you are still wearing, being careful not to touch the outside of the glove.	❑	❑	❑
8. Stretch the glove of the dominant hand up and away from your hand while turning it inside out, with the already removed glove balled up inside.	❑	❑	❑
9. Both gloves should now be removed, with the first glove inside the second glove and the second glove inside out.	❑	❑	❑
10. Discard both gloves as one unit into a biohazard waste receptacle.	❑	❑	❑

PSY PROCEDURE 17-2 Select Appropriate Personal Protective Equipment and Remove Contaminated Gloves (continued)

11. If only gloves were worn as PPE, wash your hands.	❑	❑	❑
12. If other PPE were worn (i.e., gown, mask, goggles), remove gloves following the procedure above and untie the gown carefully at the neck. Pull the neck strings of the gown toward the front of the body with the arms straight. Pull each arm out of the sleeve, making the sleeves inside out. Continue removing the gown, rolling it into a ball, touching only the uncontaminated inside of the gown with the hands. Drop the rolled gown in a biohazard waste container.	❑	❑	❑
13. Remove the googles, face shield, and/or mask. Dispose of any disposable items appropriately. If goggles are nondisposable, place in a designated area for disinfecting.	❑	❑	❑
14. Wash your hands.	❑	❑	❑

____

____

____

____

CALCULATION

Total Possible Points: __________

Total Points Earned: __________ Multiplied by 100 = __________ Divided by Total Possible Points = __________ %

PASS ❑ **FAIL** ❑ **COMMENTS:**

Student's signature ____________________ Date __________

Partner's signature ____________________ Date __________

Instructor's signature ____________________ Date __________

PSY PROCEDURE 17-3 Cleaning Biohazardous Spills

Name: ______________________ **Date:** __________ **Time:** __________ **Grade:** __________

EQUIPMENT/SUPPLIES: Commercially prepared germicide *or* 1:10 bleach solution, gloves, disposable towels, chemical absorbent, biohazardous waste bag, protective eye wear (goggles or mask and face shield), disposable shoe coverings, disposable gown or apron made of plastic or other material that is impervious to soaking up contaminated fluids

STANDARDS: Given the needed equipment and a place to work, the student will perform this skill with _____ % accuracy in a total of _____ minutes. *(Your instructor will tell you what the percentage and time limits will be before you begin.)*

KEY: 4 = Satisfactory 0 = Unsatisfactory NA = This step is not counted

PROCEDURE STEPS	SELF	PARTNER	INSTRUCTOR
1. Put on gloves. Wear protective eyewear, gown or apron, and shoe coverings if you anticipate any splashing.	❑	❑	❑
2. Apply chemical absorbent material to the spill as indicated by office policy. Clean up the spill with disposable paper towels, being careful not to splash.	❑	❑	❑
3. Dispose of paper towels and absorbent material in a biohazard waste bag.	❑	❑	❑
4. Spray the area with commercial germicide or bleach solution and wipe with disposable paper towels. Discard towels in a biohazard bag.	❑	❑	❑
5. With your gloves on, remove the protective eyewear and discard or disinfect per office policy. Remove the gown or apron and shoe coverings and put in the biohazard bag if disposable or the biohazard laundry bag for reusable linens.	❑	❑	❑
6. Place the biohazard bag in an appropriate waste receptacle for removal according to your facility's policy.	❑	❑	❑
7. Remove your gloves and wash your hands thoroughly.	❑	❑	❑

____

____

____

____

CALCULATION

Total Possible Points: __________

Total Points Earned: __________ Multiplied by 100 = __________ Divided by Total Possible Points = __________ %

PASS ❑ **FAIL** ❑ **COMMENTS:**

Student's signature ____________________ Date __________

Partner's signature ____________________ Date __________

Instructor's signature ____________________ Date __________

PSY PROCEDURE 17-4 Bloodborne Pathogen Training

Name: ______________________ **Date:** __________ **Time:** __________ **Grade:** __________

EQUIPMENT/SUPPLIES: A commercial kit that includes presentation materials with current OSHA guidelines regarding bloodborne pathogen training; Participation log documenting training including date.

STANDARDS: Given the needed equipment and a place to work, the student will perform this skill with _____ % accuracy in a total of _____ minutes. *(Your instructor will tell you what the percentage and time limits will be before you begin.)*

KEY: 4 = Satisfactory 0 = Unsatisfactory NA = This step is not counted

PROCEDURE STEPS	SELF	PARTNER	INSTRUCTOR
1. Plan ahead to attend the training as scheduled by your facility.	❑	❑	❑
2. Come to the training on time and prepared to take notes and ask questions.	❑	❑	❑
3. The training includes information about the following: **a.** Bloodborne pathogens and diseases **b.** Exposure control plan **c.** Postexposure evaluation and follow-up procedures	❑	❑	❑
4. After participating in the training, you should be able to define bloodborne pathogens and the diseases that may affect humans from these pathogens. Procedures to follow in case of an accidental exposure, and engineering and workplace controls to reduce the likelihood of contamination.	❑	❑	❑
5. Sign and date the Bloodborne Pathogen Training log to document your attendance.	❑	❑	❑

____

____

____

____

CALCULATION

Total Possible Points: __________

Total Points Earned: __________ Multiplied by 100 = __________ Divided by Total Possible Points = __________ %

PASS ❑ **FAIL** ❑ **COMMENTS:**

Student's signature ____________________ Date __________

Partner's signature ____________________ Date __________

Instructor's signature ____________________ Date __________

2. Mrs. Frank is a returning patient at Dr. Mohammad's office. She is 89 years old and needs the assistance of a wheelchair. What are some important considerations that you should make when showing Mrs. Frank to an exam room, gathering her medical history, and performing a patient assessment? How would those considerations change if the patient was a 2-year-old child?

____

____

____

____

3. Your patient is a 49-year-old female who speaks very little English. She is a returning patient, so her medical history is already on file at the office. You have called a coworker who can act as a translator, but he will not arrive at the office for an hour. Meanwhile, the patient is clearly uncomfortable. She appears sweaty and lethargic. She leans on you as you escort her to an examination room. Describe how you can determine the patient's chief complaint and present illness so that you and the physician can begin to help her.

____

____

____

____

4. Alicia, a medical assistant in Dr. Howard's office, has recorded the following in a patient assessment:
"CC: Pt. c/o fatigue, depressed mood, and inability to stay asleep at night. He has taken Tylenol PM for two nights with "no effect" on sleep and has not eaten for 2 days because of lack of appetite, which is likely caused by his depression. His face is pale and his skin clammy."
Was there anything in this documentation that should not have been recorded? Explain your answer.

5. Giles is a medical assistant in Dr. Yardley's office. Giles enters the examination room to interview a patient. Giles notices that the patient is lying on the examination table, holding his abdomen. He is holding a black trash bin that contains a small amount of his vomit. The patient is flushed and sweating. Before even speaking to the patient, Giles has realized some of the patient's signs and symptoms of illness. Explain the significance of signs and symptoms and then fill in this patient's signs and symptoms in the chart below.

Signs	**Symptoms**
a.	**a.**
b.	**b.**
c.	**c.**

6. There are two patients waiting in examination rooms to see the physician. Patient A is a new patient, and Patient B is coming into the office for a complete physical examination. When sorting these patients to determine who should be taken back to the exam room first, what factors should be considered?

7. What are your ethical and legal responsibilities as a medical assistant concerning a patient's medical history records?

8. Your patient is a 17-year-old male. His symptoms are shortness of breath and fatigue. During the interview, you learn that his father and older brother are obese. You also learn that both of his grandfathers died of complications resulting from heart disease. Although this patient is not overweight, he tells you that he does not have time to exercise but would like to avoid gaining weight, especially when he enters college this fall. What changes does the patient needs to make in his lifestyle in order to improve his health and avoid obesity and heart disease? Should you make suggestions for the members of his family who are obese? Why or why not?

9. Ms. Butler, 20 years old, received a pregnancy test during a visit to the physician's office. A week later, Mr. Gordon, a 25-year-old male, comes into the office demanding to see the results of Ms. Butler's test. He tells you that he is her boyfriend and that if Ms. Butler is pregnant, he deserves to know. What would you say to Mr. Gordon?

10. On your way to the exam room, you notice a coworker weighing another patient on the scales located in the hallway. As the patient steps onto the scale, your coworker moves the weights on the scale and then reads the patient's weight out loud. The patient appears embarrassed. What would you say, if anything, to your coworker? Why or why not?

PSY PROCEDURE 18-1 Obtain and Record a Patient History

Name: ______________________ **Date:** __________ **Time:** __________ **Grade:** __________

EQUIPMENT/SUPPLIES: Paper medical history form or questionnaire, black or blue pen

STANDARDS: Given the needed equipment and a place to work, the student will perform this skill with _____ % accuracy in a total of _____ minutes. *(Your instructor will tell you what the percentage and time limits will be before you begin.)*

KEY: 4 = Satisfactory 0 = Unsatisfactory NA =This step is not counted

PROCEDURE STEPS	SELF	PARTNER	INSTRUCTOR
1. Gather the supplies.	❑	❑	❑
2. Review the medical history form for completeness.	❑	❑	❑
3. Take the patient to a private area or the examination room and assist him or her with completing the form.	❑	❑	❑
4. Sit across from the patient at eye level and maintain eye contact.	❑	❑	❑
5. Introduce yourself and explain the purpose of the interview.	❑	❑	❑
6. Using language the patient can understand, ask the appropriate questions, and document the patient's responses. Be sure to determine the patient's CC and PI.	❑	❑	❑
7. Use feedback techniques including: **a.** Reflection. **b.** Restatement. **c.** Clarification.	❑	❑	❑
8. Regardless of the confidences shared by the patient, avoid projecting a judgmental attitude with words or actions.	❑	❑	❑
9. AFF Explain how to respond to a patient who does not speak English.	❑	❑	❑
10. AFF Explain to the patient what to expect during examinations or procedures at that visit.	❑	❑	❑
11. Review the history form for completion and accuracy.	❑	❑	❑
12. Thank the patient for cooperating during the interview, and offer to answer any questions.	❑	❑	❑
13. Describe examples of applying local, state, and federal health care legislation and regulation in the medical office.	❑	❑	❑

____

____

____

____

PROCEDURE 18-1 Obtain and Record a Patient History
(continued)

CALCULATION

Total Possible Points: __________

Total Points Earned: __________ Multiplied by 100 = __________ Divided by Total Possible Points = __________ %

PASS ❑ **FAIL** ❑ **COMMENTS:**

Student's signature ____________________ Date __________

Partner's signature ____________________ Date __________

Instructor's signature ____________________ Date __________

PSY PROCEDURE 18-2 Document a Chief Complaint and Present Illness

Name: ______________________________ **Date:** __________ **Time:** __________ **Grade:** __________

EQUIPMENT/SUPPLIES: A paper or electronic medical record including a cumulative problem list or progress notes form, black or blue ink pen

STANDARDS: Given the needed equipment and a place to work, the student will perform this skill with _____ % accuracy in a total of _____ minutes. *(Your instructor will tell you what the percentage and time limits will be before you begin.)*

KEY: 4 = Satisfactory 0 = Unsatisfactory NA = This step is not counted

PROCEDURE STEPS	SELF	PARTNER	INSTRUCTOR
1. Gather the supplies including the medical record containing the cumulative problem list or progress note form.	❑	❑	❑
2. Review the new or established patient's medical history form.	❑	❑	❑
3. Greet and identify the patient while escorting him or her to the examination room. Close the door.	❑	❑	❑
4. Use open-ended questions to find out why the patient is seeking medical care; maintain eye contact.	❑	❑	❑
5. When reviewing medical history including medications with patient, pronounce all terms and medications accurately.	❑	❑	❑
6. AFF Explain how to respond to a patient who has dementia and whose facial expression shows confusion.	❑	❑	❑
7. Determine the PI using open-ended and closed-ended questions.	❑	❑	❑
8. Document the CC and PI correctly on the cumulative problem list or progress report form.	❑	❑	❑
______________________________ ______________________________ ______________________________ ______________________________			
9. How would you respond to a patient who is moving to another town and asks about having his or her medical records transferred to a physician in another town?	❑	❑	❑
10. Thank the patient for cooperating, and explain that the physician will soon be in to examine the patient.	❑	❑	❑

PSY PROCEDURE 18-2 Document a Chief Complaint and Present Illness (continued)

CALCULATION

Total Possible Points: __________

Total Points Earned: __________ Multiplied by 100 = __________ Divided by Total Possible Points = __________ %

PASS **FAIL** **COMMENTS:**

❑ ❑

Student's signature ____________________ Date __________

Partner's signature ____________________ Date __________

Instructor's signature ____________________ Date __________

PSY PROCEDURE 19-1 Measure and Record a Patient's Weight

Name: ______________________________ **Date:** __________ **Time:** __________ **Grade:** __________

EQUIPMENT/SUPPLIES: Calibrated balance beam scale, digital scale or dial scale; paper towel

STANDARDS: Given the needed equipment and a place to work, the student will perform this skill with _____ % accuracy in a total of _____ minutes. *(Your instructor will tell you what the percentage and time limits will be before you begin.)*

KEY: 4 = Satisfactory 0 = Unsatisfactory NA = This step is not counted

PROCEDURE STEPS	SELF	PARTNER	INSTRUCTOR
1. Wash your hands.	❑	❑	❑
2. Ensure that the scale is properly balanced at zero.	❑	❑	❑
3. Greet and identify the patient. Explain the procedure.	❑	❑	❑
4. Escort the patient to the scale and place a paper towel on the scale.	❑	❑	❑
5. Have the patient remove shoes and heavy outerwear and put down purse.	❑	❑	❑
6. Assist patient onto the scale facing forward and standing on paper towel without touching or holding on to anything if possible, while watching for difficulties with balance.	❑	❑	❑
7. Weigh the patient: **A.** Balance beam scale: Slide counterweights on bottom and top bars (start with heavier bars) from zero to approximate weight. Each counterweight should rest securely in the notch with indicator mark at proper calibration. To obtain measurement, balance bar must hang freely at exact midpoint. To calculate weight, add top reading to bottom one. (Example: If bottom counterweight reads 100 and lighter one reads 16 plus three small lines, record weight as 116 3/4 pounds). **B.** Digital scale: Read and record weight displayed on digital screen. **C.** Dial scale: Indicator arrow rests at patient's weight. Read this number directly above the dial.	❑	❑	❑
8. Return the bars on the top and bottom to zero.	❑	❑	❑
9. Assist the patient from the scale if necessary and discard the paper towel.	❑	❑	❑
10. Record the patient's weight.	❑	❑	❑
11. AFF Explain how to respond to a patient who is visually impaired.	❑	❑	❑

____

____

____

____

PSY PROCEDURE 19-1 Measure and Record a Patient's Weight
(continued)

CALCULATION

Total Possible Points: __________

Total Points Earned: __________ Multiplied by 100 = __________ Divided by Total Possible Points = __________ %

PASS ❑ **FAIL** ❑ **COMMENTS:**

Student's signature ____________________ Date __________

Partner's signature ____________________ Date __________

Instructor's signature ____________________ Date __________

PSY PROCEDURE 19-2 Measure and Record a Patient's Height

Name: ______________________ **Date:** __________ **Time:** __________ **Grade:** __________

EQUIPMENT/SUPPLIES: A scale with a ruler

STANDARDS: Given the needed equipment and a place to work, the student will perform this skill with _____ % accuracy in a total of _____ minutes. *(Your instructor will tell you what the percentage and time limits will be before you begin.)*

KEY: 4 = Satisfactory 0 = Unsatisfactory NA =This step is not counted

PROCEDURE STEPS	SELF	PARTNER	INSTRUCTOR
1. Wash your hands if this procedure is not done at the same time as the weight.	❑	❑	❑
2. Have the patient remove shoes and stand straight and erect on the scale, with heels together and eyes straight ahead. (Patient may face the ruler, but a better measurement is made with the patient's back to the ruler.)	❑	❑	❑
3. With the measuring bar perpendicular to the ruler, slowly lower it until it firmly touches the patient's head. Press lightly if the hair is full or high	❑	❑	❑
4. Read the measurement at the point of movement on the ruler. If measurements are in inches, convert to feet and inches (e.g., if the bar reads 65 plus two smaller lines, read it at 65 1/2. Remember that 12 inches equals 1 foot; therefore, the patient is 5 feet, 5 1/2 inches tall).	❑	❑	❑
5. Assist the patient from the scale if necessary; watch for signs of difficulty with balance.	❑	❑	❑
6. Record the weight and height measurements in the medical record.	❑	❑	❑
7. AFF Explain how to respond to a patient who has dementia.	❑	❑	❑

____

____

____

____

CALCULATION

Total Possible Points: __________

Total Points Earned: __________ Multiplied by 100 = __________ Divided by Total Possible Points = __________ %

PASS ❑ **FAIL** ❑ **COMMENTS:**

Student's signature ____________________ Date __________

Partner's signature ____________________ Date __________

Instructor's signature ____________________ Date __________

PSY PROCEDURE 19-3 Measure and Record a Rectal Temperature

Name: ______________________ **Date:** __________ **Time:** __________ **Grade:** __________

EQUIPMENT/SUPPLIES: Electronic thermometer with rectal probe; tissues or cotton balls; disposable plastic sheaths; surgical lubricant; biohazard waste container; gloves.

STANDARDS: Given the needed equipment and a place to work, the student will perform this skill with _____ % accuracy in a total of _____ minutes. *(Your instructor will tell you what the percentage and time limits will be before you begin.)*

KEY: 4 = Satisfactory 0 = Unsatisfactory NA = This step is not counted

PROCEDURE STEPS	SELF	PARTNER	INSTRUCTOR
1. Wash your hands and assemble the necessary supplies.	❏	❏	❏
2. Insert the thermometer into a plastic sheath.	❏	❏	❏
3. Spread lubricant onto a tissue and then from the tissue onto the sheath of the thermometer.	❏	❏	❏
4. Greet and identify the patient and explain the procedure.	❏	❏	❏
5. Ensure the patient's privacy by placing the patient in a side-lying position facing the examination room door and draping appropriately.	❏	❏	❏
6. Apply gloves and visualize the anus by lifting the top buttock with your nondominant hand.	❏	❏	❏
7. Gently insert the thermometer past the sphincter muscle about 1 1/2 inches for an adult, 1 inch for a child, and 1/2 inch for an infant.	❏	❏	❏
8. Release the upper buttock and hold the thermometer in place with your dominant hand for 3 minutes. Replace the drape without moving the dominant hand.	❏	❏	❏
9. The electronic thermometer will signal when the reading is obtained. Discard the sheath into an appropriate waste container and note the reading.	❏	❏	❏
10. Replace the electronic thermometer into the charger as necessary.	❏	❏	❏
11. Remove your gloves and wash your hands.	❏	❏	❏
12. Record the procedure and mark the letter R next to the reading, indicating that the temperature was taken rectally.	❏	❏	❏
13. AFF Explain how to respond to a patient who is developmentally challenged.	❏	❏	❏

____

____

____

____

PSY PROCEDURE 19-3 Measure and Record a Rectal Temperature (continued)

CALCULATION

Total Possible Points: __________

Total Points Earned: __________ Multiplied by 100 = __________ Divided by Total Possible Points = __________ %

PASS ❑ **FAIL** ❑ **COMMENTS:**

Student's signature ____________________ Date __________

Partner's signature ____________________ Date __________

Instructor's signature ____________________ Date __________

PSY PROCEDURE 19-4 Measure and Record an Axillary Temperature

Name: ________________ **Date:** ________ **Time:** ________ **Grade:** ________

EQUIPMENT/SUPPLIES: Electronic thermometer (oral or rectal); tissues or cotton balls; disposable plastic sheaths; biohazard waste container.

STANDARDS: Given the needed equipment and a place to work, the student will perform this skill with _____ % accuracy in a total of _____ minutes. *(Your instructor will tell you what the percentage and time limits will be before you begin.)*

KEY: 4 = Satisfactory 0 = Unsatisfactory NA =This step is not counted

PROCEDURE STEPS	SELF	PARTNER	INSTRUCTOR
1. Wash your hands and assemble the necessary supplies.	❑	❑	❑
2. Insert the electronic thermometer probe into a plastic sheath.	❑	❑	❑
3. Expose the patient's axilla without exposing more of the chest or upper body than is necessary.	❑	❑	❑
4. Place the tip of the thermometer deep in the axilla and bring the patient's arm down, crossing the forearm over the chest. Drape the patient as appropriate for privacy.	❑	❑	❑
5. The electronic thermometer will signal when the reading is obtained. Discard the sheath into an appropriate waste container and note the reading.	❑	❑	❑
6. Replace the electronic thermometer into the charger as necessary.	❑	❑	❑
7. Wash your hands.	❑	❑	❑
8. Record the procedure and mark a letter A next to the reading, indicating that the reading is axillary.	❑	❑	❑
9. AFF Explain how to respond to a patient who is from a different generation.	❑	❑	❑

____

____

____

____

PSY PROCEDURE 19-4 Measure and Record an Axillary Temperature (continued)

CALCULATION

Total Possible Points: __________

Total Points Earned: __________ Multiplied by 100 = __________ Divided by Total Possible Points = __________ %

PASS ❑ **FAIL** ❑ **COMMENTS:**

Student's signature ____________________ Date __________

Partner's signature ____________________ Date __________

Instructor's signature ____________________ Date __________

PSY PROCEDURE 19-5 Measure and Record a Patient's Oral Temperature Using an Electronic Thermometer

Name: ______________________ **Date:** __________ **Time:** __________ **Grade:** __________

EQUIPMENT/SUPPLIES: Electronic thermometer with oral or rectal probe, disposable probe covers, biohazard waste container, gloves for taking an oral temperature

STANDARDS: Given the needed equipment and a place to work, the student will perform this skill with _____ % accuracy in a total of _____ minutes. *(Your instructor will tell you what the percentage and time limits will be before you begin.)*

KEY: 4 = Satisfactory 0 = Unsatisfactory NA = This step is not counted

PROCEDURE STEPS	SELF	PARTNER	INSTRUCTOR
1. Wash your hands and assemble the necessary supplies.	❑	❑	❑
2. Greet and identify the patient and explain the procedure.	❑	❑	❑
3. Attach the appropriate probe to the battery-powered unit.	❑	❑	❑
4. Insert the probe into a probe cover.	❑	❑	❑
5. Position the thermometer appropriately for the method. To take an oral temperature, place the end of the thermometer under the patient's tongue to either side of the frenulum.	❑	❑	❑
6. Wait for the electronic thermometer unit to "beep" when it senses no signs of the temperature rising further. This usually occurs within 20 to 30 seconds.	❑	❑	❑
7. After the beep, remove the probe and note the reading on the digital display screen on the unit before replacing the probe into the unit.	❑	❑	❑
8. Discard the probe cover by pressing a button, usually on the end of the probe, while holding the probe over a biohazard container. After noting the temperature, replace the probe into the unit.	❑	❑	❑
9. Remove your gloves, if used, wash your hands, and record the procedure	❑	❑	❑
10. Return the unit and probe to the charging base.	❑	❑	❑
11. AFF Explain how to respond to a patient who is hearing impaired.	❑	❑	❑

____

____

____

____

PSY PROCEDURE 19-5 Measure and Record a Patient's Oral Temperature Using an Electronic Thermometer (continued)

CALCULATION

Total Possible Points: __________

Total Points Earned: __________ Multiplied by 100 = __________ Divided by Total Possible Points = __________ %

PASS FAIL COMMENTS:

❑ ❑

Student's signature ____________________ Date __________

Partner's signature ____________________ Date __________

Instructor's signature __________________ Date __________

PSY PROCEDURE 19-6 Measure and Record a Patient's Temperature Using a Tympanic Thermometer

Name: ______________________ **Date:** __________ **Time:** __________ **Grade:** __________

EQUIPMENT/SUPPLIES: Tympanic thermometer, disposable probe covers, biohazard waste container

STANDARDS: Given the needed equipment and a place to work, the student will perform this skill with _____ % accuracy in a total of _____ minutes. *(Your instructor will tell you what the percentage and time limits will be before you begin.)*

KEY: 4 = Satisfactory 0 = Unsatisfactory NA = This step is not counted

PROCEDURE STEPS	SELF	PARTNER	INSTRUCTOR
1. Wash your hands and assemble the necessary supplies.	❑	❑	❑
2. Greet and identify the patient and explain the procedure.	❑	❑	❑
3. Insert the ear probe into a probe cover.	❑	❑	❑
4. Place the end of the ear probe into the patient's ear canal with your dominant hand while straightening out the ear canal with your nondominant hand.	❑	❑	❑
5. With the ear probe properly placed in the ear canal, press the button on the thermometer. The reading is displayed on the digital display screen in about 2 seconds.	❑	❑	❑
6. Remove the probe and note the reading. Discard the probe cover into an appropriate waste container.	❑	❑	❑
7. Wash your hands and record the procedure.	❑	❑	❑
8. Return the unit to the charging base.	❑	❑	❑
9. AFF Explain how to respond to a patient who is deaf.	❑	❑	❑

____

____

____

____

CALCULATION

Total Possible Points: __________

Total Points Earned: __________ Multiplied by 100 = __________ Divided by Total Possible Points = __________ %

PASS ❑ **FAIL** ❑ **COMMENTS:**

Student's signature ____________________ Date __________

Partner's signature ____________________ Date __________

Instructor's signature ____________________ Date __________

PSY PROCEDURE 19-7 Measure and Record a Patient's Temperature Using a Temporal Artery Thermometer

Name: ______________________ **Date:** __________ **Time:** __________ **Grade:** __________

EQUIPMENT/SUPPLIES: Temporal artery thermometer, antiseptic wipes

STANDARDS: Given the needed equipment and a place to work, the student will perform this skill with _____ % accuracy in a total of _____ minutes. *(Your instructor will tell you what the percentage and time limits will be before you begin.)*

KEY: 4 = Satisfactory 0 = Unsatisfactory NA = This step is not counted

PROCEDURE STEPS	SELF	PARTNER	INSTRUCTOR
1. Wash your hands and assemble the necessary supplies.	❑	❑	❑
2. Greet and identify the patient and explain the procedure.	❑	❑	❑
3. Place the probe end of the hand-held unit on the forehead of the patient. Make sure the patient's skin is dry.	❑	❑	❑
4. With the thermometer against the forehead, depress the on/off button, move the thermometer across and down the forehead, and release the on/off button with the unit over the temporal artery.	❑	❑	❑
5. The reading is displayed on the digital display screen in 1 to 2 seconds.	❑	❑	❑
6. Properly disinfect the end of the thermometer according to manufacturer instructions	❑	❑	❑
7. Wash your hands and record the procedure.	❑	❑	❑
8. Return the unit to the charging base.	❑	❑	❑
9. AFF Explain how to respond to a patient who is visually impaired.	❑	❑	❑

____

____

____

____

CALCULATION

Total Possible Points: __________

Total Points Earned: __________ Multiplied by 100 = __________ Divided by Total Possible Points = __________ %

PASS ❑ **FAIL** ❑ **COMMENTS:**

Student's signature ____________________ Date __________

Partner's signature ____________________ Date __________

Instructor's signature ____________________ Date __________

PSY PROCEDURE 19-8 Measure and Record a Patient's Radial Pulse

Name: ______________________ **Date:** __________ **Time:** __________ **Grade:** __________

EQUIPMENT/SUPPLIES: A watch with a sweeping second hand

STANDARDS: Given the needed equipment and a place to work, the student will perform this skill with _____ % accuracy in a total of _____ minutes. *(Your instructor will tell you what the percentage and time limits will be before you begin.)*

KEY: 4 = Satisfactory 0 = Unsatisfactory NA = This step is not counted

PROCEDURE STEPS	SELF	PARTNER	INSTRUCTOR
1. Wash your hands.	❑	❑	❑
2. Greet and identify the patient and explain the procedure.	❑	❑	❑
3. Position the patient with the arm relaxed and supported either on the lap of the patient or on a table.	❑	❑	❑
4. With the index, middle, and ring fingers of your dominant hand, press with your fingertips firmly enough to feel the pulse but gently enough not to obliterate it	❑	❑	❑
5. If the pulse is regular, count it for 30 seconds, watching the second hand of your watch. Multiply the number of pulsations by 2 since the pulse is always recorded as beats per minute. If the pulse is irregular, count it for a full 60 seconds.	❑	❑	❑
6. Record the rate in the medical record with the other vital signs. Also note the rhythm if irregular and the volume if thready or bounding.	❑	❑	❑
7. AFF Explain how to respond to a patient who is developmentally challenged.	❑	❑	❑

____

____

____

____

CALCULATION

Total Possible Points: __________

Total Points Earned: __________ Multiplied by 100 = __________ Divided by Total Possible Points = __________ %

PASS ❑ **FAIL** ❑ **COMMENTS:**

Student's signature ____________________ Date __________

Partner's signature ____________________ Date __________

Instructor's signature ____________________ Date __________

PSY PROCEDURE 19-9 Measure and Record a Patient's Respirations

Name: ______________________ **Date:** __________ **Time:** __________ **Grade:** __________

EQUIPMENT/SUPPLIES: A watch with a sweeping second hand

STANDARDS: Given the needed equipment and a place to work, the student will perform this skill with _____ % accuracy in a total of _____ minutes. *(Your instructor will tell you what the percentage and time limits will be before you begin.)*

KEY: 4 = Satisfactory 0 = Unsatisfactory NA = This step is not counted

PROCEDURE STEPS	SELF	PARTNER	INSTRUCTOR
1. Wash your hands.	❑	❑	❑
2. Greet and identify the patient and explain the procedure.	❑	❑	❑
3. After counting the radial pulse and still watching your second hand, count a complete rise and fall of the chest as one respiration. Note: Some patients have abdominal movement rather than chest movement during respirations. Observe carefully for the easiest area to assess for the most accurate reading	❑	❑	❑
4. If the breathing pattern is regular, count the respiratory rate for 30 seconds and multiply by 2. If the pattern is irregular, count for a full 60 seconds.	❑	❑	❑
5. Record the respiratory rate in the medical record with the other vital signs. Also, note whether the rhythm is irregular, along with any unusual or abnormal sounds such as wheezing.	❑	❑	❑
6. AFF Explain how to respond to a patient who has dementia.	❑	❑	❑

____

____

____

____

CALCULATION

Total Possible Points: __________

Total Points Earned: __________ Multiplied by 100 = __________ Divided by Total Possible Points = __________ %

PASS ❑ **FAIL** ❑ **COMMENTS:**

Student's signature ____________________ Date __________

Partner's signature ____________________ Date __________

Instructor's signature ____________________ Date __________

PSY PROCEDURE 19-10 Measure and Record a Patient's Blood Pressure

Name: ______________________ **Date:** __________ **Time:** __________ **Grade:** __________

EQUIPMENT/SUPPLIES: Sphygmomanometer, stethoscope

STANDARDS: Given the needed equipment and a place to work, the student will perform this skill with _____ % accuracy in a total of _____ minutes. *(Your instructor will tell you what the percentage and time limits will be before you begin.)*

KEY: 4 = Satisfactory 0 = Unsatisfactory NA = This step is not counted

PROCEDURE STEPS	SELF	PARTNER	INSTRUCTOR
1. Wash your hands.	❑	❑	❑
2. Greet and identify the patient and explain the procedure.	❑	❑	❑
3. Position the patient with the arm to be used supported with the forearm on the lap or a table and slightly flexed, with the palm upward. The upper arm should be level with the patient's heart.	❑	❑	❑
4. Expose the patient's upper arm.	❑	❑	❑
5. Palpate the brachial pulse in the antecubital area and center the deflated cuff directly over the brachial artery. The lower edge of the cuff should be 1 to 2 inches above the antecubital area.	❑	❑	❑
6. Wrap the cuff smoothly and snugly around the arm and secure it with the Velcro edges.	❑	❑	❑
7. With the air pump in your dominant hand and the valve between your thumb and the forefinger, turn the screw clockwise to tighten. Do not tighten it to the point that it will be difficult to release.	❑	❑	❑
8. While palpating the brachial pulse with your nondominant hand, inflate the cuff and note the point or number on the dial or mercury column at which you no longer feel the brachial pulse	❑	❑	❑
9. Deflate the cuff by turning the valve counterclockwise. Wait at least 30 seconds before reinflating the cuff.	❑	❑	❑
10. Place the stethoscope earpieces in your ears with the openings pointed slightly forward. Stand about 3 feet from the manometer with the gauge at eye level. Your stethoscope tubing should hang freely without touching or rubbing against any part of the cuff.	❑	❑	❑
11. Place the diaphragm of the stethoscope against the brachial artery and hold it in place with the nondominant hand without pressing too hard.	❑	❑	❑
12. With your dominant hand, turn the screw on the valve just enough to close the valve; inflate the cuff. Pump the valve bulb to about 30 mm Hg above the number felt during Step 8.	❑	❑	❑

PSY PROCEDURE 19-10 Measure and Record a Patient's Blood Pressure (continued)

13. Once the cuff is appropriately inflated, turn the valve counter-clockwise to release air at about 2 to 4 mm Hg per second.	❑	❑	❑
14. Listening carefully, note the point on the gauge at which you hear the first clear tapping sound. This is the systolic sound, or Korotkoff I	❑	❑	❑
15. Maintaining control of the valve screw, continue to listen and deflate the cuff. When you hear the last sound, note the reading and quickly deflate the cuff. Note: Never immediately reinflate the cuff if you are unsure of the reading. Totally deflate the cuff and wait 1 to 2 minutes before repeating the procedure.	❑	❑	❑
16. Remove the cuff and press the air from the bladder of the cuff.	❑	❑	❑
17. If this is the first recording or a new patient, the physician may also want a reading in the other arm or in another position.	❑	❑	❑
18. Put the equipment away and wash your hands.	❑	❑	❑
19. Record the reading with the systolic over the diastolic pressure, noting which arm was used (120/80 LA). Also, record the patient's position if other than sitting.	❑	❑	❑
20. AFF Explain how to respond to a patient who is from a different culture.	❑	❑	❑

____

____

____

____

CALCULATION

Total Possible Points: __________

Total Points Earned: __________ Multiplied by 100 = __________ Divided by Total Possible Points = __________ %

PASS **FAIL** **COMMENTS:**

❑ ❑

Student's signature ____________________ Date __________

Partner's signature ____________________ Date __________

Instructor's signature ____________________ Date __________

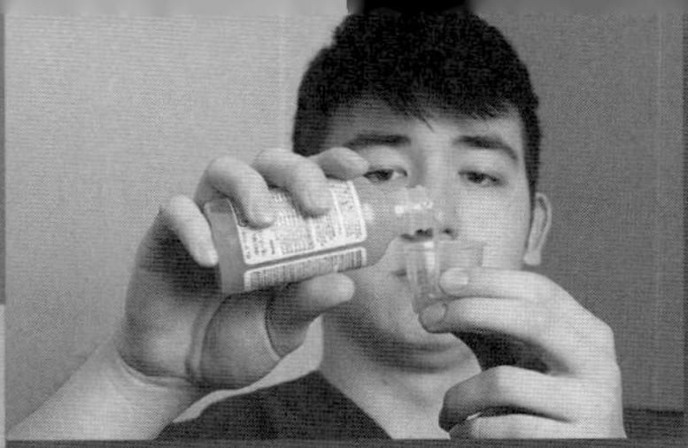

CHAPTER

20 Assisting with the Physical Examination

Learning Outcomes

COG Cognitive Domain

1. Spell and define the key terms
2. Identify and state the use of the basic and specialized instruments and supplies used in the physical examination
3. Describe the four methods used to examine the patient
4. State your responsibilities before, during, and after the physical examination
5. List the basic sequence of the physical examination
6. Describe the normal function of each body system

PSY Psychomotor Domain

1. Assist with the adult physical examination (Procedure 20-1)
2. Assist provider with a patient exam
3. Coach patients appropriately considering cultural diversity, developmental life stages, and communication barriers
4. Document accurately in the medical record

AFF Affective Domain

1. Incorporate critical thinking skills when performing patient assessment
2. Show awareness of a patient's concerns related to the procedure being performed
3. Explain to a patient the rationale for performance of a procedure
4. Demonstrate empathy, active listening, and nonverbal communication
5. Demonstrate respect for individual diversity including gender, race, religion, age, economic status, and appearance
6. Protect the integrity of the medical record

ABHES Competencies

1. Prepare and maintain examination and treatment area
2. Prepare patient for examinations and treatments
3. Assist physician with routine and specialty examinations and treatments

7. You are assisting a physician during a genital and pelvic examination on a female disabled patient who cannot be placed into the lithotomy position. What is the correct course of action?

____

____

____

____

PSY PROCEDURE 20-1 Assisting with the Adult Physical Examination

Name: ______________________ **Date:** __________ **Time:** __________ **Grade:** __________

EQUIPMENT/SUPPLIES: A variety of instruments and supplies, including the stethoscope, ophthalmoscope, otoscope, penlight, tuning fork, nasal speculum, tongue blade, percussion hammer, gloves, water-soluble lubricant, an examinations light, and patient gown and draping supplies

STANDARDS: Given the needed equipment and a place to work, the student will perform this skill with _____ % accuracy in a total of _____ minutes. *(Your instructor will tell you what the percentage and time limits will be before you begin.)*

KEY: 4 = Satisfactory 0 = Unsatisfactory NA = This step is not counted

PROCEDURE STEPS	SELF	PARTNER	INSTRUCTOR
1. Wash your hands.	❑	❑	❑
2. Prepare the examination room and assemble the equipment.	❑	❑	❑
3. Greet the patient by name and escort him or her to the examining room.	❑	❑	❑
4. Explain the procedure.	❑	❑	❑
5. Obtain and record the medical history and chief complaint.	❑	❑	❑
6. Take and record the vital signs, height, weight, and visual acuity.	❑	❑	❑
7. If anticipated, instruct the patient to obtain a urine specimen and escort him or her to the bathroom.	❑	❑	❑
8. Once inside the examination room, instruct the patient in disrobing including directions on how to put the gown on (open in the front or back). Leave the room unless the patient needs assistance.	❑	❑	❑
9. AFF Explain how to respond to a patient who has cultural or religious beliefs and is uncomfortable about disrobing.	❑	❑	❑
10. Assist patient into a sitting position on the edge of the examination table. Cover the lap and legs with a drape.	❑	❑	❑
11. AFF Place the medical record outside the examination room and notify the physician that the patient is ready. If your office uses an electronic medical record, assure you have entered and updated all information necessary and log off the computer before leaving the room.	❑	❑	❑
12. Assist the physician by handing him or her the instruments as needed and positioning the patient appropriately.	❑	❑	❑
13. Help the patient return to a sitting position.	❑	❑	❑

PSY PROCEDURE 20-1 Assisting with the Adult Physical Examination (continued)

14. Perform any follow-up procedures or treatments.	❑	❑	❑
15. Leave the room while the patient dresses unless assistance is needed.	❑	❑	❑
16. Return to the examination room after the patient has dressed to: **a.** answer questions. **b.** reinforce instructions. **c.** provide patient education.	❑	❑	❑
17. Escort the patient to the front desk.	❑	❑	❑
18. Properly clean or dispose of all used equipment and supplies.	❑	❑	❑
19. Clean the room with a disinfectant and prepare for the next patient.	❑	❑	❑
20. Wash your hands. **a.** Record any instructions that were ordered for the patient. **b.** Note if any specimens were obtained. **c.** Indicate the results of the test or note the laboratory where the specimens are being sent for testing.	❑	❑	❑

____

____

____

____

CALCULATION

Total Possible Points: __________

Total Points Earned: __________ Multiplied by 100 = __________ Divided by Total Possible Points = __________ %

PASS ❑ **FAIL** ❑ **COMMENTS:**

Student's signature ____________________ Date __________

Partner's signature ____________________ Date __________

Instructor's signature ____________________ Date __________

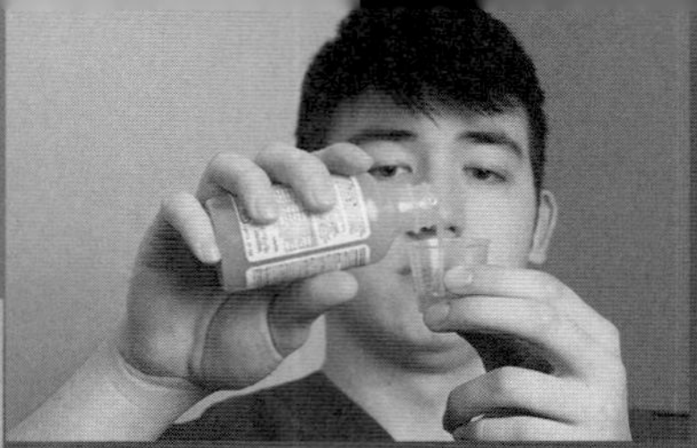

CHAPTER

21 Sterilization and Surgical Instruments

Learning Outcomes

COG Cognitive Domain

1. Spell and define the key terms
2. Define the following as practiced within an ambulatory care setting: surgical asepsis
3. Identify quality assurance practices in health care.
4. Describe several methods of sterilization
5. Categorize surgical instruments based on use and identify each by its characteristics
6. Identify surgical instruments specific to designated specialties
7. State the difference between reusable and disposable instruments
8. Explain how to handle and store instruments, equipment, and supplies
9. Describe the necessity and steps for maintaining documents and records of maintenance for instruments and equipment

PSY Psychomotor Domain

1. Sanitize equipment and instruments (Procedure 21-1)
2. Prepare items for autoclaving
3. Properly wrap instruments for autoclaving (Procedure 21-2)
4. Perform sterilization procedures
5. Perform sterilization technique and operate an autoclave (Procedure 21-3)
6. Perform a quality control measure

ABHES Competencies

1. Wrap items for autoclaving
2. Practice quality control
3. Use standard precautions
4. Perform sterilization techniques

6. Your office uses formaldehyde to sterilize some instruments. While transporting the instruments soaking in formaldehyde, you accidentally spill the formaldehyde. You are in a hurry and consider leaving the small amount of chemical on the floor until later. Would this be an appropriate action to take? Why or why not? How would you clean up this spill?

____

____

____

____

PSY PROCEDURE 21-1 Sanitize Equipment and Instruments

Name: ______________________ **Date:** __________ **Time:** __________ **Grade:** __________

EQUIPMENT/SUPPLIES: Instruments or equipment to be sanitized, gloves, eye protection, impervious gown, soap and water, small hand-held scrub brush

STANDARDS: Given the needed equipment and a place to work, the student will perform this skill with _____ % accuracy in a total of _____ minutes. *(Your instructor will tell you what the percentage and time limits will be before you begin.)*

KEY: 4 = Satisfactory 0 = Unsatisfactory NA = This step is not counted

PROCEDURE STEPS	SELF	PARTNER	INSTRUCTOR
1. Put on gloves, gown, and eye protection.	❑	❑	❑
2. For equipment that requires assembly, take removable sections apart.	❑	❑	❑
3. Check the operation and integrity of the equipment.	❑	❑	❑
4. Rinse the instrument with cool water.	❑	❑	❑
5. Force streams of soapy water through any tubular or grooved instruments.	❑	❑	❑
6. Use a hot, soapy solution to dissolve fats or lubricants left on the surface.	❑	❑	❑
7. Soak 5 to 10 minutes. **a.** Use friction (brush or gauze) to wipe down the instruments. **b.** Check jaws or scissors/forceps to ensure that all debris has been removed.	❑	❑	❑
8. Rinse well.	❑	❑	❑
9. Dry well before autoclaving if sterilizing or soaking in disinfecting solution.	❑	❑	❑
10. Items (brushes, gauze, solution) used in sanitation process must be disinfected or discarded.	❑	❑	❑

CALCULATION

Total Possible Points: __________

Total Points Earned: __________ Multiplied by 100 = __________ Divided by Total Possible Points = __________ %

PASS ❑ **FAIL** ❑ **COMMENTS:**

Student's signature ____________________ Date __________

Partner's signature ____________________ Date __________

Instructor's signature ____________________ Date __________

PSY PROCEDURE 21-2 Properly Wrap Instruments for Autoclaving

Name: ______________________ **Date:** __________ **Time:** __________ **Grade:** __________

EQUIPMENT/SUPPLIES: Sanitized and wrapped instruments or equipment, distilled water, autoclave operating manual

STANDARDS: Given the needed equipment and a place to work, the student will perform this skill with _____ % accuracy in a total of _____ minutes. *(Your instructor will tell you what the percentage and time limits will be before you begin.)*

KEY: 4 = Satisfactory 0 = Unsatisfactory NA = This step is not counted

PROCEDURE STEPS	SELF	PARTNER	INSTRUCTOR
1. Assemble the equipment and supplies.	❑	❑	❑
2. Check the instruments being wrapped for working order. Explain what to do if an instrument is found not to be in good working order.	❑	❑	❑
3. Obtain correct material for wrapping instruments to be autoclaved.	❑	❑	❑
4. Tear off 1 to 2 pieces of autoclave tape. On one piece, label the contents of the pack, the date, and your initials.	❑	❑	❑
5. Lay the wrap diagonally on a flat, clean, dry surface. **a.** Place the instrument in the center, with ratchets or handles in open position. **b.** Include a sterilization indicator.	❑	❑	❑
6. Fold the first flap up at the bottom of the diagonal wrap. Fold back the corner to make a tab.	❑	❑	❑
7. Fold left corner of the wrap toward the center. Fold back the corner to make a tab.	❑	❑	❑
8. Fold right corner of the wrap toward the center. Fold back the corner to make a tab.	❑	❑	❑
9. Fold the top corner down, making the tab tuck under the material.	❑	❑	❑
10. Secure the package with labeled autoclave tape.	❑	❑	❑

CALCULATION

Total Possible Points: __________

Total Points Earned: __________ Multiplied by 100 = __________ Divided by Total Possible Points = __________ %

PASS ❑ **FAIL** ❑ **COMMENTS:**

Student's signature ____________________ Date __________

Partner's signature ____________________ Date __________

Instructor's signature ____________________ Date __________

PSY PROCEDURE 21-3 Perform Sterilization Technique and Operate an Autoclave

Name: ______________________ **Date:** __________ **Time:** __________ **Grade:** __________

EQUIPMENT/SUPPLIES: Sanitized and wrapped instruments or equipment, distilled water, autoclave, autoclave operating manual

STANDARDS: Given the needed equipment and a place to work, the student will perform this skill with _____ % accuracy in a total of _____ minutes. *(Your instructor will tell you what the percentage and time limits will be before you begin.)*

KEY: 4 = Satisfactory 0 = Unsatisfactory NA = This step is not counted

PROCEDURE STEPS	SELF	PARTNER	INSTRUCTOR
1. Assemble the equipment, including the wrapped articles with a sterilization indicator in each package according to office policy.	❑	❑	❑
2. Check the water level of the autoclave reservoir and add more if needed.	❑	❑	❑
3. Add water to the internal chamber of the autoclave to the fill line.	❑	❑	❑
4. Properly load the autoclave.	❑	❑	❑
5. Read the instructions, close the door, and secure or lock it. Turn the machine on.	❑	❑	❑
6. Set the timer at the appropriate time and for the proper length of time.	❑	❑	❑
7. When the timer indicates that the cycle is over, vent the chamber.	❑	❑	❑
8. When the load has cooled, remove the items. Check the separately wrapped sterilization indicator, if used, for proper sterilization.	❑	❑	❑
9. Store the items in a clean, dry, dust-free area.	❑	❑	❑
10. Explain how to clean the autoclave.	❑	❑	❑

CALCULATION

Total Possible Points: __________

Total Points Earned: __________ Multiplied by 100 = __________ Divided by Total Possible Points = __________ %

PASS ❑ **FAIL** ❑ **COMMENTS:**

Student's signature ____________________ Date __________

Partner's signature ____________________ Date __________

Instructor's signature ____________________ Date __________

8. A 15-year-old patient has a mole on her face that needs to be removed. She feels anxious about having to wear a large dressing to cover the wound on her face while it heals. In addition, she is nervous about the possibilities of scarring, and she is worried that the mole is cancerous. How would you handle this situation? What would you say to her to ease her mind before and after the procedure?

____

____

____

____

9. You are working with another medical assistant to prepare a sterile field for surgery. You are almost finished setting up the sterile field when your coworker sneezes over the sterile field. She says that it's only allergies and that she's not contagious, so the field isn't contaminated. She assures you that you don't need to start your work over again. How would you handle this situation? What would you say to your coworker? What should you do next?

____

____

____

____

PSY PROCEDURE 22-1 Opening Sterile Surgical Packs

Name: ______________________ **Date:** __________ **Time:** __________ **Grade:** __________

EQUIPMENT/SUPPLIES: Surgical pack, surgical or Mayo stand

STANDARDS: Given the needed equipment and a place to work, the student will perform this skill with _____ % accuracy in a total of _____ minutes. *(Your instructor will tell you what the percentage and time limits will be before you begin.)*

KEY: 4 = Satisfactory 0 = Unsatisfactory NA =This step is not counted

PROCEDURE STEPS	SELF	PARTNER	INSTRUCTOR
1. Wash your hands.	❑	❑	❑
2. Verify the procedure to be performed and remove the appropriate tray or item from the storage area. Check the label for contents and expiration date. Check the package for tears and moisture.	❑	❑	❑
3. Place the package, with the label facing up, on a clean, dry, flat surface such as a Mayo or surgical stand.	❑	❑	❑
4. Without tearing the wrapper, carefully remove the sealing tape. With commercial packages, carefully remove the outer protective wrapper.	❑	❑	❑
5. Loosen the first flap of the folded wrapper by pulling it up, out, and away; let it fall over the far side of the table or stand.	❑	❑	❑
6. Open the side flaps in a similar manner, using your left hand for the left flap and your right hand for the right flap. Touch only the unsterile outer surface; do not touch the sterile inner surface.	❑	❑	❑
7. Pull the remaining flap down and toward you by grasping the outside surface only. The outer surface of the wrapper is now against the surgical stand; the sterile inside of the wrapper forms the sterile field.	❑	❑	❑
8. Open the side flaps in a similar manner. Do not touch the sterile inner surface.	❑	❑	❑
9. Pull the remaining flap down and toward you.	❑	❑	❑
10. Repeat steps 4 through 6 for packages with a second or inside wrapper.	❑	❑	❑
11. If you must leave the area after opening the field, cover the tray with a sterile drape.	❑	❑	❑

PSY PROCEDURE 22-1 Opening Sterile Surgical Packs (continued)

CALCULATION

Total Possible Points: __________

Total Points Earned: __________ Multiplied by 100 = __________ Divided by Total Possible Points = __________ %

PASS **FAIL** **COMMENTS:**

❑ ❑

Student's signature ____________________ Date __________

Partner's signature ____________________ Date __________

Instructor's signature __________________ Date __________

PSY PROCEDURE 22-2 Using Sterile Transfer Forceps

Name: ______________________ **Date:** __________ **Time:** __________ **Grade:** __________

EQUIPMENT/SUPPLIES: Sterile transfer forceps in a container with sterilization solution, sterile field, sterile items to be transferred

STANDARDS: Given the needed equipment and a place to work, the student will perform this skill with _____ % accuracy in a total of _____ minutes. *(Your instructor will tell you what the percentage and time limits will be before you begin.)*

KEY: 4 = Satisfactory 0 = Unsatisfactory NA =This step is not counted

PROCEDURE STEPS	SELF	PARTNER	INSTRUCTOR
1. Slowly lift the forceps straight up and out of the container without touching the inside above the level of the solution or outside of the container.	❑	❑	❑
2. Hold the forceps with the tips down at all times.	❑	❑	❑
3. Keep the forceps above waist level.	❑	❑	❑
4. With the forceps, pick up the articles to be transferred and drop them onto the sterile field, but do not let the forceps come into contact with the sterile field.	❑	❑	❑
5. Carefully place the forceps back into the sterilization solution.	❑	❑	❑

CALCULATION

Total Possible Points: __________

Total Points Earned: __________ Multiplied by 100 = __________ Divided by Total Possible Points = __________ %

PASS ❑ **FAIL** ❑ **COMMENTS:**

Student's signature ____________________ Date __________

Partner's signature ____________________ Date __________

Instructor's signature ____________________ Date __________

PSY PROCEDURE 22-3 Adding Sterile Solution to a Sterile Field

Name: ______________________ **Date:** __________ **Time:** __________ **Grade:** __________

EQUIPMENT/SUPPLIES: Sterile setup, container of sterile solution, sterile bowl or cup

STANDARDS: Given the needed equipment and a place to work, the student will perform this skill with _____ % accuracy in a total of _____ minutes. *(Your instructor will tell you what the percentage and time limits will be before you begin.)*

KEY: 4 = Satisfactory 0 = Unsatisfactory NA = This step is not counted

PROCEDURE STEPS	SELF	PARTNER	INSTRUCTOR
1. Identify the correct solution by carefully reading the label.	❑	❑	❑
2. Check the expiration date on the label.	❑	❑	❑
3. If adding medications into the solution, show medication label to the physician.	❑	❑	❑
4. Remove the cap or stopper; avoid contamination of the inside of the cap.	❑	❑	❑
5. If it is necessary to put the cap down, place on side table with opened end facing up.	❑	❑	❑
6. Retain bottle to track amount added to field.	❑	❑	❑
7. Grasp container with label against the palm of your hand.	❑	❑	❑
8. Pour a small amount of the solution into a separate container or waste receptacle.	❑	❑	❑
9. Slowly pour the desired amount of solution into the sterile container.	❑	❑	❑
10. Recheck the label for the contents and expiration date and replace the cap.	❑	❑	❑
11. Return the solution to its proper storage area or discard the container after rechecking the label again.	❑	❑	❑

CALCULATION

Total Possible Points: __________

Total Points Earned: __________ Multiplied by 100 = __________ Divided by Total Possible Points = __________ %

PASS **FAIL** **COMMENTS:**

❑ ❑

Student's signature ____________________ Date __________

Partner's signature ____________________ Date __________

Instructor's signature ____________________ Date __________

PSY PROCEDURE 22-4 Performing Skin Preparation and Hair Removal

Name: ______________________ **Date:** __________ **Time:** __________ **Grade:** __________

EQUIPMENT/SUPPLIES: Nonsterile gloves; shave cream, lotion, or soap; new disposable razor; gauze or cotton balls; warm water; antiseptic; sponge forceps

STANDARDS: Given the needed equipment and a place to work, the student will perform this skill with _____ % accuracy in a total of _____ minutes. *(Your instructor will tell you what the percentage and time limits will be before you begin.)*

KEY: 4 = Satisfactory 0 = Unsatisfactory NA = This step is not counted

PROCEDURE STEPS	SELF	PARTNER	INSTRUCTOR
1. Wash your hands.	❑	❑	❑
2. Assemble the equipment.	❑	❑	❑
3. Greet and identify the patient; explain the procedure and answer any questions.	❑	❑	❑
4. Put on gloves.	❑	❑	❑
5. Prepare the patient's skin.	❑	❑	❑
6. If the patient's skin is to be shaved, apply shaving cream or soapy lather. **a.** Pull the skin taut and shave in the direction of hair growth. **b.** Rinse and pat the shaved area thoroughly dry using a gauze square.	❑	❑	❑
7. If the patient's skin is not to be shaved, wash with soap and water; rinse well and pat the area thoroughly dry using a gauze square.	❑	❑	❑
8. Apply antiseptic solution to the operative area using sterile gauze sponges. **a.** Wipe skin in circular motions starting at the operative site and working outward. **b.** Discard each sponge after a complete sweep has been made. **c.** If circles are not appropriate, the sponge may be wiped straight outward from the operative site and discarded. **d.** Repeat the procedure until the entire area has been thoroughly cleaned.	❑	❑	❑
9. Instruct the patient not to touch or cover the prepared area.	❑	❑	❑
10. Explain how to respond to a patient who is developmentally challenged.	❑	❑	❑

PSY **PROCEDURE 22-4 Performing Skin Preparation and Hair Removal** (continued)

____

____

____

____

11. Remove your gloves and wash your hands.	❑	❑	❑
12. Inform the physician that the patient is ready for the surgical procedure.	❑	❑	❑
13. Drape the prepared area with a sterile drape if the physician will be delayed more than 10 or 15 minutes.	❑	❑	❑

CALCULATION

Total Possible Points: __________

Total Points Earned: __________ Multiplied by 100 = __________ Divided by Total Possible Points = __________ %

PASS **FAIL** **COMMENTS:**

❑ ❑

Student's signature ____________________ Date __________

Partner's signature ____________________ Date __________

Instructor's signature ____________________ Date __________

PSY PROCEDURE 22-5 Applying Sterile Gloves

Name: ______________________ **Date:** __________ **Time:** __________ **Grade:** __________

EQUIPMENT/SUPPLIES: One package of sterile gloves in the appropriate size

STANDARDS: Given the needed equipment and a place to work, the student will perform this skill with _____ % accuracy in a total of _____ minutes. *(Your instructor will tell you what the percentage and time limits will be before you begin.)*

KEY: 4 = Satisfactory 0 = Unsatisfactory NA = This step is not counted

PROCEDURE STEPS	SELF	PARTNER	INSTRUCTOR
1. Remove rings and other jewelry.	❑	❑	❑
2. Wash your hands.	❑	❑	❑
3. Place prepackaged gloves on a clean, dry, flat surface with the cuffed end toward you. **a.** Pull the outer wrapping apart to expose the sterile inner wrap. **b.** With the cuffs toward you, fold back the inner wrap to expose the gloves.	❑	❑	❑
4. Grasping the edges of the outer paper, open the package out to its fullest.	❑	❑	❑
5. Use your nondominant hand to pick up the dominant hand glove. **a.** Grasp the folded edge of the cuff and lift it up and away from the paper. **b.** Curl your fingers and thumb together and insert them into the glove. **c.** Straighten your fingers and pull the glove on with your non-dominant hand still grasping the cuff.	❑	❑	❑
6. Unfold the cuff by pinching the inside surface and pull it toward your wrist.	❑	❑	❑
7. Place the fingers of your gloved hand under the cuff of the remaining glove. **a.** Lift the glove up and away from the wrapper. **b.** Slide your ungloved hand carefully into the glove with your fingers and thumb curled together. **c.** Straighten your fingers and pull the glove up and over your wrist by carefully unfolding the cuff.	❑	❑	❑
8. Settle the gloves comfortably onto your fingers by lacing your fingers together.	❑	❑	❑
9. Remove contaminated sterile gloves and discard them appropriately. Wash your hands.	❑	❑	❑

PSY PROCEDURE 22-5 Applying Sterile Gloves (continued)

CALCULATION

Total Possible Points: __________

Total Points Earned: __________ Multiplied by 100 = __________ Divided by Total Possible Points = __________ %

PASS ❑ **FAIL** ❑ **COMMENTS:**

Student's signature ____________________ Date __________

Partner's signature ____________________ Date __________

Instructor's signature ____________________ Date __________

PSY PROCEDURE 22-6 Applying a Sterile Dressing

Name: ______________________ **Date:** __________ **Time:** __________ **Grade:** __________

EQUIPMENT/SUPPLIES: Sterile gloves, sterile gauze dressings, scissors, bandage tape, any medication to be applied to the dressing if ordered by the physician

STANDARDS: Given the needed equipment and a place to work, the student will perform this skill with _____ % accuracy in a total of _____ minutes. *(Your instructor will tell you what the percentage and time limits will be before you begin.)*

KEY: 4 = Satisfactory 0 = Unsatisfactory NA = This step is not counted

PROCEDURE STEPS	SELF	PARTNER	INSTRUCTOR
1. Wash your hands.	❑	❑	❑
2. Assemble the equipment and supplies.	❑	❑	❑
3. Greet and identify the patient.	❑	❑	❑
4. Ask about any tape allergies before deciding on what type of tape to use.	❑	❑	❑
5. Cut or tear lengths of tape to secure the dressing.	❑	❑	❑
6. Explain the procedure and instruct the patient to remain still; avoid coughing, sneezing, or talking until the procedure is complete.	❑	❑	❑
7. Open the dressing pack to create a sterile field, maintaining sterile asepsis. **a.** If sterile gloves are to be used, open and place near dressing pack. **b.** If using a sterile transfer forceps, place it near the other supplies.	❑	❑	❑
8. Apply topical medication to the sterile dressing that will cover the wound.	❑	❑	❑
9. Apply the number of dressings necessary to properly cover and protect the wound.	❑	❑	❑
10. Apply sufficient cut lengths of tape over the dressing to secure.	❑	❑	❑
11. Remove contaminated gloves and discard in the proper receptacle. Wash your hands.	❑	❑	❑
12. Provide patient education and supplies as appropriate.	❑	❑	❑
13. AFF Explain how to respond to a patient who is visually impaired.	❑	❑	❑

PROCEDURE 22-6 Applying a Sterile Dressing (continued)

____

____

____

____

14. Clean and sanitize the room and equipment.	❏	❏	❏
15. Record the procedure.	❏	❏	❏

CALCULATION

Total Possible Points: ________

Total Points Earned: ________ Multiplied by 100 = ________ Divided by Total Possible Points = ________ %

PASS ❏ **FAIL** ❏ **COMMENTS:**

Student's signature ________________ Date ________

Partner's signature ________________ Date ________

Instructor's signature ________________ Date ________

PSY PROCEDURE 22-7 Changing an Existing Sterile Dressing

Name: ______________________ **Date:** __________ **Time:** __________ **Grade:** __________

EQUIPMENT/SUPPLIES: Sterile gloves, nonsterile gloves, sterile dressing, prepackaged skin antiseptic swabs (or sterile antiseptic solution poured into a sterile basin and sterile cotton balls or gauze), tape, approved biohazard containers

STANDARDS: Given the needec equipment and a place to work, the student will perform this skill with _____ % accuracy in a total of _____ minutes. *(Your instructor will tell you what the percentage and time limits will be before you begin.)*

KEY: 4 = Satisfactory 0 = Unsatisfactory NA = This step is not counted

PROCEDURE STEPS	SELF	PARTNER	INSTRUCTOR
1. Wash your hands.	❑	❑	❑
2. Assemble the equipment and supplies.	❑	❑	❑
3. Greet and identify the patient; explain the procedure and answer any questions.	❑	❑	❑
4. Prepare a sterile field including opening sterile dressings.	❑	❑	❑
5. Open a sterile basin and use the inside of the wrapper as the sterile field. **a.** Flip the sterile gauze or cotton balls into the basin. **b.** Pour antiseptic solution appropriately into the basin. **c.** If using prepackaged antiseptic swabs, carefully open an adequate number. **d.** Set swabs aside without contaminating them.	❑	❑	❑
6. Instruct the patient not to talk, cough, sneeze, laugh, or move during the procedure.	❑	❑	❑
7. AFF Explain how to respond to a patient who has dementia.	❑	❑	❑
____________________ ____________________ ____________________ ____________________			
8. Wear clean gloves and carefully remove tape from the wound dressing by pulling it toward the wound. **a.** Remove the old dressing. **b.** Discard the soiled dressing into a biohazard container.	❑	❑	❑
9. Inspect wound for the degree of healing, amount and type of drainage, and appearance of wound edges.	❑	❑	❑

PSY PROCEDURE 22-7 Changing an Existing Sterile Dressing (continued)

10. Observing medical asepsis, remove and discard your gloves.	❑	❑	❑
11. Using proper technique, apply sterile gloves.	❑	❑	❑
12. Clean the wound with the antiseptic solution ordered by the physician.	❑	❑	❑
13. Clean in a straight motion with the cotton or gauze or the pre-packaged antiseptic swab. Discard the wipe (cotton ball, swab) after each use.	❑	❑	❑
14. Remove your gloves and wash your hands.	❑	❑	❑
15. Change the dressing using the procedure for sterile dressing application (Procedure 22-6) and using sterile gloves (Procedure 22-5) or sterile transfer forceps (Procedure 22-2).	❑	❑	❑
16. Record the procedure.	❑	❑	❑

CALCULATION

Total Possible Points: __________

Total Points Earned: __________ Multiplied by 100 = __________ Divided by Total Possible Points = __________ %

PASS ❑ **FAIL** ❑ **COMMENTS:**

Student's signature ____________________ Date __________

Partner's signature ____________________ Date __________

Instructor's signature ____________________ Date __________

PSY PROCEDURE 22-8 Assisting with Excisional Surgery

Name: ________________ **Date:** __________ **Time:** __________ **Grade:** __________

EQUIPMENT/SUPPLIES: Sterile gloves, local anesthetic, antiseptic wipes, adhesive tape, specimen container with completed laboratory request; *On the field:* basin for solutions, gauze sponges and cotton balls, antiseptic solution, sterile drape, dissecting scissors, disposable scalpel, blade of physician's choice, mosquito forceps, tissue forceps, needle holder, suture and needle of physician's choice

STANDARDS: Given the needed equipment and a place to work, the student will perform this skill with _____ % accuracy in a total of _____ minutes. *(Your instructor will tell you what the percentage and time limits will be before you begin.)*

KEY: 4 = Satisfactory 0 = Unsatisfactory NA = This step is not counted

PROCEDURE STEPS	SELF	PARTNER	INSTRUCTOR
1. Wash your hands.	❑	❑	❑
2. Assemble the equipment appropriate for the procedure and according to physician preference.	❑	❑	❑
3. Greet and identify the patient; explain the procedure and answer any questions.	❑	❑	❑
4. Set up a sterile field on a surgical stand with additional equipment close at hand.	❑	❑	❑
5. Cover the field with a sterile drape until the physician arrives.	❑	❑	❑
6. Position the patient appropriately.	❑	❑	❑
7. Put on sterile gloves (Procedure 22-5) or use sterile transfer forceps (Procedure 22-2) and cleanse the patient's skin (Procedure 22-4).	❑	❑	❑
8. Be ready to assist during the procedure: adding supplies as needed, assisting the physician, and comforting the patient.	❑	❑	❑
9. Assist with collecting tissue specimen in an appropriate container.	❑	❑	❑
10. At the end of the procedure, wash your hands and dress the wound using sterile technique (Procedure 22-6).	❑	❑	❑
11. Thank the patient and give appropriate instructions.	❑	❑	❑
12. AFF Explain how to respond to a patient who is hearing impaired.	❑	❑	❑

PSY PROCEDURE 22-8 Assisting with Excisional Surgery (continued)

____

____

____

____

13. Sanitize the examining room in preparation for the next patient.	❑	❑	❑
14. Discard all disposables in the appropriate biohazard containers.	❑	❑	❑
15. Record the procedure.	❑	❑	❑

CALCULATION

Total Possible Points: __________

Total Points Earned: __________ Multiplied by 100 = __________ Divided by Total Possible Points = __________ %

PASS ❑ **FAIL** ❑ **COMMENTS:**

Student's signature ____________________ Date __________

Partner's signature ____________________ Date __________

Instructor's signature ____________________ Date __________

PSY PROCEDURE 22-9 Assisting with Incision and Drainage

Name: ________________ **Date:** __________ **Time:** __________ **Grade:** __________

EQUIPMENT/SUPPLIES: Sterile gloves, local anesthetic, antiseptic wipes, adhesive tape, sterile dressings, packing gauze, a culture tube if the wound may be cultured; *On the field:* basin for solutions, gauze sponges and cotton balls, antiseptic solution, sterile drape, syringes and needles for local anesthetic, commercial I&D sterile setup *or* scalpel, dissecting scissors, hemostats, tissue forceps, 4 × 4 gauze sponges, probe (optional)

STANDARDS: Given the needed equipment and a place to work, the student will perform this skill with _____ % accuracy in a total of _____ minutes. *(Your instructor will tell you what the percentage and time limits will be before you begin.)*

KEY: 4 = Satisfactory 0 = Unsatisfactory NA = This step is not counted

PROCEDURE STEPS	SELF	PARTNER	INSTRUCTOR
1. Wash your hands.	❑	❑	❑
2. Assemble the equipment appropriate for the procedure and according to physician preference.	❑	❑	❑
3. Greet and identify the patient. Explain the procedure and answer any questions.	❑	❑	❑
4. Set up a sterile field on a surgical stand with additional equipment close at hand	❑	❑	❑
5. Cover the field with a sterile drape until the physician arrives.	❑	❑	❑
6. Position the patient appropriately.	❑	❑	❑
7. Put on sterile gloves (Procedure 22-5) or use sterile transfer forceps (Procedure 22-2) and cleanse the patient's skin (Procedure 22-4).	❑	❑	❑
8. Be ready to assist during the procedure: adding supplies as needed, assisting the physician, comforting the patient.	❑	❑	❑
9. Assist with collecting culturette specimen for culture and sensitivity.	❑	❑	❑
10. At the end of procedure, remove gloves, wash your hands, and dress the wound using sterile technique (Procedure 22-6).	❑	❑	❑
11. Thank the patient and give appropriate instructions.	❑	❑	❑
12. Sanitize the examining room in preparation for the next patient.	❑	❑	❑
13. Discard all disposables in appropriate biohazard containers.	❑	❑	❑
14. Record the procedure.	❑	❑	❑

PSY PROCEDURE 22-9 Assisting with Incision and Drainage
(continued)

CALCULATION

Total Possible Points: __________

Total Points Earned: __________ Multiplied by 100 = __________ Divided by Total Possible Points = __________ %

PASS ❑ **FAIL** ❑ **COMMENTS:**

Student's signature ____________________ Date __________

Partner's signature ____________________ Date __________

Instructor's signature ____________________ Date __________

PSY PROCEDURE 22-10 Removing Sutures

Name: ______________________ **Date:** __________ **Time:** __________ **Grade:** __________

EQUIPMENT/SUPPLIES: Skin antiseptic, sterile gloves, prepackaged suture removal kit or thumb forceps, suture scissors, gauze

STANDARDS: Given the needed equipment and a place to work, the student will perform this skill with _____ % accuracy in a total of _____ minutes. *(Your instructor will tell you what the percentage and time limits will be before you begin.)*

KEY: 4 = Satisfactory 0 = Unsatisfactory NA = This step is not counted

PROCEDURE STEPS	SELF	PARTNER	INSTRUCTOR
1. Wash your hands and apply clean examination gloves.	❑	❑	❑
2. Assemble the equipment.	❑	❑	❑
3. Greet and identify the patient; explain the procedure and answer any questions.	❑	❑	❑
4. If dressings have not been removed previously, remove them from the wound area. **a.** Properly dispose of the soiled dressings in the biohazard trash container. **b.** Remove your gloves and wash your hands.	❑	❑	❑
5. Cover the field with a sterile drape until the physician arrives.	❑	❑	❑
6. Open suture removal packet using sterile asepsis.	❑	❑	❑
7. Put on sterile gloves. **a.** With the thumb forceps, grasp the end of the knot closest to the skin surface and lift it slightly and gently up from the skin. **b.** Cut the suture below the knot as close to the skin as possible. **c.** Use the thumb forceps to pull the suture out of the skin with a smooth motion.	❑	❑	❑
8. Place the suture on the gauze sponge; repeat the procedure for each suture to be removed.	❑	❑	❑
9. Clean the site with an antiseptic solution and cover it with a sterile dressing.	❑	❑	❑
10. Thank the patient.	❑	❑	❑
11. AFF Explain how to respond to a patient who is developmentally challenged.	❑	❑	❑

PSY PROCEDURE 22-10 Removing Sutures (continued)

____

____

____

____

12. Properly dispose of the equipment and supplies.	❑	❑	❑
13. Clean the work area, remove your gloves, and wash your hands.	❑	❑	❑
14. Record the procedure, including the time, location of sutures, the number removed, and the condition of the wound.	❑	❑	❑

CALCULATION

Total Possible Points: __________

Total Points Earned: __________ Multiplied by 100 = __________ Divided by Total Possible Points = __________ %

PASS ❑ **FAIL** ❑ **COMMENTS:**

Student's signature ____________________ Date __________

Partner's signature ____________________ Date __________

Instructor's signature ____________________ Date __________

PSY PROCEDURE 22-11 Removing Staples

Name: ______________________ **Date:** __________ **Time:** __________ **Grade:** __________

EQUIPMENT/SUPPLIES: Antiseptic solution or wipes, gauze squares, sponge forceps, prepackaged sterile staple removal instrument, examination gloves, sterile gloves

STANDARDS: Given the needed equipment and a place to work, the student will perform this skill with _____ % accuracy in a total of _____ minutes. *(Your instructor will tell you what the percentage and time limits will be before you begin.)*

KEY: 4 = Satisfactory 0 = Unsatisfactory NA = This step is not counted

PROCEDURE STEPS	SELF	PARTNER	INSTRUCTOR
1. Wash your hands.	❑	❑	❑
2. Assemble the equipment.	❑	❑	❑
3. Greet and identify the patient; explain the procedure and answer any questions.	❑	❑	❑
4. If the dressing has not been removed, put on clean examination gloves and do so.	❑	❑	❑
5. Dispose of the dressing properly in a biohazard container.	❑	❑	❑
6. Clean the incision with antiseptic solution.	❑	❑	❑
7. Pat dry using dry sterile gauze sponges.	❑	❑	❑
8. Put on sterile gloves.	❑	❑	❑
9. Gently slide the end of the staple remover under each staple to be removed; press the handles together to lift the ends of the staple out of the skin and remove the staple.	❑	❑	❑
10. Place each staple on a gauze square as it is removed.	❑	❑	❑
11. When all staples are removed, clean the incision as instructed for all procedures.	❑	❑	❑
12. Pat dry and dress the site if ordered to do so by the physician.	❑	❑	❑
13. Thank the patient and properly care for, or dispose of, all equipment and supplies.	❑	❑	❑
14. AFF Explain how to respond to a patient who is visually impaired.	❑	❑	❑

PSY PROCEDURE 22-11 Removing Staples (continued)

____

____

____

____

15. Clean the work area, remove your gloves, and wash your hands.	❑	❑	❑
16. Record the procedure.	❑	❑	❑

CALCULATION

Total Possible Points: __________

Total Points Earned: __________ Multiplied by 100 = __________ Divided by Total Possible Points = __________ %

PASS ❑ **FAIL** ❑ **COMMENTS:**

Student's signature ____________________ Date __________

Partner's signature ____________________ Date __________

Instructor's signature ____________________ Date __________

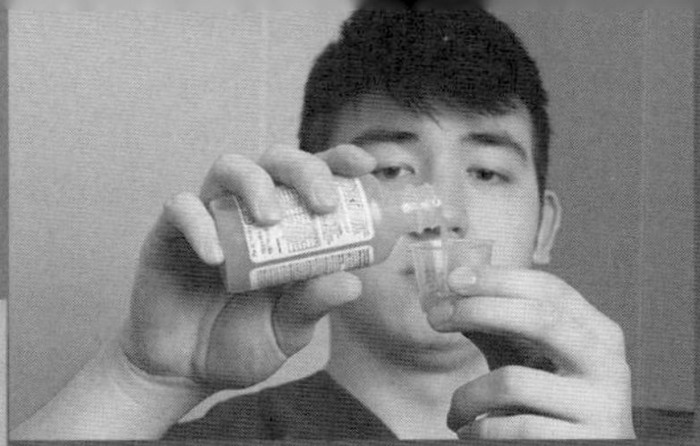

CHAPTER 23 Pharmacology

Learning Outcomes

COG Cognitive Domain

1. Spell and define key terms
2. Describe the relationship between anatomy and physiology of all body systems and medications used for treatment in each
3. Identify chemical, trade, and generic drug names
4. Discuss all levels of governmental legislation and regulation as they apply to medical assisting practice, including FDA and DEA regulations
5. Explain the various drug actions and interactions including pharmacodynamics and pharmacokinetics
6. Identify the classifications of medications, including indications for use, desired effects, side effects, and adverse reactions
7. Name the sources for locating information on pharmacology

AFF Affective Domain

1. Properly utilize PDR, drug handbook, and other drug references to identify a drug's classification, usual dosage, usual side effects, and contradictions
2. Identify and define common abbreviations that are accepted in prescription writing
3. Understand legal aspects of writing prescriptions, including federal and state laws

ABHES Competencies

1. Properly utilize *Physicians' Desk Reference,* drug handbook, and other drug references to identify a drug's classification, usual dosage, usual side effects, and contradictions
2. Identify and define common abbreviations that are accepted in prescription writing
3. Understand legal aspects of writing prescriptions, including federal and state laws

COG AFF CASE STUDIES FOR CRITICAL THINKING

Grade: ___________

1. You are doing an inventory of the controlled substances in your office and notice that the office's supply of morphine is off count. You double-check all written records of medications given for administration and still cannot account for the missing morphine. After realizing this, you immediately tell the physician. The physician tells you not to worry about it. Three weeks later you notice that more morphine is missing. What do you do?

____

____

____

____

2. A patient just received a shot of penicillin. Before the shot was administered, you advised the patient that she needs to remain in the physician's office for 30 minutes before leaving. However, the patient just remembers that she must pick her mother up for an appointment that her mother needs to attend. The patient is adamant that she must leave right away so as not to be late. How would you respond to this patient?

____

____

____

____

3. You have an elderly patient who is taking Lasix for his high blood pressure. This patient has recently called in to the office complaining of muscle weakness. What classification is the drug Lasix? What is possibly causing the patients' muscle weakness? How would you respond to this patient?

____

____

____

____

4. You have a patient with hepatic disease. After she consults with the physician, she asks you some general questions to clarify how her body processes medication. Think about the pharmacokinetic effects of drugs on her body. What processes would you discuss with her about her condition and medications?

____

____

____

____

5. Your patient tells you that she feels like she is coming down with a cold and has had a sore throat since yesterday. She also tells you that her friend gave her some leftover antibiotics that she did not finish when she had strep throat last month. How would you respond to this patient? Is this important information for the physician to know? Why or why not?

____

____

____

____

6. Louise asks Mr. Fujiwara about his medical history and if he has any allergies to any medications. Mr. Fujiwara says that he has an allergy to aspirin. Louise marks Mr. Fujiwara's drug allergy prominently on the front of his medication record before giving the record to the physician. What else should the medical assistant do?

____

____

____

____

COG AFF CASE STUDIES FOR CRITICAL THINKING

Grade: ______

1. The parent of an 18-month old insists that you give the IM immunization in the child's "hip." How would you respond to the parent's request?

______

______

______

______

2. The patient you are monitoring is receiving intravenous fluids for rehydration. Unfortunately, the insertion site in the left anterior forearm has developed complications and must be removed. How would you respond to the patient who does not understand why the IV must be removed?

______

______

______

______

3. One of the physicians in your medical office would like to change office policy so that no abbreviations are used in the patients' medical charts for fear of potentially harmful errors. The office is divided on the issue. What is your opinion and why?

______

______

______

______

4. You are directed to give a Z-track IM injection to a patient. The patient's spouse observes you deliberately draw a bubble into the syringe and panics because you are about to inject air into the patient. How do you address the spouse's concerns?

______

______

______

______

PSY PROCEDURE 24-1 Administer Oral Medications

Name: ____________________ **Date:** __________ **Time:** __________ **Grade:** __________

EQUIPMENT/SUPPLIES: Physician's order, oral medication, disposable calibrated cup, glass of water, patient's medical record

STANDARDS: Given the needed equipment and a place to work, the student will perform this skill with _____ % accuracy in a total of _____ minutes. *(Your instructor will tell you what the percentage and time limits will be before you begin.)*

KEY: 4 = Satisfactory 0 = Unsatisfactory NA = This step is not counted

PROCEDURE STEPS	SELF	PARTNER	INSTRUCTOR
1. Wash your hands.	❑	❑	❑
2. Review the physician's medication order and select the correct oral medication. **a.** Compare the label with the physician's instructions. **b.** Note the expiration date. **c.** Check the label three times: when taking it from the shelf, while pouring, and when returning to the shelf.	❑	❑	❑
3. Calculate the correct dosage to be given if necessary.	❑	❑	❑
4. If using a multidose container, remove cap from container. For single-dose medications, obtain the correct amount of medication.	❑	❑	❑
5. Remove the correct dose of medication. **a.** For solid medications: **(1)** Pour the capsule/tablet into the bottle cap. **(2)** Transfer the medication to a disposable cup. **b.** For liquid medications: **(1)** Open the bottle lid: place it on a flat surface with open end up. **(2)** Palm the label to prevent liquids from dripping onto the label. **(3)** With opposite hand, place the thumbnail at the correct calibration. **(4)** Pour the medication until the proper amount is in the cup.	❑	❑	❑
6. Greet and identify the patient. Explain the procedure.	❑	❑	❑
7. Ask the patient about medication allergies that might not be noted on the chart.	❑	❑	❑
8. Give the patient a glass of water, unless contraindicated. Hand the patient the disposable cup containing the medication or pour the tablets or capsules into the patient's hand.	❑	❑	❑
9. Remain with the patient to be sure that all of the medication is swallowed. **a.** Observe any unusual reactions and report them to the physician.	❑	❑	❑
10. Thank the patient and give any appropriate instructions.	❑	❑	❑

PSY PROCEDURE 24-1 Administer Oral Medications (continued)

11. AFF Explain how to respond to a patient who is hearing impaired.	❑	❑	❑
______________________________			
12. Wash your hands.	❑	❑	❑
13. AFF Log into the Electronic Medical Record (EMR) using your username and secure password OR obtain the paper medical record from a secure location and assure it is kept away from public access. Record the procedure noting the date, time, name of medication, dose administered, route of administration, and your name.	❑	❑	❑
14. When finished, log out of the EMR and/or replace the paper medical record in an appropriate and secure location.	❑	❑	❑

CALCULATION

Total Possible Points: __________

Total Points Earned: __________ Multiplied by 100 = __________ Divided by Total Possible Points = __________ %

PASS ❑ **FAIL** ❑ **COMMENTS:**

Student's signature ____________________ Date __________

Partner's signature ____________________ Date __________

Instructor's signature ____________________ Date __________

PSY PROCEDURE 24-2 Prepare Injections

Name: ______________________ **Date:** __________ **Time:** __________ **Grade:** __________

EQUIPMENT/SUPPLIES: Physician's order, medication for injection in ampule or vial, antiseptic wipes, gloves, appropriate-size needle and syringe, small gauze pad, biohazard sharps container, patient's medical record

STANDARDS: Given the needed equipment and a place to work, the student will perform this skill with _____ % accuracy in a total of _____ minutes. *(Your instructor will tell you what the percentage and time limits will be before you begin.)*

KEY: 4 = Satisfactory 0 = Unsatisfactory NA = This step is not counted

PROCEDURE STEPS	SELF	PARTNER	INSTRUCTOR
1. Wash your hands.	❑	❑	❑
2. Review the physician's medication order and select the correct medication. **a.** Compare the label with the physician's instructions. Note the expiration date. **b.** Check the label three times: when taking it from the shelf, while drawing it up into the syringe, and when returning to the shelf.	❑	❑	❑
3. Calculate the correct dosage to be given, if necessary.	❑	❑	❑
4. Choose the needle and syringe according to the route of administration, type of medication, and size of the patient.	❑	❑	❑
5. Open the needle and syringe package. Assemble if necessary. Secure the needle to the syringe.	❑	❑	❑
6. Withdraw the correct amount of medication: **a.** From an ampule: **(1)** Tap the stem of the ampule lightly. **(2)** Place a piece of gauze around the ampule neck. **(3)** Grasp the gauze and ampule firmly. Snap the stem off the ampule. **(4)** Dispose of the ampule top in a biohazard sharps container. **(5)** Insert the needle lumen below the level of the medication. **(6)** Withdraw the medication. **(7)** Dispose of the ampule in a biohazard sharps container. **(8)** Remove any air bubbles in the syringe. **(9)** Draw back on the plunger to add a small amount of air; then gently push the plunger forward to eject the air out of the syringe.	❑	❑	❑

PSY PROCEDURE 24-2 Prepare Injections (continued)

b. From a vial: **(1)** Using the antiseptic wipe, cleanse the rubber stopper of the vial. **(2)** Pull air into the syringe with the amount equivalent to the amount of medication to be removed from the vial. **(3)** Insert the needle into the vial top. Inject the air from the syringe. **(4)** With the needle inside the vial, invert the vial. **(5)** Hold the syringe at eye level. **(6)** Aspirate the desired amount of medication into the syringe. **(7)** Displace any air bubbles in the syringe by gently tapping the barrel. **(8)** Remove the air by pushing the plunger slowly and forcing the air into the vial.	❑	❑	❑
7. Carefully recap the needle using one-hand technique.	❑	❑	❑

____

____

____

____

CALCULATION

Total Possible Points: __________

Total Points Earned: __________ Multiplied by 100 = __________ Divided by Total Possible Points = __________ %

PASS **FAIL** **COMMENTS:**

❑ ❑

Student's signature ____________________ Date __________

Partner's signature ____________________ Date __________

Instructor's signature ____________________ Date __________

PSY PROCEDURE 24-3 Administer an Intradermal Injection

Name: ______________________ **Date:** __________ **Time:** __________ **Grade:** __________

EQUIPMENT/SUPPLIES: Physician's order, medication for injection in ampule or vial, antiseptic wipes, gloves, appropriate-size needle and syringe, small gauze pad, biohazard sharps container, patient's medical record

STANDARDS: Given the needed equipment and a place to work, the student will perform this skill with _____ % accuracy in a total of _____ minutes. *(Your instructor will tell you what the percentage and time limits will be before you begin.)*

KEY: 4 = Satisfactory 0 = Unsatisfactory NA = This step is not counted

PROCEDURE STEPS	SELF	PARTNER	INSTRUCTOR
1. Wash your hands. **a.** Review the physician's medication order and select the correct medication. **b.** Compare the label with the physician's instructions. Note the expiration date. **c.** Check the label three times: when taking it from the shelf, while drawing it up into the syringe, and when returning it to the shelf.	❏	❏	❏
2. Prepare the injection according to the steps in Procedure 24-2.	❏	❏	❏
3. Greet and identify the patient. Explain the procedure.	❏	❏	❏
4. Ask patient about medication allergies.	❏	❏	❏
5. Select the appropriate site for the injection.	❏	❏	❏
6. Prepare the site by cleansing with an antiseptic wipe.	❏	❏	❏
7. Put on gloves. Remove the needle guard.	❏	❏	❏
8. Using your nondominant hand, pull the patient's skin taut.	❏	❏	❏
9. With the bevel of the needle facing upward, insert needle at a 10- to 15-degree angle into the upper layer of the skin. **a.** When the bevel of the needle is under the skin, stop inserting the needle. **b.** The needle will be slightly visible below the surface of the skin. **c.** It is not necessary to aspirate when performing an intradermal injection.	❏	❏	❏
10. Inject the medication slowly by depressing the plunger. **a.** A wheal will form as the medication enters the dermal layer of the skin. **b.** Hold the syringe steady for proper administration.	❏	❏	❏
11. Remove the needle from the skin at the same angle at which it was inserted. **a.** Do not use an antiseptic wipe or gauze pad over the site. **b.** Do not press or massage the site. Do not apply an adhesive bandage.	❏	❏	❏

PSY PROCEDURE 24-3 Administer an Intradermal Injection
(continued)

12. Do not recap the needle.	❑	❑	❑
13. Dispose of the needle and syringe in an approved biohazard sharps container.	❑	❑	❑
14. AFF Explain how to respond to a patient with dementia.	❑	❑	❑
______________________________ ______________________________ ______________________________ ______________________________			
15. Remove your gloves, and wash your hands.	❑	❑	❑
16. Depending upon the type of skin test administered, the length of time required for the body tissues to react, and the policies of the medical office, perform one of the following: **a.** Read the test results. Inspect and palpate the site for the presence and amount of induration. **b.** Tell the patient when to return (date and time) to the office to have the results read. **c.** Instruct the patient to read the results at home. **d.** Make sure the patient understands the instructions.	❑	❑	❑
17. AFF Log into the Electronic Medical Record (EMR) using your username and secure password OR obtain the paper medical record from a secure location and assure it is kept away from public access. Record the procedure noting the date, time, name of medication, dose administered, route of administration, patient instructions, and your name.	❑	❑	❑
18. When finished, log out of the EMR and/or replace the paper medical record in an appropriate and secure location.	❑	❑	❑

CALCULATION

Total Possible Points: __________

Total Points Earned: __________ Multiplied by 100 = __________ Divided by Total Possible Points = __________ %

PASS ❑ **FAIL** ❑ **COMMENTS:**

Student's signature ____________________ Date __________

Partner's signature ____________________ Date __________

Instructor's signature ____________________ Date __________

PSY PROCEDURE 24-4 Administer a Subcutaneous Injection

Name: ______________________ **Date:** __________ **Time:** __________ **Grade:** __________

EQUIPMENT/SUPPLIES: Physician's order, medication for injection in ampule or vial, antiseptic wipes, gloves, appropriate-size needle and syringe, small gauze pad, biohazard sharps container, patient's medical record

STANDARDS: Given the needed equipment and a place to work, the student will perform this skill with _____ % accuracy in a total of _____ minutes. *(Your instructor will tell you what the percentage and time limits will be before you begin.)*

KEY: 4 = Satisfactory 0 = Unsatisfactory NA = This step is not counted

PROCEDURE STEPS	SELF	PARTNER	INSTRUCTOR
1. Wash your hands. **a.** Review the physician's medication order and select the correct medication. **b.** Compare the label with the physician's instructions. Note the expiration date. **c.** Check the label three times: when taking it from the shelf, while drawing it up into the syringe, and when returning it to the shelf.	❑	❑	❑
2. Prepare the injection according to the steps in Procedure 24-2.	❑	❑	❑
3. Greet and identify the patient. Explain the procedure.	❑	❑	❑
4. Ask the patient about medication allergies.	❑	❑	❑
5. Select the appropriate site for the injection.	❑	❑	❑
6. Prepare the site by cleansing with an antiseptic.	❑	❑	❑
7. Put on gloves.	❑	❑	❑
8. Using your nondominant hand, hold the skin surrounding the injection site.	❑	❑	❑
9. With a firm motion, insert the needle into the tissue at a 45-degree angle to the skin surface.	❑	❑	❑
10. Hold the barrel between the thumb and the index finger of your dominant hand.	❑	❑	❑
11. Insert the needle completely to the hub.	❑	❑	❑
12. Remove your nondominant hand from the skin.	❑	❑	❑
13. Holding the syringe steady, pull back on the syringe gently. If blood appears in the hub or the syringe, do not inject the medication; remove the needle and prepare a new injection.	❑	❑	❑
14. Inject the medication slowly by depressing the plunger.	❑	❑	❑

PSY PROCEDURE 24-4 Administer a Subcutaneous Injection (continued)

15. Place a gauze pad over the injection site and remove the needle. **a.** Gently massage the injection site with the gauze pad. **b.** Do not recap the used needle; place it in the biohazard sharps container. **c.** Apply an adhesive bandage if needed.	❑	❑	❑
16. Remove your gloves and wash your hands.	❑	❑	❑
17. AFF Explain how to respond to a patient who is deaf.	❑	❑	❑
18. An injection given for allergy desensitization requires: **a.** Keeping the patient in the office for at least 30 minutes for observation. **b.** Notifying the doctor of any reaction. (Be alert, anaphylaxis is possible.)	❑	❑	❑
19. AFF Log into the Electronic Medical Record (EMR) using your username and secure password OR obtain the paper medical record from a secure location and assure it is kept away from public access. Record the procedure noting the date, time, name of medication, dose administered, route of administration, and your name.	❑	❑	❑
20. When finished, log out of the EMR and/or replace the paper medical record in an appropriate and secure location.	❑	❑	❑

CALCULATION

Total Possible Points: __________

Total Points Earned: __________ Multiplied by 100 = __________ Divided by Total Possible Points = __________ %

PASS ❑ **FAIL** ❑ **COMMENTS:**

Student's signature ____________________ Date __________

Partner's signature ____________________ Date __________

Instructor's signature ____________________ Date __________

PSY PROCEDURE 24-5 Administer an Intramuscular Injection

Name: ______________ **Date:** ________ **Time:** ________ **Grade:** ________

EQUIPMENT/SUPPLIES: Physician's order, medication for injection in ampule or vial, antiseptic wipes, gloves, appropriate-size needle and syringe, small gauze pad, biohazard sharps container, patient's medical record

STANDARDS: Given the needed equipment and a place to work, the student will perform this skill with _____ % accuracy in a total of _____ minutes. *(Your instructor will tell you what the percentage and time limits will be before you begin.)*

KEY: 4 = Satisfactory 0 = Unsatisfactory NA = This step is not counted

PROCEDURE STEPS	SELF	PARTNER	INSTRUCTOR
1. Wash your hands. **a.** Review the physician's order and select the correct medication. **b.** Compare the label with the physician's instructions. Note the expiration date. **c.** Check the label three times: when taking it from the shelf, while drawing it up into the syringe, and when returning to the shelf.	❑	❑	❑
2. Prepare the injection according to the steps in Procedure 24-2.	❑	❑	❑
3. Greet and identify the patient. Explain the procedure.	❑	❑	❑
4. Ask the patient about medication allergies.	❑	❑	❑
5. Select the appropriate site for the injection.	❑	❑	❑
6. Prepare the site by cleansing with an antiseptic wipe.	❑	❑	❑
7. Put on gloves.	❑	❑	❑
8. Using your nondominant hand, hold the skin surrounding the injection site.	❑	❑	❑
9. While holding the syringe like a dart, use a quick, firm motion to insert the needle at a 90-degree angle to the skin surface. Hold the barrel between the thumb and the index finger of the dominant hand and insert the needle completely to the hub.	❑	❑	❑
10. Holding the syringe steady, pull back on the syringe gently. If blood appears in the hub or the syringe, do not inject the medication; remove the needle and prepare a new injection.	❑	❑	❑
11. Inject the medication slowly by depressing the plunger.	❑	❑	❑
12. Place a gauze pad over the injection site and remove the needle. **a.** Gently massage the injection site with the gauze pad. **b.** Do not recap the used needle. Place in biohazard sharps container. **c.** Apply an adhesive bandage if needed.	❑	❑	❑
13. AFF Explain how to respond to a patient who is visually impaired.	❑	❑	❑

PSY PROCEDURE 24-5 Administer an Intramuscular Injection (continued)

____

____

____

____

14. Remove your gloves, and wash your hands.	❑	❑	❑
15. Notify the doctor of any reaction. (Be alert, anaphylaxis is possible.)	❑	❑	❑
16. AFF Log into the Electronic Medical Record (EMR) using your username and secure password OR obtain the paper medical record from a secure location and assure it is kept away from public access. Record the procedure noting the date, time, name of medication, dose administered, route of administration, and your name.	❑	❑	❑
17. When finished, log out of the EMR and/or replace the paper medical record in an appropriate and secure location.	❑	❑	❑

CALCULATION

Total Possible Points: __________

Total Points Earned: __________ Multiplied by 100 = __________ Divided by Total Possible Points = __________ %

PASS **FAIL** **COMMENTS:**

❑ ❑

Student's signature ____________________ Date __________

Partner's signature ____________________ Date __________

Instructor's signature ____________________ Date __________

PSY PROCEDURE 24-6 Administer an Intramuscular Injection Using the Z-Track Method

Name: ______________________ **Date:** __________ **Time:** __________ **Grade:** __________

EQUIPMENT/SUPPLIES: Physician's order, medication for injection in ampule or vial, antiseptic wipes, gloves, appropriate-size needle and syringe, small gauze pad, biohazard sharps container, patient's medical record

STANDARDS: Given the needed equipment and a place to work, the student will perform this skill with _____ % accuracy in a total of _____ minutes. *(Your instructor will tell you what the percentage and time limits will be before you begin.)*

KEY: 4 = Satisfactory 0 = Unsatisfactory NA = This step is not counted

PROCEDURE STEPS	SELF	PARTNER	INSTRUCTOR
1. Follow steps 1 through 7 as described in Procedure 24-5.	❑	❑	❑
2. Pull the top layer of skin to the side and hold it with your nondominant hand throughout the injection.	❑	❑	❑
3. While holding the syringe like a dart, use a quick, firm motion to insert the needle at a 90-degree angle to the skin surface. **a.** Hold the barrel between the thumb and index finger of the dominant hand. **b.** Insert the needle completely to the hub.	❑	❑	❑
4. Aspirate by withdrawing the plunger slightly. **a.** If no blood appears, push the plunger in slowly and steadily. **b.** Count to 10 before withdrawing the needle.	❑	❑	❑
5. Place a gauze pad over the injection site and remove the needle. **a.** Gently massage the injection site with the gauze pad. **b.** Do not recap the used needle. Place in the biohazard sharps container. **c.** Apply an adhesive bandage if needed.	❑	❑	❑
6. Remove your gloves, and wash your hands.	❑	❑	❑
7. Notify the doctor of any reaction. (Be alert, anaphylaxis is possible.)	❑	❑	❑
8. AFF Log into the Electronic Medical Record (EMR) using your username and secure password OR obtain the paper medical record from a secure location and assure it is kept away from public access. Record the procedure noting the date, time, name of medication, dose administered, route of administration, and your name. If instructions were given to the patient, document these also.	❑	❑	❑
9. When finished, log out of the EMR and/or replace the paper medical record in an appropriate and secure location.	❑	❑	❑

PSY PROCEDURE 24-6 Administer an Intramuscular Injection Using the Z-Track Method (continued)

CALCULATION

Total Possible Points: __________

Total Points Earned: __________ Multiplied by 100 = __________ Divided by Total Possible Points = __________ %

PASS ❑ **FAIL** ❑ **COMMENTS:**

Student's signature ____________________ Date __________

Partner's signature ____________________ Date __________

Instructor's signature ____________________ Date __________

PSY PROCEDURE 24-7 Apply Transdermal Medications

Name: ________________________________ **Date:** __________ **Time:** __________ **Grade:** __________

EQUIPMENT/SUPPLIES: Physician's order, medication, gloves, patient's medical record

STANDARDS: Given the needed equipment and a place to work, the student will perform this skill with _____ % accuracy in a total of _____ minutes. *(Your instructor will tell you what the percentage and time limits will be before you begin.)*

KEY: 4 = Satisfactory 0 = Unsatisfactory NA = This step is not counted

PROCEDURE STEPS	SELF	PARTNER	INSTRUCTOR
1. Wash your hands.	❑	❑	❑
2. Review the physician's medication order and select the correct medication. **a.** Compare the label with the physician's instructions. Note the expiration date. **b.** Check the label three times: when taking it from the shelf, before taking it into the patient exam room, and before applying it to the patient's skin.	❑	❑	❑
3. Greet and identify the patient. Explain the procedure.	❑	❑	❑
4. Ask the patient about medication allergies that might not be noted on the medical record.	❑	❑	❑
5. Select the appropriate site and perform any necessary skin preparation. The sites are usually the upper arm, the chest or back surface, or behind the ear. **a.** Ensure that the skin is clean, dry, and free from any irritation. **b.** Do not shave areas with excessive hair; trim the hair closely with scissors.	❑	❑	❑
6. If there is a transdermal patch already in place, remove it carefully while wearing gloves. Discard the patch in the trash container. Inspect the site for irritation.	❑	❑	❑
7. Open the medication package by pulling the two sides apart. Do not touch the area of medication.	❑	❑	❑
8. Apply the medicated patch to the patient's skin, following the manufacturer's directions. **a.** Press the adhesive edges down firmly all around, starting at the center and pressing outward. **b.** If the edges do not stick, fasten with tape.	❑	❑	❑
9. AFF Explain how to respond to a patient who is uncomfortable exposing skin on areas such as the chest or arms due to cultural or religious beliefs.	❑	❑	❑

PSY PROCEDURE 24-7 Apply Transdermal Medications (continued)

10. Wash your hands.	❑	❑	❑
11. AFF Log into the Electronic Medical Record (EMR) using your username and secure password OR obtain the paper medical record from a secure location and assure it is kept away from public access. Record the procedure noting the date, time, name of medication, dose administered, route of administration, site of the new patch, and your name.	❑	❑	❑
12. When finished, log out of the EMR and/or replace the paper medical record in an appropriate and secure location.	❑	❑	❑

CALCULATION

Total Possible Points: __________

Total Points Earned: __________ Multiplied by 100 = __________ Divided by Total Possible Points = __________ %

PASS **FAIL** **COMMENTS:**

❑ ❑

Student's signature ____________________ Date __________

Partner's signature ____________________ Date __________

Instructor's signature ____________________ Date __________

PSY PROCEDURE 24-8 Complete an Incident Report Related to an Error in Patient Care

Name: ______________________ **Date:** __________ **Time:** __________ **Grade:** __________

EQUIPMENT/SUPPLIES: An incident form

STANDARDS: Given the needed equipment and a place to work, the student will perform this skill with _____ % accuracy in a total of _____ minutes. *(Your instructor will tell you what the percentage and time limits will be before you begin.)*

KEY: 4 = Satisfactory 0 = Unsatisfactory NA = This step is not counted

PROCEDURE STEPS	SELF	PARTNER	INSTRUCTOR
1. Recognize the error in patient care (i.e., medication administration) and notify the physician immediately after assessing the patient and providing emergency procedures if appropriate.	❑	❑	❑
2. Once the patient is assessed and necessary interventions taken as per physician instructions, complete an incident report form.	❑	❑	❑
3. Sign and date the incident report form and file with the office or practice manager.	❑	❑	❑
4. AFF Advise the patient on any follow-up procedures as instructed by the physician.	❑	❑	❑

CALCULATION

Total Possible Points: __________

Total Points Earned: __________ Multiplied by 100 = __________ Divided by Total Possible Points = __________ %

PASS ❑ **FAIL** ❑ **COMMENTS:**

Student's signature ____________________ Date __________

Partner's signature ____________________ Date __________

Instructor's signature ____________________ Date __________

Great Falls Medical Center Physician Offices

Employee Incident/Injury Report Form

Employee Name:	Title:
Location:	Date and Time of Injury/Illness:
Person or Employee the Injury/Illness Reported to:	Title of Person or Employee Injury or Illness Reported to:
Describe the details of your accident, injury, or illness. Be as specific as possible:	
Explain what you were doing at the time of your accident, injury, or illness:	
For injuries, list the part or parts of your body that were injured. Be specific (i.e., right index finger, left ankle, etc…):	
If there was a delay in reporting the injury or illness, explain the reason for this delay:	
Names and Titles of Any Witnesses to your Injury or Illness:	
Employee Signature:	Date:

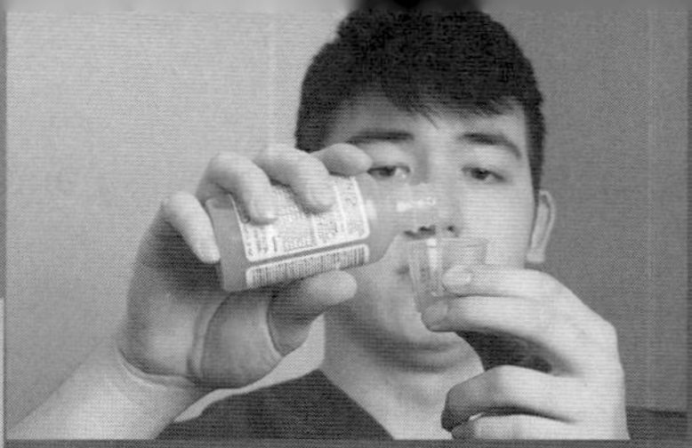

CHAPTER

25 Diagnostic Imaging

Learning Outcomes

COG Cognitive Domain

1. Spell and define the key terms
2. Explain the theory and function of x-rays and x-ray machines
3. State the principles of radiology
4. Describe routine and contrast media, fluoroscopy, computed tomography, sonography, magnetic resonance imaging, nuclear medicine, and mammographic examinations
5. Explain the role of the medical assistant in radiologic procedures
6. Describe body planes, directional terms, quadrants, and cavities
7. Identify critical information required for scheduling patient procedures

PSY Psychomotor Domain

1. Assist with x-ray procedures (Procedure 25-1)

AFF Affective Domain

1. Incorporate critical thinking skills when performing patient care
2. Show awareness of a patient's concerns related to the procedure being performed
3. Demonstrate respect for individual diversity including gender, race, religion, age, economic status, appearance
4. Explain to a patient the rationale for performance of a procedure
5. Demonstrate empathy, active listening, nonverbal communication
6. Protect the integrity of the medical record

ABHES Competencies

1. Assist the physician with the regimen of diagnostic and treatment modalities as they relate to each body system
2. Comply with federal, state, and local health laws and regulations
3. Communicate on the recipient's level of comprehension
4. Serve as a liaison between the physician and others
5. Show empathy and impartiality when dealing with patients

Name: ______________________________ Date: __________ Grade: __________

OG MULTIPLE CHOICE

Circle the letter preceding the correct answer.

1. Which term below means lying face downward?
a. Supine
b. Prone
c. Decubitus
d. Recumbent
e. Relaxed

2. Which of the following is a form of nuclear medicine?
a. Radiopaque
b. Barium
c. Iodine
d. Radionuclides
e. Radiolucent

3. Noises heard during an x-ray exposure may come from:
a. the x-ray tube.
b. x-rays.
c. the positioning aid.
d. high voltage.
e. the sheet of film.

4. Which of the following is an example of radiopaque tissue?
a. Lungs
b. Bone
c. Muscle
d. Fat
e. Veins

5. A minimum of two x-rays should be taken at:
a. 180 degrees of each other.
b. 30 degrees of each other.
c. 70 degrees of each other.
d. 90 degrees of each other.
e. 50 degrees of each other.

6. A type of radiography that creates cross-sectional images of the body is:
a. fluoroscopy.
b. echogram.
c. computerized tomography.
d. ultrasound.
e. mammography.

7. Which of the following form of radiography does not use x-rays?
a. MRI
b. Nuclear medicine
c. Fluoroscopy
d. Teleradiology
e. Tomography

8. Which procedure creates an image that depends on the chemical makeup of the body?
a. Tomography
b. Fluoroscopy
c. MRI
d. Mammography
e. Nuclear medicine

9. Sonograms create images using:
a. radioactive material.
b. contrast media.
c. magnetic resonance.
d. chemotherapy.
e. sound waves.

10. X-rays can be harmful to infants and young children because:
a. their immune systems are not fully developed.
b. their cells divide at a rapid pace.
c. they have less muscle mass than adults.
d. they have a smaller body mass.
e. they have less body fat than adults.

11. Which of the following procedures may be done in a confined space?
a. MRI
b. Nuclear medicine
c. Fluoroscopy
d. Teleradiology
e. Tomography

12. A physician who specializes in interpreting the images on the processed film is a(n):
a. pulmonologist.
b. internist.
c. immunologist.
d. ophthalmologist.
e. radiologist.

Scenario for questions 13 and 14: A patient has come in for an x-ray. The physician wants you to get a clear image of the patient's liver.

13. What is another possible way to view the patient's liver without injections?
a. Mammography
b. Sonography
c. Fluoroscopy
d. Teleradiology
e. Tomography

14. Which position would allow the best images of the liver?
a. Supine
b. Decubitus
c. Posterior
d. Left anterior oblique
e. Right anterior oblique

15. Who owns the x-ray film after it has been developed?
a. The patient
b. The physician who ordered the x-rays
c. The physician who will use the x-rays
d. The lab that developed the film
e. The site where the film was taken and developed.

16. You should wear a dosimeter to:
a. lower the level of radiation.
b. protect against radiation effects.
c. monitor personal radiation exposure.
d. enhance radiography images.
e. collect data on different procedures.

17. Why do some tests require patients to be NPO before an administration of barium PO?
a. Gastric juices may interfere with the readings.
b. A full stomach may distort or alter an image.
c. Patients are not allowed to relieve themselves.
d. Undigested food might counteract contrast media.
e. Instruments might become soiled during the procedure.

18. Images that partially block x-rays are called:
a. radiographs.
b. radiolucent.
c. radiopaque.
d. radionuclides.
e. radiograms.

19. Why is radiology used as a form of cancer treatment?
a. X-rays show the exact location of cancer.
b. Radioactive cells produce more white blood cells.
c. Radiation can destroy or weaken cancer cells.
d. Radiation makes cancerous tumors benign.
e. Chemotherapy is not as effective as radiation.

20. When explaining procedures to patients:
a. let the physician go into detail.
b. answer all the questions they ask.
c. do not worry them with potential risk.
d. soothe their fears without telling them anything.
e. allow only the nurse to explain the procedure.

COG MATCHING

Grade: _______

Match each key term with its definition.

Key Terms

21. _____ cassette
22. _____ contrast medium
23. _____ film
24. _____ fluoroscopy
25. _____ magnetic resonance imaging
26. _____ nuclear medicine
27. _____ radiograph
28. _____ radiography
29. _____ radiologist
30. _____ radiology
31. _____ radiolucent
32. _____ radionuclide
33. _____ radiopaque
34. _____ teleradiology
35. _____ tomography
36. _____ ultrasound
37. _____ x-rays

Definitions

a. invisible electromagnetic radiation waves used in diagnosis and treatment of various disorders
b. a lightproof holder in which film is exposed
c. imaging technique that uses a strong magnetic field
d. a radioactive material with a short life that is used in small amounts in nuclear medicine studies
e. physician who interprets images to provide diagnostic information
f. imaging technique that uses sound waves to diagnose or monitor various body structures
g. not permeable to passage of x-rays
h. processed film that contains a visible image
i. a substance ingested or injected into the body to facilitate imaging of internal structures
j. the use of computed imaging and information systems to transmit diagnostic images to distant locations
k. a procedure in which the x-ray tube and film move in relation to each other during exposure, blurring out all structures except those in the focal plane

Key Terms	Definitions
	l. a raw material on which x-rays are projected through the body; prior to processing, this does not contain a visible image
	m. permitting the passage of x-rays
	n. a special x-ray technique for examining a body part by immediate projection onto a fluorescent screen
	o. the branch of medicine involving diagnostic and therapeutic applications of x-rays
	p. a branch of medicine that uses radioactive isotopes to diagnose and treat disease
	q. the art and science of producing diagnostic images with x-rays

COG MATCHING

Grade: ______

Match the different types of radiography techniques with their individual characteristics.

Techniques	Characteristics
38. ______ Fluoroscopy	**a.** the image depends on the chemical makeup of the body, commonly used in prenatal testing
39. ______ Tomography	**b.** can create three-dimensional images, so that organs can be viewed from all angles
40. ______ Mammography	**c.** the area of the body exposed must be defined exactly so that each treatment is identical
41. ______ Ultrasound	**d.** used as an aid to other types of treatment, such as reducing fractures and implanting devices such as pacemakers
42. ______ Magnetic resonance imaging	**e.** a vital adjunct to biopsy
43. ______ Radiation therapy	**f.** designed to concentrate on specific areas of the body

COG SHORT ANSWER

Grade: ______

44. List the four processes by which radiographic film is produced.

______

______

______

______

45. List five radiation safety procedures for patients.

______

______

______

______

46. Fill in the full names for the abbreviations below.

a. PET ______

b. SPECT ______

c. ALARA ______

47. Name two contrast mediums.

48. What are the three ways contrast media may be introduced into the body?

49. Name four types of interventional radiological procedures.

50. List five side effects of radiation therapy.

51. What is the difference between radiolucent and radiopaque tissues? How do these tissues appear differently on a radiograph? Give an example of each.

52. Why do x-ray examinations require a minimum of two exposures?

53. Why is it imperative to have an esophagogastroduodenoscopy done before other barium studies?

54. Compare and contrast fluoroscopy with tomography. How do these procedures use movement?

____

____

____

____

55. You have a patient who will have a radiographic exam using contrast media next week. You find out this patient has an allergy to shellfish. What should you do?

____

____

____

____

COG TRUE OR FALSE?

Grade: ____________

Indicate whether the statements are true or false by placing the letter T (true) or F (false) on the line preceding the statement.

56. ______________ A patient may hear noises during an x-ray procedure.

57. ______________ A mammogram is a minimally invasive procedure.

58. ______________ You need to be proficient in the operation of your facility's equipment.

59. ______________ The best way to explain procedures to a patient is with lots of detail.

COG AFF CASE STUDIES FOR CRITICAL THINKING

Grade: ____________

1. Mrs. Kay has had several radiographic and contrast media studies over the past 5 years. She is now moving to another state and wants to know how to get copies of the films and reports to her new physician. What will you tell her about transferring these records?

____

____

____

____

2. You have a patient with a fear of enclosed spaces who is not able to have an open MRI at your outpatient radiographic center. How would you console this patient and explain x-ray procedures?

____

____

____

____

3. You have a patient coming in for radiation therapy who has been experiencing side effects such as weight loss, loss of appetite, and hair loss. She has concerns about the radiation therapy that she has been receiving and feels that it may be too much for her body. What would you say to her to help her better understand the situation?

____

____

____

____

4. You have a patient who has had radiographs taken with a referring physician. This patient has already spoken to his referral physician about the finding in his x-rays and would now like to consult with his primary care physician. However, the referring physician has not yet sent a summary of findings. Your patient is very anxious. What should you say?

____

____

____

____

PSY PROCEDURE 25-1 Assist with x-Ray Procedures

Name: ______________________ **Date:** __________ **Time:** __________ **Grade:** __________

EQUIPMENT/SUPPLIES: Patient gown and drape

STANDARDS: Given the needed equipment and a place to work, the student will perform this skill with _____ % accuracy in a total of _____ minutes. *(Your instructor will tell you what the percentage and time limits will be before you begin.)*

KEY: 4 = Satisfactory 0 = Unsatisfactory NA = This step is not counted

PROCEDURE STEPS	SELF	PARTNER	INSTRUCTOR
1. Wash your hands.	❑	❑	❑
2. Greet the patient by name, introduce yourself, and escort him or her to the room where the x-ray equipment is maintained.	❑	❑	❑
3. Ask female patients about the possibility of pregnancy. If the patient is unsure or indicates pregnancy in any trimester, consult with the physician before proceeding with the x-ray procedure.	❑	❑	❑
4. AFF Explain how to respond to a patient who speaks English as a second language.	❑	❑	❑
____ ____ ____ ____			
5. After explaining what clothing should be removed, if any, give the patient a gown and privacy.	❑	❑	❑
6. Notify the x-ray technician or physician that the patient is ready for the x-ray procedure. Stay behind the lead-lined wall during the x-ray procedure to avoid exposure to x-rays during the procedure.	❑	❑	❑
7. After the x-ray, ask the patient to remain in the room until the film has been developed and checked for accuracy and readability.	❑	❑	❑
8. Once you have determined that the exposed film is adequate for the physician to view for diagnosis, have the patient get dressed and escort him or her to the front desk.	❑	❑	❑

PSY PROCEDURE 25-1 Assist with x-Ray Procedures (continued)

9. AFF Log into the Electronic Medical Record (EMR) using your username and secure password OR obtain the paper medical record from a secure location and assure it is kept away from public access.	❑	❑	❑
10. When finished, log out of the EMR and/or replace the paper medical record in an appropriate and secure location.	❑	❑	❑

CALCULATION

Total Possible Points: __________

Total Points Earned: __________ Multiplied by 100 = __________ Divided by Total Possible Points = __________ %

PASS ❑ **FAIL** ❑ **COMMENTS:**

Student's signature ____________________ Date __________

Partner's signature ____________________ Date __________

Instructor's signature ____________________ Date __________

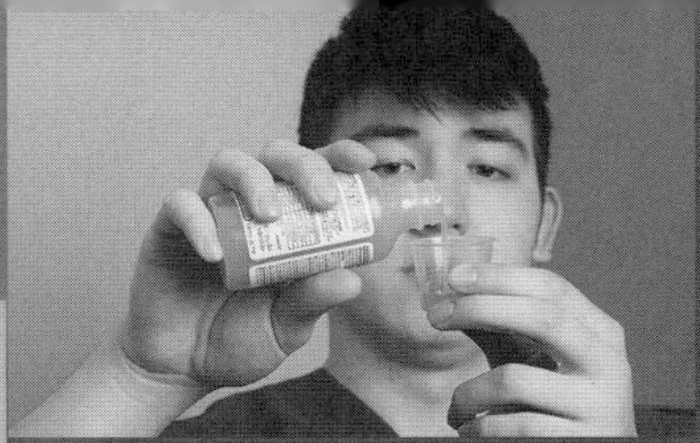

CHAPTER

26 Medical Office Emergencies

Learning Outcomes

COG Cognitive Domain

1. Spell and define key terms
2. List principles and steps of professional/provider CPR
3. Describe basic principles of first aid as they pertain to the ambulatory health care setting.
4. Identify the five types of shock and the management of each
5. Describe how burns are classified and managed
6. Explain the management of allergic reactions
7. Describe the management of poisoning and the role of the poison control center
8. List the three types of hyperthermic emergencies and the treatment for each type
9. Discuss the treatment of hypothermia
10. Describe the role of the medical assistant in managing psychiatric emergencies

PSY Psychomotor Domain

1. Administer oxygen (Procedure 26-1)
2. Perform cardiopulmonary resuscitation (Procedure 26-2)
3. Use an automatic external defibrillator (Procedure 26-3)
4. Manage a foreign body airway obstruction (Procedure 26-4)
5. Control bleeding (Procedure 26-5)
6. Respond to medical emergencies other than bleeding, cardiac/respiratory arrest, or foreign body airway obstruction (Procedure 26-6)
7. Document patient care accurately in the medical record

AFF Affective Domain

1. Incorporate critical thinking skills in performing patient assessment
2. Incorporate critical thinking skills in performing patient care
3. Show awareness of patients' concerns related to the procedure being performed
4. Demonstrate empathy, active listening, nonverbal communication
5. Demonstrate respect for individual diversity including gender, race, religion, age, economic status, and appearance
6. Explain to a patient the rationale for performance of a procedure
7. Protect the integrity of the medical record
8. Demonstrate self-awareness in responding to an emergency situation

ABHES Competencies

1. Document accurately
2. Recognize and respond to verbal and nonverbal communication
3. Adapt to individualized needs
4. Apply principles of aseptic techniques and infection control
5. Recognize emergencies and treatments and minor office surgical procedures
6. Use standard precautions
7. Perform first aid and CPR
8. Demonstrate professionalism by exhibiting a positive attitude and sense of responsibility

Name: ______________________________ Date: __________ Grade: __________

COG MULTIPLE CHOICE

Circle the letter preceding the correct answer.

1. During a primary assessment, you should check:
   a. AVPU.
   b. pupils.
   c. responsiveness.
   d. vital signs.
   e. patient identification.

2. What signs and symptoms are consistent with heat stroke?
   a. Cyanotic skin
   b. Pale wet skin
   c. Ecchymosis
   d. Dry, flushed skin
   e. Waxy, gray skin

3. Superficial burns are categorized as:
   a. first degree.
   b. second degree.
   c. third degree.
   d. partial thickness.
   e. full thickness.

4. Which is an example of a closed wound?
   a. Abrasion
   b. Avulsion
   c. Contusion
   d. Laceration
   e. Ecchymosis

5. What is the BSA of the anterior portion of an adult's trunk?
   a. 1%
   b. 9%
   c. 13.5%
   d. 18%
   e. 36%

6. A patient with pneumonia is at risk for:
   a. hypothermia.
   b. hypovolemic shock.
   c. septic shock.
   d. seizures.
   e. hyperthermia.

7. The first step to take when discovering an unresponsive patient is to:
   a. begin CPR.
   b. check circulation.
   c. establish an airway.
   d. go find help.
   e. identify the patient.

8. During a physical examination of an emergency patient's abdomen, check for:
   a. cerebral fluid.
   b. distal pulses.
   c. paradoxical movement.
   d. tenderness, rigidity, and distension.
   e. lethargy and slow movements.

9. A potential complication from a splint could be:
   a. compartment syndrome.
   b. dislocation.
   c. hematoma.
   d. injury from sharp bone fragments.
   e. tissue ischemia and infarction.

10. Circulation after splinting can be tested using:
    a. blood pressure.
    b. brachial pulse.
    c. carotid pulse.
    d. distal pulse.
    e. femoral pulse.

Scenario for questions 11 and 12: A patient complains about tightness in the chest, a feeling of warmth, and itching. After a minute, the patient's breathing is labored.

11. You are most likely watching the early warning signs of:
    a. an allergic reaction.
    b. cardiogenic shock.
    c. a myocardial infarction.
    d. poisoning.
    e. ecchymosis.

12. What action is contraindicated should this patient go into shock?
    a. Cardiac monitoring
    b. Epinephrine (1:1,000)
    c. Establishing an IV line
    d. Intubation
    e. Providing high-flow oxygen

13. If a patient is having a seizure, you should:
    a. force something into the patient's mouth to protect the tongue.
    b. maintain spine immobilization.
    c. protect the patient from injury.
    d. restrain the patient.
    e. assist patient to supine position.

14. What is the difference between an emotional crisis and a psychiatric emergency?
a. A psychiatric emergency results from substance abuse.
b. A patient in a psychiatric emergency poses a physical threat to himself or others.
c. An emotional crisis is a case of bipolar disorder.
d. A psychiatric emergency involves a patient diagnosed with a psychiatric disorder.
e. An emotional crisis does not include delusions.

15. A patient suffering hypothermia should be given:
a. alcohol to promote circulation.
b. hot chocolate to provide sugar.
c. IV fluids for rehydration.
d. warm coffee to raise his or her level of consciousness.
e. dry heat to warm the surface.

16. What agency should be contacted first when a patient is exposed to a toxic substance?
a. AMAA
b. EMS
c. MSDS
d. Centers for Disease Control
e. Poison Control Center

17. Which form of shock is an acute allergic reaction?
a. Neurogenic shock
b. Anaphylactic shock
c. Cardiogenic shock
d. Septic shock
e. Hypovolemic shock

18. What does the "V" in AVPU stand for?
a. Vocalization
b. Vital signs
c. Viscosity
d. Voice recognition
e. Verbal response

19. To manage open soft tissue injuries, you should:
a. leave them open to the air.
b. wrap loosely in bandages.
c. immediately stitch closed.
d. elevate the wound.
e. apply direct pressure.

20. Which of the following items should be included in an emergency kit?
a. Alcohol wipes
b. Syringe
c. Penicillin
d. Oscilloscope
e. Sample containers

COG MATCHING

Grade: ______

Match each key term with its definition.

Key Terms	Definitions
21. ____ allergen	**a.** an abnormal discharge of electrical activity in the brain, resulting in erratic muscle movements, strange sensations, or a complete loss of consciousness
22. ____ anaphylactic shock	**b.** black, tarry stools caused by digested blood from the gastrointestinal tract
23. ____ cardiogenic shock	**c.** severe allergic reaction within minutes to hours after exposure to a foreign substance
24. ____ contusion	**d.** an emergency where the body cannot compensate for elevated temperatures
25. ____ ecchymosis	**e.** a bruise or collection of blood under the skin or in damaged tissue
26. ____ full-thickness burn	**f.** a burn limited to the epidermis
27. ____ heat cramps	**g.** any device used to immobilize a sprain, strain, fracture, or dislocated limb
28. ____ heat stroke	**h.** shock that results from dysfunction of the nervous system following a spinal cord injury
29. ____ hematoma	**i.** muscle cramping that follows a period of physical exertion and profuse sweating in a hot environment
30. ____ hyperthermia	**j.** a penetrating burn that has destroyed all skin layers
31. ____ hypothermia	**k.** a characteristic black and blue mark from blood accumulation
32. ____ hypovolemic shock	**l.** below-normal body temperature
33. ____ infarction	**m.** the general condition of excessive body heat
34. ____ ischemia	**n.** a blood clot that forms at an injury site
35. ____ melena	**o.** a burn that involves epidermis and varying levels of the dermis
36. ____ neurogenic shock	
37. ____ partial-thickness burn	
38. ____ seizure	
39. ____ septic shock	

Key Terms	Definitions
40. ______ shock	p. a decrease in oxygen to tissue
41. ______ splint	q. a substance that causes manifestations of an allergy
42. ______ superficial burn	r. shock that results from general infection in the bloodstream
	s. shock caused by loss of blood or other body fluids
	t. death of tissue due to lack of oxygen
	u. condition resulting from the lack of oxygen to individual cells of the body
	v. type of shock in which the left ventricle fails to pump enough blood for the body to function

COG IDENTIFICATION

Grade: ______

43. As a medical assistant, you may be called on to assist during an emergency. Review the list of tasks below and determine which tasks you may be responsible for as a medical assistant. Place a check mark in the "Yes" column for those duties you might assist with as a medical assistant and place a check mark in the "No" column for those tasks that not be the responsibility of the medical assistant.

Task	Yes	No
a. Obtain important patient information.		
b. Perform CPR.		
c. Set and splint bone fractures.		
d. Remove foreign body airway obstructions.		
e. Remain calm and react competently and professionally during a psychiatric crisis.		
f. Coordinate multiple ongoing events while rendering patient care in a cardiac emergency.		
g. Negotiate with or attempt to calm a violent patient during a psychiatric crisis.		
h. Know what emergency system is used in the community.		
i. Provide immediate care to the patient while the physician is notified.		
j. Perform rapid sequence intubation (RSI) on a patient who is suffering respiratory failure.		
k. Administer first aid.		
l. Document all actions taken.		
m. Complete routine scheduled tasks.		
n. Assist EMS personnel as necessary.		
o. Examine the patient for EMS personnel.		
p. Direct care of the patient for EMS personnel.		
q. Remove any obstacles that prevent speedy evacuation of the patient by stretcher.		
r. Direct family members to the reception area or a private room.		

44. Identify the type of shock described in the following scenarios.

a. A very ill patient has been complaining of increasing pain in the pelvis and legs. Blood is present in the urine. The patient's temperature was elevated but is dropping.

____

b. An elderly patient falls on her back while attempting to get out of bed. Her heart rate becomes rapid and thready, and her blood pressure drops quickly.

____

c. A patient presents with fluid in the lungs, difficulty breathing, and chest pain.

____

d. A patient presents with labored breathing, grunting, wheezing, and swelling followed by fainting.

____

e. A child is brought in for diarrhea. She has poor skin turgor and capillary refill. Her mental status appears to be deteriorating.

____

45. Put a check mark on the line next to the correct signs and symptoms of shock.

a. ____________ low blood pressure

b. ____________ high blood pressure

c. ____________ calm or lethargic

d. ____________ restlessness or signs of fear

e. ____________ thirst

f. ____________ polyuria

g. ____________ hunger

h. ____________ nausea

i. ____________ hot, sweaty skin

j. ____________ cool, clammy skin

k. ____________ pale skin with cyanosis (bluish color) at the lips and earlobes

l. ____________ flushed skin

m. ____________ rapid and weak pulse

n. ____________ bounding pulse

46. Classify the type, severity, and coverage of the burns in each of these scenarios.

a. A contractor installing medical equipment accidentally touches exposed wires. He has burns on his right arm, but no sensation of pain.

- Type:

____

- Severity:

____

- Coverage:

____

b. A child spills bleach on one leg. The leg is blistering and causing severe pain.

- Type:

____

- Severity:

____

- Coverage:

____

c. A man watches a welder installs handrails on your office's handicapped ramp. Now his face is red and painful, and his eyes have a painful itching sensation.

- Type:

____

- Severity:

____

- Coverage:

____

d. A patient spills hot coffee while driving to your office, painfully blistering his genital area.

- Type:

____

- Severity:

____

- Coverage:

____

47. Identify the hyperthermic and hypothermic emergencies from the list below and match them with the proper treatment. Place the number preceding the correct treatment on the line next to the heat or cold emergency.

a. ______________ heat cramps

b. ______________ frostbite

c. ______________ heat stroke

d. ______________ hypothermia

1. Remove wet clothing.
Cover the patient.
Give warm fluids by mouth if the patient is alert and oriented.

2. Move the patient to a cool area.
Remove clothing that may be keeping in the heat.
Place cool, wet clothes or a wet sheet on the scalp, neck, axilla, and groin.
Administer oxygen as directed by the physician and apply a cardiac monitor.
Notify the EMS for transportation to the hospital as directed by the physician.

3. Immerse the affected tissue in lukewarm water (41°C, 105°F) until the area becomes pliable and the color and sensation return.
Do not apply dry heat.
Do not massage the area; massage may cause further tissue damage.
Avoid breaking any blisters that may form.
Notify the EMS for transportation to a hospital.

4. Move the patient to a cool area.
Give fluids (commercial electrolyte solution) by mouth if uncomplicated.
Give IV fluids if patient presents with nausea.

48. What are your responsibilities for managing an allergic reaction? Circle the letter preceding all tasks that apply.

a. Leave the patient to bring the emergency kit or cart, oxygen, and to get a physician to evaluate the patient.

b. Assist the patient to a supine position.

c. Scrub the patient's skin to remove allergens and urticaria.

d. Assess the patient's respiratory and circulatory status by obtaining the blood pressure, pulse, and respiratory rates.

e. Observe skin color and warmth.

f. If the patient complains of being cold or is shivering, cover with a blanket.

g. Intubate the patient.

h. Upon the direction of the physician, start an intravenous line and administer oxygen.

i. Administer medications as ordered by the physician.

j. Document vital signs and any medications and treatments given, noting the time each set of vital signs is taken or medications are administered.

k. Communicate relevant information to the EMS personnel, including copies of the progress notes or medication record as needed.

COG SHORT ANSWER

Grade: _______

49. List nine interventions or steps to manage burns.

____

____

____

____

50. A sullen and moody patient suddenly becomes threatening. Name three things the medical assistant should do.

____

____

____

____

51. What six pieces of information should be included in your office's emergency plan?

____

____

____

____

52. What are the elements of the AVPU scale for assessing a patient's level of consciousness?

A	
V	
P	
U	

53. List the first three steps you should use to control bleeding from an open wound.

____

____

____

____

54. You enter an exam room and unexpectedly find someone sprawled on the floor. What four things do you check on your primary assessment?

____

____

____

____

55. At what point do you assess the general appearance of the patient?

____

____

____

____

56. A patient is found unconscious. You do not suspect trauma. In what order would you perform the physical examination?

____

____

____

57. An examination of the eyes can be done according to the acronym "PEARL," meaning *P*upils *E*qual *A*nd *R*eactive to *L*ight. What does this examination reveal?

____

____

____

58. A 55-year-old male begins complaining about nausea. He is clearly anxious or agitated. What could this be an early symptom of?

____

____

____

COG TRUE OR FALSE?

Grade: __________

Indicate whether the statements are true or false by placing the letter T (true) or F (false) on the line preceding the statement.

59. __________ During a primary assessment, you find a patient has inadequate respirations. You should proceed to the secondary assessment and physical examination to find out why.

60. __________ An impaled object should not be removed but requires careful immobilization of the patient and the injured area of the body.

61. __________ An allergic reaction will be evident immediately after exposure to an allergen.

62. __________ Closed wounds are not life threatening.

COG AFF CASE STUDY FOR CRITICAL THINKING

Grade: ___________

1. A male older adult falls in an exam room. He is conscious, but agitated and anxious. You are the first to discover him struggling on the floor. What is the only duty you will perform until others arrive, and why?

____

____

____

____

2. A patient in your office is in respiratory arrest. The physician is attending this patient. You have collected notes on the patient's vitals and SAMPLE history (signs and symptoms, allergies, medications, past pertinent history, last oral intake, and the events that led to the problem). A family member of the patient is present and is growing upset and intrusive. The EMTs arrive on the scene. What is your immediate responsibility? Explain.

____

____

____

____

3. A teenage patient is given an instant coldpack for an injury to the mouth. A few minutes later you discover the teenager misunderstood, and drank the contents of the cold pack. What information do you need to collect to prepare for a call to the poison control center?

____

____

____

____

4. Dante commutes to your office by public transportation. On a particularly cold day, Dante arrives late with cool, pale skin. He is lethargic and confused, with slow and shallow respirations and a slow and faint pulse. Describe what actions are appropriate.

____

____

____

____

5. You have just had a patient suffer anaphylactic shock and respiratory arrest due to an unsuspected penicillin allergy. EMS has transported the patient to a local hospital. The following week, the patient calls to ask what she can do to prevent this from happening in the future. What would you tell this patient? Are there any future precautions this patient should take? If so, what?

____

____

____

____

6. You have a 35-year-old patient who has religious reservations about some medical procedures. Normally, you and the physician carefully explain procedures to this patient so she has the opportunity to make informed consent decisions. Now she is lying unconscious in front of you with a medical emergency. How do you handle informed consent with an unconscious patient?

____

____

____

____

7. You have an elderly patient with a "do not resuscitate" order, because he does not want to receive CPR in the event of a heart attack. During treatment for another condition, he collapses in apparent anaphylactic shock. Do you provide emergency medical assistance?

____

____

____

____

PSY PROCEDURE 26-1 Administer Oxygen

Name: ______________________ **Date:** ________ **Time:** ________ **Grade:** ________

EQUIPMENT/SUPPLIES: Oxygen tank with a regulator and flow meter, an oxygen delivery system (nasal cannula or mask)

STANDARDS: Given the needed equipment and a place to work, the student will perform this skill with _____ % accuracy in a total of _____ minutes. *(Your instructor will tell you what the percentage and time limits will be before you begin.)*

KEY: 4 = Satisfactory 0 = Unsatisfactory NA = This step is not counted

PROCEDURE STEPS	SELF	PARTNER	INSTRUCTOR
1. Wash your hands.	❑	❑	❑
2. Check the physician order for the amount of oxygen and the delivery method (nasal cannula, mask).	❑	❑	❑
3. Obtain the oxygen tank and nasal cannula or mask.	❑	❑	❑
4. Greet and identify the patient.	❑	❑	❑
5. AFF Explain how to respond to a patient who has dementia.	❑	❑	❑
6. Connect the distal end of the nasal cannula or mask tubing to the adapter on the oxygen tank regulator, which is attached to the oxygen tank.	❑	❑	❑
7. Place the oxygen delivery device into the patient's nares (nasal cannula) or over the patient's nose and mouth (mask).	❑	❑	❑
8. Turn the regulator dial to the liters per minute ordered by the physician.	❑	❑	❑
9. AFF Log into the Electronic Medical Record (EMR) using your username and secure password OR obtain the paper medical record from a secure location and assure it is kept away from public access.	❑	❑	❑
10. Record the procedure in the patient's medical record.	❑	❑	❑
11. When finished, log out of the EMR and/or replace the medical record in an appropriate and secure location to protect patient privacy.	❑	❑	❑

PSY PROCEDURE 26-1 Administer Oxygen (continued)

CALCULATION

Total Possible Points: __________

Total Points Earned: __________ Multiplied by 100 = __________ Divided by Total Possible Points = __________ %

PASS ❑ **FAIL** ❑ **COMMENTS:**

Student's signature ____________________ Date __________

Partner's signature ____________________ Date __________

Instructor's signature ____________________ Date __________

PSY PROCEDURE 26-2 Perform Cardiopulmonary Resuscitation (Adult)

Name: ______________________ **Date:** __________ **Time:** __________ **Grade:** __________

EQUIPMENT/SUPPLIES: CPR mannequin, mouth-to-mouth barrier device, gloves

STANDARDS: Given the needed equipment and a place to work, the student will perform this skill with _____ % accuracy in a total of _____ minutes. *(Your instructor will tell you what the percentage and time limits will be before you begin.)*

NOTE: All health care professionals should receive training for proficiency in CPR in an approved program. This skill sheet is not intended to substitute for proficiency training with a mannequin and structured protocol.

KEY: 4 = Satisfactory 0 = Unsatisfactory NA = This step is not counted

PROCEDURE STEPS	SELF	PARTNER	INSTRUCTOR
1. Determine unresponsiveness by shaking the patient and shouting "Are you okay?"	❑	❑	❑
2. Instruct another staff member to get the physician, emergency cart/supplies, and AED.	❑	❑	❑
3. Put on clean exam gloves.	❑	❑	❑
4. If the patient does not respond, assess for cardiac function by feeling for a pulse using the carotid artery at the side of the patient's neck.	❑	❑	❑
5. If no pulse is present, follow the protocol for chest compressions according to the standards for training provided by an approved basic life support provider.	❑	❑	❑
6. After 30 compressions, check for airway patency and respiratory effort using the head-tilt, chin-lift maneuver with the patient in the supine position.	❑	❑	❑
7. After opening the airway, begin rescue breathing by placing a mask over the patient's mouth and nose and giving two slow breaths, causing the chest to rise without overfilling the lungs.	❑	❑	❑
8. Continue chest compressions and rescue breathing at a ratio of 30:1 until relieved by another health care provider or EMS arrives.	❑	❑	❑
9. Utilize the recovery position if the patient regains consciousness or a pulse and adequate breathing.	❑	❑	❑
10. Document the procedure and copy any records necessary for transport with EMS.	❑	❑	❑

PSY PROCEDURE 26-2 Perform Cardiopulmonary Resuscitation (Adult) (continued)

CALCULATION

Total Possible Points: __________

Total Points Earned: __________ Multiplied by 100 = __________ Divided by Total Possible Points = __________ %

PASS **FAIL** **COMMENTS:**

❑ ❑

Student's signature ____________________ Date __________

Partner's signature ____________________ Date __________

Instructor's signature __________________ Date __________

PSY PROCEDURE 26-3 Use an Automatic External Defibrillator (Adult)

Name: ______________________ **Date:** __________ **Time:** __________ **Grade:** __________

EQUIPMENT/SUPPLIES: Practice mannequin, training automatic external defibrillator with chest pads and connection cables, scissors, gauze, gloves

STANDARDS: Given the needed equipment and a place to work, the student will perform this skill with _____ % accuracy in a total of _____ minutes. *(Your instructor will tell you what the percentage and time limits will be before you begin.)*

NOTE: All health care professionals should receive training for proficiency in CPR and using an AED in an approved program. This skill sheet is not intended to substitute for proficiency training with a mannequin and structured protocol.

KEY: 4 = Satisfactory 0 = Unsatisfactory NA = This step is not counted

PROCEDURE STEPS	SELF	PARTNER	INSTRUCTOR
1. Determine unresponsiveness by shaking the patient and shouting "Are you okay?"	❏	❏	❏
2. Instruct another staff member to get the physician, emergency cart/supplies, and AED.	❏	❏	❏
3. While the other staff member continues CPR, remove the patient's shirt and prepare the chest for the AED electrodes: **a.** If there are medication patches on the chest where the electrodes will be placed, remove them and wipe away any excess medication with a towel. **b.** If there is excess hair on the chest that will prevent the AED electrodes from sticking, apply one set of electrodes and quickly remove, pulling any hair from the chest. **c.** If the chest is wet, dry with a towel or other cloth before applying the electrodes.	❏	❏	❏
4. After removing the paper on the back of the AED electrodes, apply the electrodes to the chest area, one to the upper right chest area and the other on the lower left chest area.	❏	❏	❏
5. Explain what should be done in the event the patient has an implantable device in the area where the chest electrodes should be applied.	❏	❏	❏
6. With the electrodes securely on the chest, connect the wire from the electrodes to the AED unit and turn the AED on.	❏	❏	❏
7. Advise everyone to not touch the patient while the AED is analyzing the heart rhythm.	❏	❏	❏
8. If no shock is advised by the AED, resume CPR.	❏	❏	❏
9. If a shock is advised by the AED, make sure no one is touching the patient before pressing the appropriate button on the AED.	❏	❏	❏
10. After a shock is delivered by the AED, resume CPR until the AED advises you that the heart rhythm is being analyzed again.	❏	❏	❏

PSY PROCEDURE 26-3 Use an Automatic External Defibrillator (Adult) (continued)

11. Do not touch the patient while the heart rhythm is being reanalyzed at any point during the procedure.	❑	❑	❑
12. Continue to follow the instructions given by the AED and the physician until EMS has been notified and has arrived.	❑	❑	❑
13. Document the procedure and copy any records necessary for transport with EMS.	❑	❑	❑

CALCULATION

Total Possible Points: ________

Total Points Earned: ________ Multiplied by 100 = ________ Divided by Total Possible Points = ________ %

PASS ❑ **FAIL** ❑ **COMMENTS:**

Student's signature ____________________ Date __________

Partner's signature ____________________ Date __________

Instructor's signature ____________________ Date __________

PSY PROCEDURE 26-4 Manage a Foreign Body Airway Obstruction (Adult)

Name: ______________ **Date:** __________ **Time:** __________ **Grade:** __________

EQUIPMENT/SUPPLIES: Practice mannequin, mouth-to-mouth barrier device, gloves

STANDARDS: Given the needed equipment and a place to work, the student will perform this skill with _____ % accuracy in a total of _____ minutes. *(Your instructor will tell you what the percentage and time limits will be before you begin.)*

NOTE: All health care professionals should receive training for proficiency in managing a foreign body airway obstruction in an approved program. This skill sheet is not intended to substitute for proficiency training with a mannequin and structured protocol.

KEY: 4 = Satisfactory 0 = Unsatisfactory NA = This step is not counted

PROCEDURE STEPS	SELF	PARTNER	INSTRUCTOR
1. If the patient is conscious and appears to be choking, ask the patient, "Are you choking?"	❑	❑	❑
2. Do not perform abdominal thrusts if the patient can speak or cough because these are signs that the obstruction is not complete.	❑	❑	❑
3. If the patient cannot speak or cough but has indicated thate he or she is choking, move behind the patient, wrapping your arms around his or her abdomen.	❑	❑	❑
4. Place the fist of your dominant hand with the thumb against the patient's abdomen, between the navel and xiphoid process.	❑	❑	❑
5. Put your other hand against your dominant hand and give quick, upward thrusts, forceful enough to dislodge the obstruction in the airway.	❑	❑	❑
6. If the patient is obese or pregnant, place your hands against the middle of the sternum, above the xiphoid process and proceed with quick thrusts inward.	❑	❑	❑
7. Continue with the abdominal thrusts until the object is expelled and the patient can breathe or the patient becomes unconscious.	❑	❑	❑
8. If the patient becomes unconscious or is found unconscious, open the airway and give two rescue breaths.	❑	❑	❑
9. If rescue breaths are obstructed, reposition the head, and try again.	❑	❑	❑
10. If rescue breaths continue to be obstructed after repositioning, begin abdominal thrusts by placing your palm against the patient's abdomen with your fingers facing his or her head (you may need to straddle the patient's hips). The palm of the hand should be located between the navel and the xiphoid process.	❑	❑	❑

PSY PROCEDURE 26-4 Manage a Foreign Body Airway Obstruction (Adult) (continued)

11. Lace the fingers of the other hand into the fingers of the hand on the abdomen and give five abdominal thrusts.	❑	❑	❑
12. After five abdominal thrusts, open the patient's mouth using a tongue-jaw lift maneuver and do a finger- sweep of the mouth, removing any objects that may have been dislodged.	❑	❑	❑
13. If an item has been dislodged and can be removed easily, remove the object and attempt rescue breaths. Continue rescue breaths and chest compressions as necessary and appropriate.	❑	❑	❑
14. If the item has not been dislodged, attempt rescue breaths. If rescue breaths are successful, continue rescue breathing and chest compressions as necessary and appropriate.	❑	❑	❑
15. If the item has not been dislodged and rescue breaths are not successful, continue with abdominal thrusts.	❑	❑	❑
16. Repeat the pattern of abdominal thrusts, finger -sweep, and rescue breaths and follow the physician's orders until EMS is notified and arrives.	❑	❑	❑
17. Document the procedure and copy any records necessary for transport with EMS.	❑	❑	❑

CALCULATION

Total Possible Points: __________

Total Points Earned: __________ Multiplied by 100 = __________ Divided by Total Possible Points = __________ %

PASS **FAIL** **COMMENTS:**

❑ ❑

Student's signature ____________________ Date __________

Partner's signature ____________________ Date __________

Instructor's signature ____________________ Date __________

PSY

PROCEDURE 26-5 Control Bleeding

Name: ______________________ **Date:** __________ **Time:** __________ **Grade:** __________

EQUIPMENT/SUPPLIES: Gloves, sterile gauze pads

STANDARDS: Given the needed equipment and a place to work, the student will perform this skill with _____ % accuracy in a total of _____ minutes. *(Your instructor will tell you what the percentage and time limits will be before you begin.)*

KEY: 4 = Satisfactory 0 = Unsatisfactory NA = This step is not counted

PROCEDURE STEPS	SELF	PARTNER	INSTRUCTOR
1. Identify the patient and assess the extent of the bleeding and type of accident.	❑	❑	❑
2. Take the patient to an examination room and notify the physician if appropriate.	❑	❑	❑
3. Give the patient some gauze pads and have him or her apply pressure to the area while you put on a pair of clean examination gloves and open additional sterile gauze pads.	❑	❑	❑
4. Observe the patient for signs of dizziness or lightheadedness. Have the patient lie down.	❑	❑	❑
5. Using several sterile gauze pads, apply direct pressure to the wound.	❑	❑	❑
6. Maintain pressure until the bleeding stops.	❑	❑	❑
7. If the bleeding continues or seeps through the gauze, apply additional gauze on top of the saturated gauze while continuing to apply direct pressure.	❑	❑	❑
8. If directed by the physician to do so, apply pressure to the artery delivering blood to this area while continuing to apply direct pressure to the wound to control bleeding.	❑	❑	❑
9. Once the bleeding is controlled, prepare to assist the physician with a minor office surgical procedure to close the wound.	❑	❑	❑
10. Continue to monitor the patient for signs of shock and be prepared to treat the patient appropriately.	❑	❑	❑
11. Document the treatment in the patient's medical record.	❑	❑	❑

CALCULATION

Total Possible Points: __________

Total Points Earned: __________ Multiplied by 100 = __________ Divided by Total Possible Points = __________ %

PASS ❑ **FAIL** ❑ **COMMENTS:**

Student's signature ____________________ Date __________

Partner's signature ____________________ Date __________

Instructor's signature ____________________ Date __________

PSY PROCEDURE 26-6 Respond to Medical Emergencies Other than Bleeding, Cardiac/Respiratory Arrest, or Foreign Body Airway Obstruction

Name: ______________________ **Date:** __________ **Time:** __________ **Grade:** __________

EQUIPMENT/SUPPLIES: A medical emergency kit that contains a minimum of personal protective equipment including gloves, low-dose aspirin tablets, 2 × 2 and 4 × 4 sterile gauze pads, vinegar or acetic acid solution, blood pressure cuff and stethoscope, sterile water or saline for irrigation, ice bags, and towel or rolled gauze bandage material

STANDARDS: Given the needed equipment and a place to work, the student will perform this skill with _____ % accuracy in a total of _____ minutes. *(Your instructor will tell you what the percentage and time limits will be before you begin.)*

KEY: 4 = Satisfactory 0 = Unsatisfactory NA = This step is not counted

PROCEDURE STEPS	SELF	PARTNER	INSTRUCTOR
1. Identify the patient and assess the type of emergency involved.	❏	❏	❏
2. Escort the patient to an examination room.	❏	❏	❏
3. Have another staff member get the physician, medical emergency cart/supplies, and AED.	❏	❏	❏
4. Apply clean examination gloves and other PPE as appropriate.	❏	❏	❏
5. Assist the patient to the exam table and have him or her lie down.	❏	❏	❏
6. Treat the patient according to the physician's instructions and the most current guidelines for first aid procedures for the following: **a.** Chest pain **b.** Snakebite **c.** Jellyfish sting **d.** Dental injuries **(1) Chipped tooth** **(2) Cracked or broken tooth** **(3) Tooth removed** **(4) Broken jaw** **e.** Fracture Injuries **f.** Seizure **g.** Shock **h.** Syncope	❏	❏	❏
7. If the patient develops cardiac or respiratory arrest, follow the procedure for CPR according to the most recent standards and guidelines.	❏	❏	❏
8. Document the treatment in the patient's medical record.	❏	❏	❏

PROCEDURE 26-6 Respond to Medical Emergencies Other than Bleeding, Cardiac/Respiratory Arrest, or Foreign Body Airway Obstruction (continued)

CALCULATION

Total Possible Points: ________

Total Points Earned: ________ Multiplied by 100 = ________ Divided by Total Possible Points = ________ %

PASS ❑ **FAIL** ❑ **COMMENTS:**

Student's signature ________________ Date ________

Partner's signature ________________ Date ________

Instructor's signature ________________ Date ________

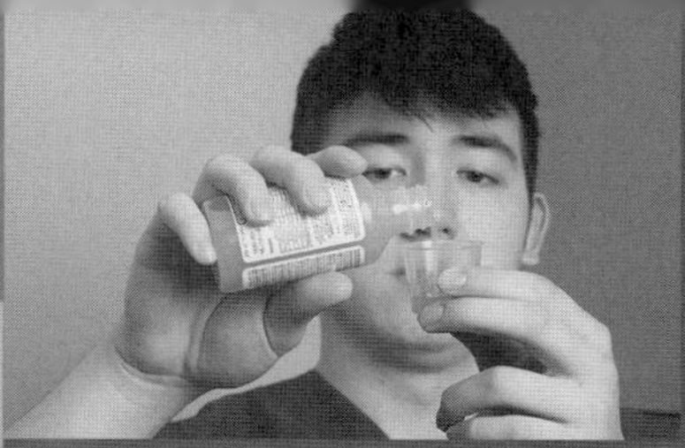

CHAPTER

27

Disaster Preparedness and the Medical Assistant

Learning Outcomes

COG Cognitive Domain

1. Spell and define the key terms
2. Describe what is meant by a disaster and disaster preparedness
3. List several types of disasters
4. Identify critical elements of an emergency plan for response to a natural disaster or other emergency
5. Describe fundamental principles for evacuation of a health care setting
6. Identify emergency preparedness plans in your community
7. Discuss potential role(s) of the medical assistant in emergency preparedness

PSY Psychomotor Domain

1. Respond to a simulated disaster (Procedure 27-1)
2. Maintain a list of community resources for emergency preparedness (Procedure 27-2)
3. Develop a personal safety plan (Procedure 27-3)

AFF Affective Domain

1. Recognize the physical and emotional effects on persons involved in an emergency situation
2. Demonstrate self-awareness in responding to an emergency situation
3. Apply active listening skills
4. Use appropriate body language and other nonverbal skills in communicating with patients, family, and staff

ABHES Competencies

1. Document accurately
2. Recognize and respond to verbal and nonverbal communication
3. Adapt to individualized needs
4. Apply principles of aseptic techniques and infection control
5. Recognize emergencies and treatments and minor office surgical procedures
6. Use standard precautions
7. Perform first aid and CPR
8. Demonstrate professionalism by exhibiting a positive attitude and sense of responsibility

Name: ______________________ Date: __________ Grade: __________

COG MULTIPLE CHOICE

Circle the letter preceding the correct answer.

1. The 2001 discovery of anthrax in an envelope to be delivered to a U.S. Congressman is an example of a(n):
   a. bioterrorist attack.
   b. epidemic.
   c. pandemic.
   d. ergonomics.
   e. ADF.

2. An effective disaster plan for the medical office should include the input of which individuals?
   a. The physician or physicians
   b. The practice manager
   c. The medical assistants
   d. The receptionist
   e. All of the above

3. Which of these is not an example of a natural disaster?
   a. Flood
   b. Tornado
   c. Air quality advisory
   d. Hurricane
   e. Earthquake

4. An emergency action plan should include all of the following except:
   a. contact information for poison control.
   b. emergency procedures.
   c. the location of the emergency supplies.
   d. patient information sheets.
   e. contact information for local hospitals.

5. A well-written emergency plan is essential to being prepared for a disaster. What qualities are inherent in a well-written emergency plan?
   a. It is easy to read and include pictures.
   b. It is flexible and easily implemented.
   c. It is based on research and has references.
   d. It should include enough information to fill a 3-inch binder.
   e. It is written based on the reading level of the office personnel.

6. A location in or near the medical office should be identified to coordinate activities in a disaster, commonly known as a/n:
   a. central activities center.
   b. common planning center.
   c. central operation center.
   d. command center.
   e. operation command center.

7. An example of a manmade disaster includes all of the following except:
   a. drought.
   b. bioterriorism.
   c. a nuclear accident.
   d. contaminating a water source chemicals.
   e. none of the above.

8. A bioterrorism agent that is easily available, can be transferred to people easily, has the potential to cause injury and death to large amounts of people and other animals is included in which category?
   a. Category A
   b. Category B
   c. Category C
   d. Category D
   e. Category E

9. A disease that infects many people in a small geographical area is known as a/n:
   a. pandemic.
   b. Category C agent.
   c. infectious pathogen.
   d. bioterrorist.
   e. epidemic.

10. The role of the medical assistant in planning for emergencies and disasters includes assisting the physician with all of the following except:
    a. performing CPR if needed.
    b. transferring patients or victims.
    c. preparing and administering medications.
    d. diagnosing and treating illness and injuries caused by the emergency.
    e. collecting information and communicating clearly with everyone involved.

Scenario for questions 11 through 15: A tornado just came through the neighborhood where you are working in a family practice office. Although your office was not hit, several businesses around your office were damaged or destroyed. People are running into your office yelling for help for other victims who cannot get to the office or they are injured and bleeding themselves.

11. Your priority in assisting patients and victims in the office includes:
a. asking nonpatients coming into the office to wait outside until the EMS arrives.
b. remaining calm and implementing the emergency plan quickly and efficiently.
c. asking the practice manager if you can leave to check on your family.
d. standing outside to direct traffic and flag down emergency medical services.
e. gathering equipment and supplies that may be needed for any injuries.

12. This is an example of which type of disaster?
a. A pandemic
b. A water emergency
c. A bioterrorism disaster
d. A manmade disaster
e. A natural disaster

13. Your role in assisting in this disaster includes which of the following:
a. Gathering medical information from patients and victims
b. Assisting the physician with procedures and treatments
c. Administering tetanus to everyone who is injured before they are seen by the physician.
d. A and B.
e. All of the above.

14. Because you are actively involved in assisting during this disaster, you are considered
a. first-level victim.
b. secondary-level victim.
c. third-level victim.
d. fourth-level victim.
e. fifth-level victim.

15. One month after the disaster, you notice your coworker is unusually irritable and is unable to concentrate on simple tasks, making mistakes throughout the day. These behaviors are not typical of her personality and may be signs of:
a. depression.
b. posttraumatic stress disorder.
c. a sleeping disorder.
d. an anxiety disorder.
e. a possible infectious disease contracted during the emergency.

COG MATCHING

Grade: ______

Match each key term with its definition.

Key Terms

16. ______ bioterrorism
17. ______ disaster
18. ______ epidemic
19. ______ pandemic
20. ______ PTSD

Definitions

a. a disease that affects numerous people within a specific geographical area
b. a sudden and unplanned event that has the potential to cause damage to property or life; may be caused by an accident or by nature including weather events such as a hurricane.
c. a condition in some individuals who are affected by acute traumatic stress.
d. intentional release of a biologic agent with the intent to harm individuals.
e. a disease that affects numerous people in many areas of the world at the same time.

COG IDENTIFICATION

Grade: ______

21. You may be called upon to assist before, during, and after a disaster. Place a check mark in the "Yes" column for those duties you might assist with as a medical assistant and place a check mark in the "No" column for those tasks that not be the responsibility of the medical assistant with regard to disaster preparedness.

Task	Yes	No
a. Obtain important patient information.		
b. Perform first aid and CPR procedures.		
c. Suture small lacerations.		
d. Obtain vital signs.		
e. Remain calm and react competently and professionally.		
f. Coordinate multiple ongoing events.		
g. Prescribe antibiotics to patients who may be infected		
h. Know what emergency system is used in the community.		
i. Provide immediate care to the patient while the physician is notified.		
j. Advise victims with minor injuries to go home and take OTC medications for discomfort		
k. Work as a law enforcement officer to manage victims exhibiting dangerous behaviors		
l. Create medical records and document all actions taken.		
m. Manage the temporary medical clinic		
n. Assist EMS personnel as necessary.		

COG SHORT ANSWER

Grade: ______

22. What six pieces of information should be included in your office's emergency plan?

____

____

____

____

23. During a disaster, medical assistants must be able to coordinate multiple ongoing events while rendering patient care. What are the key components to managing a chaotic situation during a disaster?

____

____

____

____

24. Explain the purpose of a Central Operation Center.

____

____

____

____

25. How does the CDC determine that a biologic agent is a weapon?

____

____

____

____

COG TRUE OR FALSE?

Grade: ________

Indicate whether the statements are true or false by placing the letter T (true) or F (false) on the line preceding the statement.

26. ________ A pandemic is a disease that affects many people within a very specific, localized geographic area.

27. ________ Having an alternative source of electricity is essential during a disaster.

28. ________ When evacuating an office during an emergency, you must first recognize the emergency as one that requires the removal from the area.

29. ________ Psychological first aid requires that you discuss all aspects of the disaster with coworkers and patients even if they do not wish to discuss the details.

30. ________ The primary defense mechanism used by individuals after a disaster is anxiety.

COG IDENTIFICATION

Grade: ________

31. Place a checkmark in the appropriate box to indicate whether or not the statement should be considered to develop an evacuation plan for the medical office.

Consideration for Evacuation Plan?	Yes	No
a. Assign staff members to perform surgical procedures on victims who need immediate first aid.		
b. Identify evacuation routes		
c. Make sure everyone understands they are not to discuss patient/staff illness or injury during the evacuation.		
d. Identify who is responsible for ordering the evacuation.		
e. Do not allow anyone to reenter the facility after the disaster when the safety of everyone reentering the office has been established.		

f. Determine a location to move to and a backup site.		
g. Define responsibilities of each staff member.		
h. Do not waste time making sure patients and staff are accounted for during and after the evacuation.		
i. Decide what supplies or equipment will need to be transported.		

AFF CASE STUDY FOR CRITICAL THINKING

Grade: ___________

1. You have been assigned to put together an emergency kit for the family practice office where you work. What items should you include in this kit?

____

____

____

____

2. There has just been an earthquake where you live and the medical office has stopped shaking, leaving patients and staff wondering what happened. There are items on the floor throughout the office that were shaken off the shelves and walls. What is your immediate responsibility? Explain.

____

____

____

____

3. An environmental safety plan was written for the office where you work and includes emergency procedures for all chemicals used in your office. When reviewing this plan, you notice that it does not include a plan to train employees on environmental safety guidelines. Is this important to include in the plan? Why or why not?

____

____

____

____

4. The practice manager at your office has scheduled a meeting to "test" the office emergency plan. He has asked the local fire department to assist in this training. How can you "test" an emergency plan and why would the local fire department be involved?

____

____

____

____

5. A tornado hit the community where you work 1 month ago, and there was significant property damage, injuries, and fatalities. A patient comes into the office today and complains that she is unable to sleep for more than 3 hours at a time as she "wakes up" frequently hearing tornado sirens and reliving the storm. What would you tell this patient? If so, what?

____

____

____

____

PSY PROCEDURE 27-1 Respond to a Simulated Disaster

Name: ______________________________ **Date:** __________ **Time:** __________ **Grade:** __________

EQUIPMENT/SUPPLIES: Phone, disaster drill manual for a medical office, paper medical record forms and folders, pen, portable emergency kit.

STANDARDS: Given the needed equipment and a place to work, the student will perform this skill with _____ % accuracy in a total of _____ minutes. *(Your instructor will tell you what the percentage and time limits will be before you begin.)*

KEY: 4 = Satisfactory 0 = Unsatisfactory NA = This step is not counted

PROCEDURE STEPS	SELF	PARTNER	INSTRUCTOR
1. Develop and/or review an emergency/ disaster procedure manual.	❑	❑	❑
2. Assume the role of an employee, patient, or visitor in a medical office.	❑	❑	❑
3. During a "normal" workday, a disaster occurs without warning.	❑	❑	❑
4. Follow the protocol and procedures for the disaster according to the emergency/disaster plan.	❑	❑	❑
5. After the mock disaster drill, discuss the event including the strengths and weaknesses of the emergency plan.	❑	❑	❑
6. AFF Complete a reflection paper about the mock disaster including your feelings, perceptions, and thoughts before, during, and after the mock disaster.	❑	❑	❑

CALCULATION

Total Possible Points: __________

Total Points Earned: __________ Multiplied by 100 = __________ Divided by Total Possible Points = __________ %

PASS ❑ **FAIL** ❑ **COMMENTS:**

Student's signature ____________________ Date __________

Partner's signature ____________________ Date __________

Instructor's signature ____________________ Date __________

PSY

PROCEDURE 27-2 Maintain a List of Community Resources for Emergency Preparedness

Name: ______________________ **Date:** __________ **Time:** __________ **Grade:** __________

EQUIPMENT/SUPPLIES: Phone, computer with Internet access, paper and pen, binder

STANDARDS: Given the needed equipment and a place to work, the student will perform this skill with _____ % accuracy in a total of _____ minutes. *(Your instructor will tell you what the percentage and time limits will be before you begin.)*

KEY: 4 = Satisfactory 0 = Unsatisfactory NA = This step is not counted

PROCEDURE STEPS	SELF	PARTNER	INSTRUCTOR
1. Determine the geographical area of your community including the city or town, county, and surrounding counties or towns as appropriate	❑	❑	❑
2. Complete an Internet search of the possible resources that make up your community, beginning with the local resources.	❑	❑	❑
3. Create a list of resources including the name of the agency, resources available, phone numbers, addresses, and web address if available.	❑	❑	❑
4. Organize the resources you find in a binder or other notebook for easy reference	❑	❑	❑

CALCULATION

Total Possible Points: __________

Total Points Earned: __________ Multiplied by 100 = __________ Divided by Total Possible Points = __________ %

PASS ❑ **FAIL** ❑ **COMMENTS:**

Student's signature ____________________ Date __________

Partner's signature ____________________ Date __________

Instructor's signature ____________________ Date __________

PSY PROCEDURE 27-3 Develop a Personal Safety Plan

Name: ______________________ **Date:** __________ **Time:** __________ **Grade:** __________

EQUIPMENT/SUPPLIES: Phone, computer with Internet access, paper and pen, binder.

STANDARDS: Given the needed equipment and a place to work, the student will perform this skill with _____ % accuracy in a total of _____ minutes. *(Your instructor will tell you what the percentage and time limits will be before you begin.)*

KEY: 4 = Satisfactory 0 = Unsatisfactory NA = This step is not counted

PROCEDURE STEPS	SELF	PARTNER	INSTRUCTOR
1. Download an electronic version of a family or personal safety plan template from a reputable Web site.	❑	❑	❑
2. Gather information needed for inclusion in the safety plan.	❑	❑	❑
3. Speak with family members and decide how you will contact each other in the event of a disaster. Include the location where you will go and/or meet.	❑	❑	❑
4. Once the personal or family plan is developed, keep a copy in the emergency supply kit or another safe place.	❑	❑	❑

CALCULATION

Total Possible Points: __________

Total Points Earned: __________ Multiplied by 100 = __________ Divided by Total Possible Points = __________ %

PASS ❑ **FAIL** ❑ **COMMENTS:**

Student's signature ____________________ Date __________

Partner's signature ____________________ Date __________

Instructor's signature ____________________ Date __________

UNIT FIVE CLINICAL DUTIES RELATED TO MEDICAL SPECIALTIES

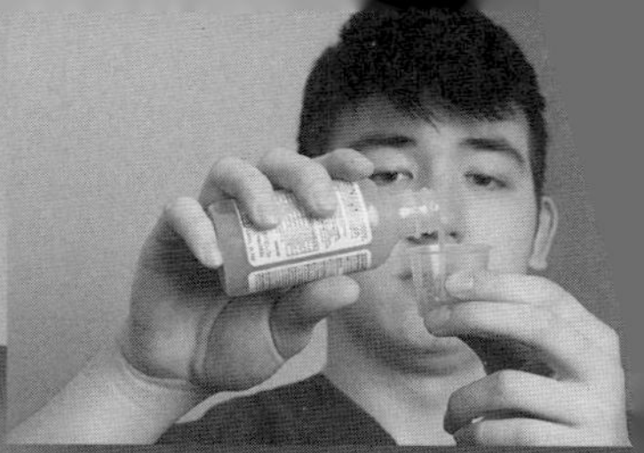

CHAPTER

28 Dermatology

Learning Outcomes

COG Cognitive Domain

1. Spell key terms
2. Define medical terms and abbreviations related to all body systems
3. Describe structural organization of the human body.
4. List major organs in each body system.
5. Identify the anatomical location of major organs in each body system.
6. Describe the normal function of each body system.
7. Identify common pathology related to each body system including signs, symptoms, and etiology.
8. Explain the difference between bandages and dressings and give the purpose of each
9. Identify the guidelines for applying bandages

PSY Psychomotor Domain

1. Apply a warm or cold compress (Procedure 28-1)
2. Assist with therapeutic soaks (Procedure 28-2)
3. Apply a tubular gauze bandage (Procedure 28-3)

AFF Affective Domain

1. Incorporate critical thinking skills when performing patient assessment
2. Incorporate critical thinking skills when performing patient care
3. Show awareness of a patient's concerns related to the procedure being performed
4. Demonstrate empathy, active listening, nonverbal communication
5. Demonstrate respect for individual diversity including gender, race, religion, age, economic status, appearance
6. Explain to a patient the rationale for performance of a procedure
7. Demonstrate sensitivity to patient rights
8. Protect the integrity of the medical record.

ABHES Competencies

1. Assist the physician with the regimen of diagnostic and treatment modalities as they relate to each body system
2. Comply with federal, state, and local health laws and regulations
3. Communicate on the recipient's level of comprehension
4. Serve as a liaison between the physician and others
5. Show empathy and impartiality when dealing with patients

Name: ______________________ Date: __________ Grade: __________

COG MULTIPLE CHOICE

Circle the letter preceding the correct answer.

1. Which of the following groups of people are most likely to develop impetigo?
   a. Older adults
   b. Women
   c. Young children
   d. Men
   e. Teenagers

2. What type of infection is herpes simplex?
   a. Bacterial
   b. Fungal
   c. Parasitic
   d. Viral
   e. Genetic

3. Public showers and swimming pools are common places to pick up fungal infections because:
   a. fungi thrive in moist conditions.
   b. areas that are highly populated increase the risk factor.
   c. sharing towels passes fungal infections from one person to another.
   d. fungi grow quickly on tile surfaces.
   e. antifungal medications do not work once they come into contact with water.

4. Which of these skin disorders may be caused by food allergies?
   a. Keloids
   b. Intertrigo
   c. Alopecia
   d. Eczema
   e. Seborrheic dermatitis

5. Which of the following statements is true about albinism?
   a. Respiratory problems are common among sufferers of albinism.
   b. Albinism is treated with benzoyl peroxide.
   c. Albinism usually occurs in exposed areas of the skin.
   d. People who suffer from albinism should have regular checkups.
   e. People who suffer from albinism should take particular care of their eyes in the sun.

6. Which statements are true about decubitus ulcers?
   a. They are frequently diagnosed in school-aged children.
   b. They are most common in aged, debilitated, and immobilized patients.
   c. They are highly contagious.
   d. They generally occur on the chin and forehead.
   e. They are effectively treated with antifungal creams.

7. When bandaging a patient, you should:
   a. fasten bandages only with safety pins.
   b. complete surgical asepsis before you begin.
   c. keep the area to be bandaged warm.
   d. leave fingers and toes exposed when possible.
   e. wrap the bandage as tightly as possible to prevent it from coming loose.

8. A person suffering from high stress levels is most likely to develop:
   a. urticaria.
   b. acne vulgaris.
   c. impetigo.
   d. leukoderma.
   e. herpes zoster.

9. How many people in the United States will typically develop malignant melanoma?
   a. 1 in 5
   b. 1 in 500
   c. 1 in 105
   d. 1 in 1,005
   e. 1 in 5,000

10. Which of the following conditions would be treated with topical antifungal cream?
    a. Folliculitis
    b. Vitiligo
    c. Tinea versicolor
    d. Urticaria
    e. Decubitus ulcers

11. What should patients do if they have an absence of melanin in their skin?
a. Avoid coming into contact with other people.
b. Protect their skin from the sun.
c. Seek immediate medical assistance.
d. Take supplementary vitamin pills.
e. Stop sharing towels and bedding.

Scenario for questions 12 and 13: A male patient comes into the physician's office to have a wart removed from his finger. While you are preparing him for the procedure, he tells you that he regularly gets verrucae on his feet.

12. How would you advise the patient to avoid further viral infections?
a. Wash all bedding and clothing at high temperatures.
b. Avoid sharing combs and toiletries with anyone.
c. Avoid coming into direct contact with skin lesions.
d. Wear comfortable footwear and avoid walking long distances.
e. Frequently wash hands with antibacterial soap.

13. The patient should look for over-the-counter wart medication that contains:
a. podophyllum resin.
b. acyclovir.
c. selenium sulfide.
d. permethrin.
e. prednisone.

14. Before you apply a bandage to an open wound, you should:
a. moisten the bandage.
b. keep the bandage at room temperature.
c. apply pressure to the wound.
d. apply a sterile dressing to the wound.
e. check to see how the patient would like the bandage fastened.

15. How can you tell that a patient is suffering from stage I decubitus ulcers?
a. The skin is blistered, peeling, or cracked.
b. Red skin does not return to normal when massaged.
c. The skin is scaly, dry, and flaky.
d. The skin is extremely itchy.
e. The patient is unable to feel pressure on the area.

16. When a physician performs a shave biopsy, he:
a. cuts the lesion off just above the skin line.
b. removes a small section from the center of the lesion.
c. removes the entire lesion for evaluation.
d. cuts the lesion off just below the skin line.
e. removes a small section from the edge of the lesion.

17. Which of these is thought to be a cause of skin cancer in areas not exposed to the sun?
a. Chemicals in toiletries
b. Pet allergies
c. Frequent irritation
d. Second-hand smoke
e. Excessive scratching

18. Treatment of impetigo involves:
a. washing the area two to three times a day followed by application of topical antibiotics.
b. cleaning with alcohol sponges twice a day.
c. washing towels, washcloths, and bed linens daily.
d. oral antibiotics for severe cases.
e. the physician removing the infected area.

19. Which of the following statements is true about nevi?
a. Nevi are usually malignant.
b. Nevi are usually found on the back or legs.
c. It is common for nevi to bleed occasionally.
d. Nevi are congenital pigmented skin blemishes.
e. Nevi are extremely rare in young patients.

20. Which part of the body is affected by tinea capitis?
a. Hands
b. Feet
c. Hair follicles
d. Groin
e. Scalp

COG MATCHING

Grade: _______

Place the letter preceding the definition on the line next to the term.

Key Terms

21. _____ alopecia
22. _____ bulla
23. _____ carbuncle
24. _____ cellulitis
25. _____ dermatophytosis
26. _____ eczema
27. _____ erythema
28. _____ folliculitis
29. _____ furuncle
30. _____ herpes simplex
31. _____ herpes zoster
32. _____ impetigo
33. _____ macule
34. _____ neoplasm
35. _____ pediculosis
36. _____ pruritus
37. _____ psoriasis
38. _____ seborrhea
39. _____ urticaria
40. _____ verruca
41. _____ vesicle
42. _____ pustule

Definitions

a. a highly infectious skin infection causing erythema and progressing to honey-colored crusts
b. redness of the skin
c. an inflammation of hair follicles
d. a small, flat discoloration of the skin
e. an abnormal growth of new tissue; tumor
f. an infection of an interconnected group of hair follicles or several furuncles forming a mass
g. an inflammation or infection of the skin and deeper tissues that may result in tissue destruction if not treated properly
h. an infection caused by the herpes simplex virus
i. hives
j. an infection caused by reactivation of varicella zoster virus, which causes chicken pox
k. a wart
l. a large blister or vesicle
m. an infestation with parasitic lice
n. baldness
o. superficial dermatitis
p. itching
q. an overproduction of sebum by the sebaceous glands
r. an infection in a hair follicle or gland; characterized by pain, redness, and swelling with necrosis of tissue in the center
s. a skin lesion that appears as a small sac containing fluid; a blister
t. a fungal infection of the skin
u. a vesicle filled with pus
v. a chronic skin disorder that appears as red patches covered with thick, dry, silvery scales

COG MATCHING

Grade: _______

Place the letter of the description on the line preceding the skin disorder.

Disorders

43. _____ vitiligo
44. _____ decubitus ulcer
45. _____ corn
46. _____ acne vulgaris
47. _____ carbuncle
48. _____ squamous cell carcinoma
49. _____ seborrheic dermatitis

Descriptions

a. a skin disease characterized by pimples, comedones, and cysts
b. a pigmentation disorder thought to be an autoimmune disorder in patients with an inherited predisposition
c. an infection in an interconnected group of hair follicles
d. a skin inflammation caused by an overproduction of sebum that affects the scalp, eyelids, face, back, umbilicus, and body folds
e. a hard, raised thickening of the stratum corneum on the toes
f. an ulcerative lesion caused by impaired blood supply and insufficient oxygen to an area
g. a type of skin cancer that is a slow-growing, malignant tumor

COG MATCHING

Grade: ________

Place the letter of the description on the line preceding the type of bandage.

Bandages

50. ______ roller bandages
51. ______ elastic bandages
52. ______ tubular gauze bandages

Descriptions

a. These bandages can be given to the patient to take home to wash and reuse. You should be careful when applying them so as not to compromise circulation.
b. These bandages are made of soft, woven materials and are available in various lengths and widths. They can be either sterile or clean.
c. These bandages are very stretchy and are used to enclose fingers, toes, arms, legs, head, and trunk.

COG MATCHING

Grade: ________

Although medical assistants do not prescribe treatments, match each of the following skin disorders with the most likely physician prescribed treatment. Place the letter of the possible treatment on the line next to the skin disorder.

Disorders

53. ______ decubitus ulcers
54. ______ basal cell carcinoma
55. ______ cellulitis
56. ______ folliculitis
57. ______ verruca
58. ______ urticaria

Treatments

a. saline soaks or compresses
b. antihistamines
c. antibiotic powder
d. surgical removal
e. keratolytic agents
f. antibiotics

PSY IDENTIFICATION

Grade: ________

59. Which of the following skin disorders cannot be treated? Circle the correct answer.

a. Impetigo

b. Folliculitis

c. Albinism

d. Malignant melanoma

e. Decubitus ulcers

60. How would a physician be able to confirm a suspected case of malignant melanoma? Circle the correct answer.

a. Wood light analysis

b. Inspection

c. Urine test

61. As a medical assistant, you'll be responsible for helping the physician perform physical examinations of the skin. Review the list of tasks below and determine which tasks you may be responsible for as a medical assistant. Place a check mark in the "Yes" column for duties that you might assist with and a check mark in the "No" column for tasks that would be completed by someone else.

Task	Yes	No
a. Assemble the equipment required by the physician.		
b. Perform a skin biopsy.		
c. Inject local anesthetic when needed.		
d. Direct specimens to the appropriate laboratories.		
e. Clean and disinfect the examination room.		
f. Diagnose and treat common skin inflammations.		
g. Reinforce the physician's instructions about caring for a skin condition at home.		

62. You are applying a bandage to a patient. Read the statements below and check the appropriate box to show whether the bandage has been applied correctly or incorrectly.

	Applied Correctly	Applied Incorrectly
a. You have fastened the bandage with adhesive tape.		
b. The area that you are about to bandage is clean and damp.		
c. You have dressed two burned fingers separately and then bandaged them together.		
d. The skin around the bandaged arm is pale and cool.		
e. You have bandaged a wounded foot by covering the toes to make it neater.		
f. You have bandaged an elbow with extra padding.		

63. Place a check mark in the appropriate box to show whether the person described is at a high risk or a low risk of developing impetigo.

	High Risk	Low Risk
a. A slightly overweight 34-year-old woman who showers twice a day		
b. A 55-year-old man who works at a hospital laundry room and does not wash his hands		
c. A 22-year-old woman with severe anorexia		

d. An 18-year-old drug addict who lives in an abandoned warehouse		
e. A 40-year-old mother of three who enjoys reading in the tub		

64. Read these descriptions of five of Dr. Marsh's patients then decide which of his patients is at the highest risk of developing malignant melanoma. Place a check mark on the line preceding the patient descriptions that are at the highest risk.

a. ______________ Mrs. Pearson, 42-year-old mother of two. Light brown hair, brown eyes, enjoys reading and watching movies.

b. ______________ Mr. Stevens, 50-year-old widower. Gray hair, brown eyes, enjoys walking and playing golf.

c. ______________ Jessica Phillips, 24-year-old college student. Red hair, blue eyes, enjoys playing volleyball and surfing.

d. ______________ Todd Andrews, 18-year-old student. Black hair, green eyes, enjoys running and swimming.

e. ______________ Mr. Archer, 39-year-old father of three. Blond hair, blue eyes, lives in Minnesota and enjoys skiing.

COG SHORT ANSWER

Grade: ____________

65. What are the symptoms of psoriasis?

____

____

____

____

66. A man brings his 85-year-old mother to the physician's office. He tells you that his mother lives in a local care home. When the physician examines the patient, you notice multiple decubitus ulcers on her body. Explain why this would be a particular cause of concern.

____

____

____

____

67. List the three types of skin biopsy performed by a physician.

____

____

____

____

68. List the three bacterial skin infections that develop in the hair follicles.

____

____

____

____

69. A patient has a band of lesions on his back made up of small red papules. What skin disorder does this person most likely have? Explain what causes the condition.

____

____

____

____

70. A father brings his 8-year-old son to the physician, who diagnoses the child with pediculosis. What advice could you give the father to ensure that no other members of the family become infected? List three things that the father could do to contain the problem.

____

____

____

____

71. What is the full version of the cancer prevention message "Slip! Slop! Slap! Wrap!"?

____

____

____

____

72. The physician suspects that a patient has ringworm. Explain what method the physician would most likely use to confirm the diagnosis?

____

____

____

____

COG TRUE OR FALSE?

Grade: ______________

73. Indicate whether the statements are true or false by placing the letter T (true) or F (false) on the line preceding the statement.

a. ______________ Before applying a bandage, you should perform surgical asepsis.

b. ______________ Young women are more likely to develop keloids than young men.

c. _____________ A wound culture is obtained by excising the wound.

d. _____________ Erythema is best treated with antihistamines.

COG AFF CASE STUDY FOR CRITICAL THINKING

Grade: __________

1. A patient has come into the physician's office for a skin biopsy on his thigh. After the physician has removed the tissue, she asks you to bandage the area. List three things you should do while you are bandaging the patient's thigh to ensure that it is both sterile and secure. Explain why they are important.

___

___

___

___

2. There are three patients waiting to be seen by a physician, and all of the appointments are slightly behind schedule. One of the patients is a young man who has clusters of wheals on his left arm. The second patient is a 7-year-old girl who has dry scaly crusts on her face and neck. The third patient is a 5-year-old boy with dried skin flakes and bald patches on his scalp. All three patients are itching, and the receptionist is concerned that they might be contagious. You have only one spare examination room. Which patient would you isolate in the examination room? Explain your answer.

___

___

___

___

3. Your patient is a 25-year-old female who has been to see the physician several times for severe sunburn. You know that her lifestyle can lead to long-term skin problems. Explain how you could educate her about staying safe in the sun. Include some of the early warning signs of skin cancer that she should keep an eye out for.

___

___

___

___

4. A mother brings her 8-year-old son to the physician's office, and the child is diagnosed with pediculosis. She insists that her child cannot possibly have lice because they live in a very clean home. The mother demands that the physician examines the child again. What do you say to the mother to calm her down? How do you reassure her?

___

___

___

___

5. A 14-year-old boy comes into the physician's office with severe acne vulgaris on his face and neck. He is embarrassed and depressed about his condition and is worried that it will never get better. He says that he has tried every over-the-counter medication and that this is his last hope. What would you say to this patient?

___

___

___

___

PSY PROCEDURE 28-1 Apply a Warm or Cold Compress

Name: ______________________ **Date:** __________ **Time:** __________ **Grade:** __________

EQUIPMENT/SUPPLIES: Warm compresses—appropriate solution (water with possible antiseptic if ordered), warmed to 110°F or recommended temperature; bath thermometer; absorbent material (cloths, gauze); waterproof barriers; hot water bottle (optional); clean or sterile basin; gloves. Cold compresses—appropriate solution; ice bag or cold pack; absorbent material (cloths, gauze); waterproof barriers; gloves

STANDARDS: Given the needed equipment and a place to work, the student will perform this skill with _____ % accuracy in a total of _____ minutes. *(Your instructor will tell you what the percentage and time limits will be before you begin.)*

KEY: 4 = Satisfactory 0 = Unsatisfactory NA = This step is not counted

PROCEDURE STEPS	SELF	PARTNER	INSTRUCTOR
1. Wash your hands and put on gloves.	❑	❑	❑
2. Check the physician's order and assemble the equipment and supplies.	❑	❑	❑
3. Pour the appropriate solution into the basin. For hot compresses, check the temperature of the warmed solution.	❑	❑	❑
4. Greet and identify the patient. Identify yourself including your title. Explain the procedure.	❑	❑	❑
5. Ask patient to remove appropriate clothing.	❑	❑	❑
6. Gown and drape accordingly.	❑	❑	❑
7. AFF Explain how to respond to a patient who is hearing impaired.	❑	❑	❑

____

____

____

____

PROCEDURE STEPS	SELF	PARTNER	INSTRUCTOR
8. Protect the examination table with a waterproof barrier.	❑	❑	❑
9. Place absorbent material or gauze into the prepared solution. Wring out excess moisture.	❑	❑	❑
10. Place the compress on the patient's skin and ask about comfort of temperature.	❑	❑	❑
11. Observe the skin for changes in color.	❑	❑	❑
12. Arrange the wet compress over the area.			

PSY PROCEDURE 28-1 Apply a Warm or Cold Compress (continued)

13. Insulate the compress with plastic or another waterproof barrier.			
14. Check the compress frequently for moisture and temperature. **a.** Hot water bottles or ice packs may be used to maintain the temperature. **b.** Rewet absorbent material as needed.			
15. After the prescribed amount of time, usually 20 to 30 minutes, remove the compress. **a.** Discard disposable materials. **b.** Disinfect reusable equipment.			
16. Remove your gloves and wash your hands.			
17. Log into the Electronic Medical Record (EMR) using your username and secure password OR obtain the paper medical record from a secure location and assure it is kept away from public access. Document the procedure including: **a.** Length of treatment, type of solution, temperature of solution **b.** Skin color after treatment, assessment of the area, and patient's reactions			
18. When finished, log out of the EMR and/or replace the paper medical record in an appropriate and secure location.			

CALCULATION

Total Possible Points: __________

Total Points Earned: __________ Multiplied by 100 = __________ Divided by Total Possible Points = __________ %

PASS ❑ **FAIL** ❑ **COMMENTS:**

Student's signature ____________________ Date __________

Partner's signature ____________________ Date __________

Instructor's signature ____________________ Date __________

PSY PROCEDURE 28-2 Assist with Therapeutic Soaks

Name: ______________________ **Date:** __________ **Time:** __________ **Grade:** __________

EQUIPMENT/SUPPLIES: Clean or sterile basin or container to comfortably contain the body part to be soaked; solution and/or medication; dry towels; bath thermometer; gloves

STANDARDS: Given the needed equipment and a place to work, the student will perform this skill with _____ % accuracy in a total of _____ minutes. *(Your instructor will tell you what the percentage and time limits will be before you begin.)*

KEY: 4 = Satisfactory 0 = Unsatisfactory NA = This step is not counted

PROCEDURE STEPS	SELF	PARTNER	INSTRUCTOR
1. Wash your hands and apply your gloves.	❑	❑	❑
2. Assemble the equipment and supplies, including the appropriately sized basin or container. Pad surfaces of container for comfort.	❑	❑	❑
3. Fill the container with solution and check the temperature with a bath thermometer. The temperature should be below 110°F.	❑	❑	❑
4. Greet and identify the patient. Identify yourself including your credentials. Explain the procedure.	❑	❑	❑
5. AFF Explain how to respond to the patient who has dementia.	❑	❑	❑

____

____

____

____

PROCEDURE STEPS	SELF	PARTNER	INSTRUCTOR
6. Slowly lower the patient's extremity or body part into the container.	❑	❑	❑
7. Arrange the part comfortably and in easy alignment.	❑	❑	❑
8. Check for pressure areas and pad the edges as needed for comfort.	❑	❑	❑
9. Check the solution every 5 to 10 minutes for proper temperature.	❑	❑	❑
10. Soak for the prescribed amount of time, usually 15 to 20 minutes.	❑	❑	❑
11. Remove the body part from the solution and carefully dry the area with a towel.	❑	❑	❑
12. Properly care for the equipment; appropriately dispose of single-use supplies and wash your hands.	❑	❑	❑

PSY PROCEDURE 28-2 Assist with Therapeutic Soaks (continued)

13. Log into the Electronic Medical Record (EMR) using your username and secure password OR obtain the paper medical record from a secure location and assure it is kept away from public access. Document the procedure including: **a.** Length of treatment, type of solution, temperature of solution **b.** Skin color after treatment, assessment of the area, and patient's reactions	❑	❑	❑
14. When finished, log out of the EMR and/or replace the paper medical record in an appropriate and secure location.	❑	❑	❑

CALCULATION

Total Possible Points: __________

Total Points Earned: __________ Multiplied by 100 = __________ Divided by Total Possible Points = __________ %

PASS ❑ **FAIL** ❑ **COMMENTS:**

Student's signature ____________________ Date __________

Partner's signature ____________________ Date __________

Instructor's signature ____________________ Date __________

PSY PROCEDURE 28-3 Apply a Tubular Gauze Bandage

Name: ______________________________ **Date:** __________ **Time:** __________ **Grade:** __________

EQUIPMENT/SUPPLIES: Tubular gauze, applicator, tape, scissors

STANDARDS: Given the needed equipment and a place to work, the student will perform this skill with _____ % accuracy in a total of _____ minutes. *(Your instructor will tell you what the percentage and time limits will be before you begin.)*

KEY: 4 = Satisfactory 0 = Unsatisfactory NA = This step is not counted

PROCEDURE STEPS	SELF	PARTNER	INSTRUCTOR
1. Wash your hands and assemble the equipment.	❑	❑	❑
2. Greet and identify the patient. Identify yourself including your credentials. Explain the procedure.	❑	❑	❑
3. AFF Explain how to respond to a patient who is visually impaired.	❑	❑	❑
______________________________ ______________________________ ______________________________ ______________________________			
4. Choose the appropriate-size tubular gauze applicator and gauze width.	❑	❑	❑
5. Select and cut or tear adhesive tape in lengths to secure the gauze ends.	❑	❑	❑
6. Place the gauze bandage on the applicator in the following manner: **a.** Be sure that the applicator is upright (open end up) and placed on a flat surface. **b.** Pull a sufficient length of gauze from the stock box, ready to cut. **c.** Open the end of the length of gauze and slide it over the upper end of the applicator. **d.** Push estimated amount of gauze needed for this procedure onto the applicator. **e.** Cut the gauze when the required amount of gauze has been transferred to the applicator.	❑	❑	❑
7. Place applicator over the distal end of the affected part. Hold it in place as you move to Step 7.	❑	❑	❑
8. Slide applicator containing the gauze up to the proximal end of the affected part.	❑	❑	❑

PSY PROCEDURE 28-3 Apply a Tubular Gauze Bandage (continued)

9. Pull the applicator 1 to 2 inches past the end of the affected part if the part is to be completely covered.	❑	❑	❑
10. Turn the applicator one full turn to anchor the bandage.	❑	❑	❑
11. Move the applicator toward the proximal part as before.	❑	❑	❑
12. Move the applicator forward about 1 inch beyond the original starting point.	❑	❑	❑
13. Repeat the procedure until the desired coverage is obtained.	❑	❑	❑
14. The final layer should end at the proximal part of the affected area. Remove the applicator.	❑	❑	❑
15. Secure the bandage in place with adhesive tape or cut the gauze into two tails and tie them at the base of the tear.	❑	❑	❑
16. Tie the two tails around the closest proximal joint.	❑	❑	❑
17. Use the adhesive tape sparingly to secure the end if not using a tie.	❑	❑	❑
18. Properly care for or dispose of equipment and supplies.	❑	❑	❑
19. Clean the work area. Wash your hands.	❑	❑	❑
20. Log into the Electronic Medical Record (EMR) using your username and secure password OR obtain the paper medical record from a secure location and assure it is kept away from public access.	❑	❑	❑
21. When finished, log out of the EMR and/or replace the paper medical record in an appropriate and secure location.	❑	❑	❑

CALCULATION

Total Possible Points: ___________

Total Points Earned: ___________ Multiplied by 100 = ___________ Divided by Total Possible Points = ___________ %

PASS ❑ **FAIL** ❑ **COMMENTS:**

Student's signature ______________________ Date ___________

Partner's signature ______________________ Date ___________

Instructor's signature ______________________ Date ___________

3. Your coworker Ben is moving some boxes from the reception area to a closet in the office. As you walk by, you observe him bending his back and lifting a box with extended arms. You know that this method of lifting could lead to serious back problems, so you decide to speak to Ben about avoiding back strain. What should you say to Ben? How would you respond if he laughs and tells you he is fine?

____

____

____

____

4. A 46-year-old patient has been advised by the physician to avoid using his strained knee. After you secure an ice pack to the patient's knee, you begin to instruct the patient in how to care for his knee at home. While you are speaking, the patient interrupts you saying that he has had this injury before and will "just throw a heating pad on there" like he has done in the past. How would you respond to the patient?

____

____

____

____

PSY PROCEDURE 29-1 Apply an Arm Sling

Name: ______________________ **Date:** __________ **Time:** __________ **Grade:** __________

EQUIPMENT/SUPPLIES: A canvas arm sling with adjustable straps.

STANDARDS: Given the needed equipment and a place to work, the student will perform this skill with _____ % accuracy in a total of _____ minutes. *(Your instructor will tell you what the percentage and time limits will be before you begin.)*

KEY: 4 = Satisfactory 0 = Unsatisfactory NA = This step is not counted

PROCEDURE STEPS	SELF	PARTNER	INSTRUCTOR
1. Wash your hands.	❑	❑	❑
2. Assemble the equipment and supplies.	❑	❑	❑
3. Greet and identify the patient and explain the procedure. Identify yourself including your credentials.	❑	❑	❑
4. AFF Explain how to respond to a patient who does not speak English.	❑	❑	❑
____			
____			
____			
____			
5. Position the affected limb with the hand at slightly less than a 90-degree angle.	❑	❑	❑
6. Place the affected arm into the sling with the elbow snugly against the back of the sling, and the arm extended through the sling with the hand and/or fingers protruding out of the opposite end of the sling.	❑	❑	❑
7. Position the strap from the back of the sling around the patient's back, over the opposite shoulder.	❑	❑	❑
8. Secure the strap by inserting the end through the two metal rings on the top of the sling and further bringing the end of the strap back, looping it through the top metal ring only.	❑	❑	❑
9. Tighten the strap so that the patient's arm in the sling is slightly elevated. Make sure the strap coming around the patient's shoulder and neck is comfortable, padding if necessary to prevent friction and pressure areas.	❑	❑	❑
10. Check the patient's level of comfort and distal extremity circulation.	❑	❑	❑

PSY PROCEDURE 29-1 Apply an Arm Sling (continued)

11. Wash your hands.			
12. AFF Log into the Electronic Medical Record (EMR) using your username and secure password OR obtain the paper medical record from a secure location and assure it is kept away from public access. Document the appliance in the patient's chart.			
13. When finished, log out of the EMR and/or replace the paper medical record in an appropriate and secure location.			

CALCULATION

Total Possible Points: __________

Total Points Earned: __________ Multiplied by 100 = __________ Divided by Total Possible Points = __________ %

PASS ❏ **FAIL** ❏ **COMMENTS:**

Student's signature ____________________ Date __________

Partner's signature ____________________ Date __________

Instructor's signature ____________________ Date __________

PSY PROCEDURE 29-2 Apply Cold Packs

Name: ______________________ **Date:** __________ **Time:** __________ **Grade:** __________

EQUIPMENT/SUPPLIES: Ice bag and ice chips or small cubes, or disposable cold pack; small towel or cover for ice pack; gauze or tape.

STANDARDS: Given the needed equipment and a place to work, the student will perform this skill with _____ % accuracy in a total of _____ minutes. *(Your instructor will tell you what the percentage and time limits will be before you begin.)*

KEY: 4 = Satisfactory 0 = Unsatisfactory NA = This step is not counted

PROCEDURE STEPS	SELF	PARTNER	INSTRUCTOR
1. Wash your hands.	❑	❑	❑
2. Assemble the equipment and supplies, checking the ice bag, if used, for leaks. If using a commercial cold pack, read the manufacturer's directions.	❑	❑	❑
3. Fill a nondisposable ice bag about two-thirds full. **a.** Press it flat on a surface to express air from the bag. **b.** Seal the container.	❑	❑	❑
4. If using a commercial chemical ice pack, activate it now.	❑	❑	❑
5. Cover the bag in a towel or other suitable cover.	❑	❑	❑
6. Greet and identify the patient. Identify yourself including your credentials. Explain the procedure.	❑	❑	❑
7. AFF Explain how to respond to a patient who has cultural or religious beliefs that prohibit disrobing.	❑	❑	❑
____			
____			
____			
____			
8. After assessing skin for color and warmth, place the covered ice pack on the area.	❑	❑	❑
9. Secure the ice pack with gauze or tape.	❑	❑	❑
10. Apply the treatment for the prescribed amount of time, but no longer than 30 minutes.	❑	❑	❑
11. During the treatment, assess the skin under the pack frequently for mottling, pallor, or redness.	❑	❑	❑

PSY PROCEDURE 29-2 Apply Cold Packs (continued)

12. Properly care for or dispose of equipment and supplies. Wash your hands.	❑	❑	❑
13. AFF Log into the Electronic Medical Record (EMR) using your username and secure password OR obtain the paper medical record from a secure location and assure it is kept away from public access.	❑	❑	❑
14. Document the procedure, the site of the application, the results including the condition of the skin after the treatment, and the patient's reactions.	❑	❑	❑
15. When finished, log out of the EMR and/or replace the paper medical record in an appropriate and secure location.	❑	❑	❑

CALCULATION

Total Possible Points: __________

Total Points Earned: __________ Multiplied by 100 = __________ Divided by Total Possible Points = __________ %

PASS ❑ **FAIL** ❑ **COMMENTS:**

Student's signature ____________________ Date __________

Partner's signature ____________________ Date __________

Instructor's signature ____________________ Date __________

PSY PROCEDURE 29-3 Use a Hot Water Bottle or Commercial Hot Pack

Name: ______________________ **Date:** __________ **Time:** __________ **Grade:** __________

EQUIPMENT/SUPPLIES: A hot water bottle or commercial hot pack, towel or other suitable covering for the hot pack

STANDARDS: Given the needed equipment and a place to work, the student will perform this skill with _____ % accuracy in a total of _____ minutes. *(Your instructor will tell you what the percentage and time limits will be before you begin.)*

KEY: 4 = Satisfactory 0 = Unsatisfactory NA = This step is not counted

PROCEDURE STEPS	SELF	PARTNER	INSTRUCTOR
1. Wash your hands.	❑	❑	❑
2. Assemble equipment and supplies, checking the hot water bottle for leaks.	❑	❑	❑
3. Fill the hot water bottle about two-thirds full with warm (110°F) water. **a.** Place the bottle on a flat surface and the opening up; "burp" it by pressing out the air. **b.** If using a commercial hot pack, follow the manufacturer's directions for activating it.	❑	❑	❑
4. Wrap and secure the pack or bottle before placing it on the patient's skin.	❑	❑	❑
5. Greet and identify the patient. Identify yourself including your credentials. Explain the procedure.	❑	❑	❑
6. AFF Explain how to respond to a patient who is from a different generation (older) than you are.	❑	❑	❑

____

____

____

____

PROCEDURE STEPS	SELF	PARTNER	INSTRUCTOR
7. After assessing the color of the skin where the treatment is to be applied, place the covered hot pack on the area.	❑	❑	❑
8. Secure the hot pack with gauze or tape.	❑	❑	❑
9. Apply the treatment for the prescribed length of time, but no longer than 30 minutes.	❑	❑	❑
10. During treatment, assess the skin every 10 minutes for pallor (an indication of rebound), excessive redness (indicates temperature may be too high), and swelling (indicates possible tissue damage).	❑	❑	❑

PSY PROCEDURE 29-3 Use a Hot Water Bottle or Commercial Hot Pack (continued)

11. Properly care for or dispose of equipment and supplies. Wash your hands.	❑	❑	❑
12. AFF Log into the Electronic Medical Record (EMR) using your username and secure password OR obtain the paper medical record from a secure location and assure it is kept away from public access.	❑	❑	❑
13. Document the procedure, the site of the application, the results including the condition of the skin after the treatment, and the patient's reactions.	❑	❑	❑
14. When finished, log out of the EMR and/or replace the paper medical record in an appropriate and secure location.	❑	❑	❑

CALCULATION

Total Possible Points: __________

Total Points Earned: __________ Multiplied by 100 = __________ Divided by Total Possible Points = __________ %

PASS ❑ **FAIL** ❑ **COMMENTS:**

Student's signature ____________________ Date __________

Partner's signature ____________________ Date __________

Instructor's signature ____________________ Date __________

PSY PROCEDURE 29-4 Measure a Patient for Axillary Crutches

Name: ______________________ **Date:** __________ **Time:** __________ **Grade:** __________

EQUIPMENT/SUPPLIES: Axillary crutches with tips, pads for the axilla, and hand rests, as needed

STANDARDS: Given the needed equipment and a place to work, the student will perform this skill with _____ % accuracy in a total of _____ minutes. *(Your instructor will tell you what the percentage and time limits will be before you begin.)*

KEY: 4 = Satisfactory 0 = Unsatisfactory NA = This step is not counted

PROCEDURE STEPS	SELF	PARTNER	INSTRUCTOR
1. Wash your hands.	❑	❑	❑
2. Assemble the equipment including the correct-size crutches.	❑	❑	❑
3. Greet and identify the patient. Identify yourself including your credentials. Explain the procedure.	❑	❑	❑
4. Ensure that the patient is wearing low-heeled shoes with safety soles.	❑	❑	❑
5. Have the patient stand erect. Support the patient as needed.	❑	❑	❑
6. AFF Explain how to respond to a patient who is hearing impaired.	❑	❑	❑
____ ____ ____ ____			
7. While standing erect, have the patient hold the crutches in the tripod position.	❑	❑	❑
8. Adjust the central support in the base. **a.** Tighten the bolts for safety when the proper height is reached. **b.** Adjust the handgrips. Tighten bolts for safety. **c.** If needed, pad axillary bars and handgrips.	❑	❑	❑
9. Wash your hands.	❑	❑	❑
10. AFF Log into the Electronic Medical Record (EMR) using your username and secure password OR obtain the paper medical record from a secure location and assure it is kept away from public access.	❑	❑	❑

PROCEDURE 29-4 Measure a Patient for Axillary Crutches (continued)

11. Record the procedure, site of the application, results including the condition of the skin after the treatment, the patient's response, the date, time, and your name/credentials.	❑	❑	❑
12. When finished, log out of the EMR and/or replace the paper medical record in an appropriate and secure location.	❑	❑	❑

CALCULATION

Total Possible Points: __________

Total Points Earned: __________ Multiplied by 100 = __________ Divided by Total Possible Points = __________ %

PASS ❑ **FAIL** ❑ **COMMENTS:**

Student's signature ____________________ Date __________

Partner's signature ____________________ Date __________

Instructor's signature ____________________ Date __________

PSY PROCEDURE 29-5 Instruct a Patient in Various Crutch Gaits

Name: ______________________ **Date:** __________ **Time:** __________ **Grade:** __________

EQUIPMENT/SUPPLIES: Axillary crutches measured appropriately for a patient

STANDARDS: Given the needed equipment and a place to work, the student will perform this skill with _____ % accuracy in a total of _____ minutes. *(Your instructor will tell you what the percentage and time limits will be before you begin.)*

KEY: 4 = Satisfactory 0 = Unsatisfactory NA =This step is not counted

PROCEDURE STEPS	SELF	PARTNER	INSTRUCTOR
1. Wash your hands.	❑	❑	❑
2. Have the patient stand up from a chair: **a.** The patient holds both crutches on the affected side. **b.** Then the patient slides to the edge of the chair. **c.** The patient pushes down on the chair arm on the unaffected side. **d.** Then the patient pushes to stand.	❑	❑	❑
3. With one crutch in each hand, rest on the crutches until balance is restored.	❑	❑	❑
4. Assist the patient to the tripod position.	❑	❑	❑
5. AFF Explain how to respond to a patient who is visually impaired.	❑	❑	❑
______________________________ ______________________________ ______________________________ ______________________________			
6. Depending upon the patient's weight-bearing ability, coordination, and general state of health, instruct the patient in one or more of the following gaits: **a.** Three-point gait **b.** Two-point gait **c.** Four-point gait **d.** Swing-through gait	❑	❑	❑
7. AFF Log into the Electronic Medical Record (EMR) using your username and secure password OR obtain the paper medical record from a secure location and assure it is kept away from public access.	❑	❑	❑

PSY PROCEDURE 29-5 Instruct a Patient in Various Crutch Gaits (continued)

8. Record the patient education and instructions.	❑	❑	❑
9. When finished, log out of the EMR and/or replace the paper medical record in an appropriate and secure location.	❑	❑	❑

CALCULATION

Total Possible Points: __________

Total Points Earned: __________ Multiplied by 100 = __________ Divided by Total Possible Points = __________ %

PASS ❑ **FAIL** ❑ **COMMENTS:**

Student's signature ____________________ Date __________

Partner's signature ____________________ Date __________

Instructor's signature ____________________ Date __________

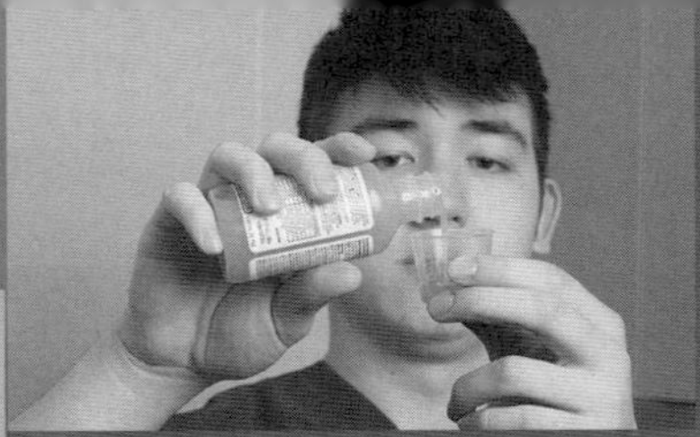

CHAPTER

30 Ophthalmology and Otolaryngology

Learning Outcomes

COG Cognitive Domain

1. Spell key terms
2. Define medical terms and abbreviations related to all body systems
3. Describe structural organization of the human body
4. List major organs in each body system
5. Identify the anatomical location of major organs in each body system
6. Describe the normal function of each body system
7. Identify common pathology related to each body system including signs, symptoms, and etiology
8. Describe patient education procedures associated with the eye, ear, nose, and throat

PSY Psychomotor Domain

1. Measure distance visual acuity with a Snellen chart (Procedure 30-1)
2. Measure color perception with an Ishihara color plate book (Procedure 30-2)
3. Instill eye medication (Procedure 30-3)
4. Irrigate the eye (Procedure 30-4)
5. Irrigate the ear (Procedure 30-5)
6. Administer an audiometric hearing test (Procedure 30-6)
7. Instill ear medication (Procedure 30-7)
8. Instill nasal medication (Procedure 30-8)

AFF Affective Domain

1. Incorporate critical thinking skills when performing patient assessment
2. Incorporate critical thinking skills when performing patient care
3. Show awareness of a patient's concerns related to the procedure being performed
4. Demonstrate empathy, active listening, nonverbal communication
5. Demonstrate respect for individual diversity including gender, race, religion, age, economic status, appearance
6. Explain to a patient the rationale for performance of a procedure
7. Demonstrate sensitivity to patient rights
8. Protect the integrity of the medical record

ABHES Competencies

1. Assist the physician with the regimen of diagnostic and treatment modalities as they relate to each body system
2. Comply with federal, state, and local health laws and regulations
3. Communicate on the recipient's level of comprehension
4. Serve as a liaison between the physician and others
5. Show empathy and impartiality when dealing with patients
6. Document accurately

Name: ______________________ Date: __________ Grade: __________

COG MULTIPLE CHOICE

Circle the letter preceding the correct answer.

1. The Ishihara method is used to test:
a. hearing.
b. color vision.
c. cataract growth.
d. corneal scarring.
e. for multiple allergies.

2. A physician who specializes in disorders of the ears, nose, and throat is an:
a. optician.
b. ophthalmologist.
c. optometrist.
d. otolaryngologist.
e. otitis externa.

3. A common cause of diminished hearing is:
a. tinnitus.
b. nasopharynx.
c. cerumen.
d. Ménière disease.
e. strabismus.

4. Epistaxis is considered severe if bleeding continues how many minutes after treatment has begun?
a. 5
b. 10
c. 15
d. 20
e. 30

5. Which of the following statements is true about preventive eye care?
a. Patients should have regular checkups to maintain healthy eyes.
b. Adults should wear UV-protected sunglasses, but children are not as susceptible.
c. Goggles do not need to be worn if you are wearing your regular glasses.
d. Patients should thoroughly wash hands before rubbing their eyes.
e. Contact lenses cause scarring, so glasses are safer to use.

6. It's important to treat sinusitis immediately because:
a. it can lead to severe cases of upper respiratory infections.
b. new allergies might develop while the nasal membrane is infected.
c. mucus may infect areas of throat, nose, and ears if left unchecked.
d. vision may be affected from pressure of sinus cavities on the eyes.
e. complications in the ear and brain may occur, causing damage.

7. One symptom of laryngitis is:
a. earache.
b. muscle soreness.
c. coughing.
d. inflamed tonsils.
e. excessive mucus.

8. An infection of any of the lacrimal glands of the eyelids is:
a. hordeolum.
b. cataract.
c. glaucoma.
d. conjunctivitis.
e. astigmatism.

9. Which of the following could the physician treat with a warm compress?
a. Nosebleed
b. Ear infection
c. Tonsillitis
d. Astigmatism
e. Tinnitus

10. The common term for *otitis externa* is:
a. pink eye.
b. nosebleed.
c. Ménière disease.
d. swimmer's ear.
e. presbycusis.

Scenario for questions 11 and 12: A patient comes in for an annual exam, and the physician diagnoses her with presbycusis and presbyopia. She complains of an intermittent, high whistling in her right ear and cloudy vision in both eyes.

11. Reading the symptoms and diagnosis above, the patient is most likely:
a. an infant or a toddler.
b. a young child to early teen.
c. an older teen to early 30s.
d. middle aged.
e. a senior citizen.

12. One possible cause of the cloudy vision is:
a. presbyopia.
b. glaucoma.
c. Ménière disease.
d. cataracts.
e. sinusitis.

13. What is a safe way to remove cerumen?
a. Gently inserting a tissue into the ear canal
b. Using a cotton swab and digging out as much as possible
c. Drops of hydrogen peroxide dropped into the ear
d. Using an otoscope to melt the earwax
e. Blowing your nose

14. It's important not to use nasal preparations more than four times a day because they:
a. severely damage your nasal cavity.
b. may become addictive.
c. dry out sinuses and cause congestion.
d. cause irritation to the throat.
e. can lead to allergies.

15. Color blindness is a result of:
a. people failing the Ishihara test.
b. patients being unable to differentiate between colors.
c. a deficiency in the number of rods in the eye.
d. a deficiency in the number of cones in the eye.
e. the size and shape of the eye.

16. What important advice can you give children when dealing with contagious diseases like pink eye?
a. Keep your hands washed and clean.
b. Do not play with children who are sick.
c. If you sneeze, immediately cover your face with your hand.
d. Do not go to school if you are sick.
e. Try to keep from touching anything others have already touched.

17. To test for pharyngitis or tonsillitis, the physician would most likely order:
a. a blood sample.
b. a urine sample.
c. a reflex test.
d. a throat culture.
e. radiology.

18. Which form of strabismus is known as *convergent eyes*, in which the eyes are crossed?
a. Esotropic
b. Exotropic
c. Hypotrophic
d. Hypertrophic
e. Nonconcomitant

19. The purpose of a hearing aid is to:
a. fully restore the ability to hear.
b. assist patients with permanent nerve damage.
c. amplify sound waves.
d. differentiate between tones.
e. permanently correct hearing disabilities.

20. A common treatment for allergic rhinitis is:
a. sleep.
b. antihistamine medication.
c. surgery.
d. antibiotics.
e. ear irrigation.

COG MATCHING

Grade: ______

Place the letter preceding the definition on the line next to the term.

Key Terms

21. ______ astigmatism
22. ______ cerumen
23. ______ decibel
24. ______ fluorescein angiography
25. ______ hyperopia
26. ______ intraocular pressure
27. ______ myopia
28. ______ myringotomy
29. ______ ophthalmologist
30. ______ ophthalmoscope
31. ______ optician
32. ______ optometrist
33. ______ otolaryngologist
34. ______ otoscope
35. ______ presbycusis
36. ______ presbyopia
37. ______ refraction
38. ______ retinal degeneration
39. ______ tinnitus
40. ______ tonometry
41. ______ hordeolum
42. ______ strabismus

Definitions

a. physician who specializes in treatment of diseases and disorders of the ears, nose, and throat
b. an extraneous noise heard in one or both ears, described as whirring, ringing, whistling, roaring, etc.; may be continuous or intermittent
c. specialist who can measure for errors of refraction and prescribe lenses but who cannot treat diseases of the eye or perform surgery
d. an instrument used for visual examination of the ear canal and tympanic membrane
e. an incision into the tympanic membrane to relieve pressure
f. unit of intensity of sound
g. an unfocused refraction of light rays on the retina
h. a misalignment of eye movements usually caused by muscle incoordination
i. loss of hearing associated with aging
j. specialist who grinds lenses to correct errors of refraction according to prescriptions
k. yellowish or brownish waxlike secretion in the external ear canal; earwax
l. physician who specializes in treatment of disorders of the eyes
m. farsightedness
n. pathological changes in the cell structure of the retina that impair or destroy its function, resulting in blindness
o. infection of any of the lacrimal glands of the eyelids
p. intravenous injection of fluorescent dye; photographing blood vessels of the eye as dye moves through the vessels
q. measurement of intraocular pressure using a tonometer
r. lighted instrument used to examine the inner surfaces of the eye
s. bending of light rays that enter the pupil to reflect exactly on the fovea centralis, the area of greatest visual acuity
t. pressure within the eyeball
u. vision change (farsightedness) associated with aging
v. nearsightedness

COG IDENTIFICATION

Grade: ______

43. Fill in the chart below with three types of vision testing charts, and when you should use each.

Type of Vision Testing Chart	When You Would Use It
a.	
b.	
c.	

44. Identify the seven causes of hearing loss.

a. ______________________________
b. ______________________________
c. ______________________________

d. ____________________

e. ____________________

f. ____________________

g. ____________________

COG SHORT ANSWER

Grade: ____________

45. List five preventive eye care tips that you may be asked to educate patients to follow.

a. ____________________

b. ____________________

c. ____________________

d. ____________________

e. ____________________

46. A patient complains of loss of vision and blurring, and cataracts are found in both eyes. How would surgery correct these symptoms?

____

____

____

____

47. What is the difference between an optometrist and an optician?

____

____

____

____

48. What is astigmatism?

____

____

____

____

49. An examination of a patient's eye reveals an irregular corneal surface. What is the method used to diagnose a corneal ulcer?

____

____

____

____

50. A patient comes in complaining of vertigo, nausea, and slight hearing loss. What might the patient be suffering from?

51. Why is otitis media so common in infants and young children?

52. What is the difference between audiometry and tympanometry?

53. List the initial therapy for common epistaxis.

54. Why is it so important to treat upper respiratory infections?

55. When is the physician likely to suggest that a patient receive a tonsillectomy?

56. What is a way to isolate the protein causing allergic reactions in a patient directly?

57. Where do nasal polyps usually occur?

____

____

____

____

COG TRUE OR FALSE?

Grade: __________

Indicate whether the statements are true or false by placing the letter T (true) or F (false) on the line preceding the statement.

58. ____________ Diagnosis of vision loss of any type is done by testing the hearing using an audiometer.

59. ____________ Swimmer's ear goes away on its own and does not need to be treated.

60. ____________ Allergic rhinitis is another name for hay fever.

61. ____________ A patient with tonsillitis should be told to rest his voice and speak as little as possible.

COG AFF CASE STUDY FOR CRITICAL THINKING

Grade: __________

1. A patient calls in to the physician's office saying that pink eye is going around her son's school.
He has not been complaining of pain in either eye, but she has noticed that his eyes are red and that he has been sniffing and coughing lately. She wants to know if she should bring him in for a checkup. What should you tell her?

____

____

____

____

2. A patient is interested in getting LASIK surgery to correct her nearsightedness. She is 24 years old, and both of her parents have strong prescriptions for nearsightedness as well. She asks you what the surgery will be like, and if there is any chance that her eyes might revert back to their previous state. What is LASIK surgery and what are the advantages and disadvantages of this procedure? Are there any side effects?

____

____

____

____

3. A middle-aged patient comes in for a routine checkup and mentions a slight loss of hearing since the last exam. What tests would most likely be ordered by the physician to check his hearing? Are there any preventative education tips that you can give him about hearing loss?

____

____

____

____

4. A swimmer comes into the office complaining of recurrent swimmer's ear. She says she has used cotton swabs in the past to clear her ear canals, and asks if there is any particular medication she can apply to help keep her ear canals clean. How would you respond to this patient?

____

____

____

____

5. A young man comes in for a routine checkup and mentions that he will soon be learning to drive. However, the physician gives him the Ishihara test, and the teen fails to differentiate between colors. What information can you give him about color blindness, and what encouragement can you give him in regard to his upcoming driving test?

____

____

____

____

6. A young boy is brought in because he is complaining of headaches in school. The physician determines that the boy needs glasses and that the headaches are from eye strain. However, the boy states that he does not want glasses because he is afraid his classmates will make fun of him. What would you say to him?

____

____

____

____

PSY PROCEDURE 30-1 Measure Distance Visual Acuity with a Snellen Chart

Name: ______________________ **Date:** __________ **Time:** __________ **Grade:** __________

EQUIPMENT/SUPPLIES: Snellen eye chart, paper cup or eye paddle

STANDARDS: Given the needed equipment and a place to work, the student will perform this skill with _____ % accuracy in a total of _____ minutes. *(Your instructor will tell you what the percentage and time limits will be before you begin.)*

KEY: 4 = Satisfactory 0 = Unsatisfactory NA = This step is not counted

PROCEDURE STEPS	SELF	PARTNER	INSTRUCTOR
1. Wash your hands.	❏	❏	❏
2. Prepare the examination area (well lit, distance marker 20 feet from the chart).	❏	❏	❏
3. Make sure the chart is at eye level.	❏	❏	❏
4. Greet and identify the patient. Identify yourself and your title. Explain the procedure.	❏	❏	❏
5. AFF Explain how to respond to a patient who is hearing impaired.	❏	❏	❏
____			
____			
____			
____			
6. Position the patient in a standing or sitting position at the 20-foot marker.	❏	❏	❏
7. If he or she is not wearing glasses, ask the patient about contact lenses. Mark results accordingly.	❏	❏	❏
8. Have the patient cover the left eye with the eye paddle.	❏	❏	❏
9. Instruct the patient not to close the left eye, but to keep both eyes open during the test.	❏	❏	❏
10. Stand beside the chart and point to each row as the patient reads aloud. **a.** Point to the lines, starting with the 20/200 line. **b.** Record the smallest line that the patient can read with no errors.	❏	❏	❏

PSY PROCEDURE 30-1 Measure Distance Visual Acuity with a Snellen Chart (continued)

11. Repeat the procedure with the right eye covered and record.	❑	❑	❑
12. Wash your hands.	❑	❑	❑
13. AFF Log into the Electronic Medical Record (EMR) using your username and secure password OR obtain the paper medical record from a secure location and assure it is kept away from public access	❑	❑	❑
14. Record the procedure.	❑	❑	❑
15. When finished, log out of the EMR and/or replace the paper medical record in an appropriate and secure location.	❑	❑	❑

CALCULATION

Total Possible Points: __________

Total Points Earned: __________ Multiplied by 100 = __________ Divided by Total Possible Points = __________ %

PASS ❑ **FAIL** ❑ **COMMENTS:**

Student's signature ____________________ Date __________

Partner's signature ____________________ Date __________

Instructor's signature ____________________ Date __________

PSY PROCEDURE 30-2 Measuring Color Perception

Name: ______________________ **Date:** __________ **Time:** __________ **Grade:** __________

EQUIPMENT/SUPPLIES: Ishihara color plates, gloves

STANDARDS: Given the needed equipment and a place to work, the student will perform this skill with _____ % accuracy in a total of _____ minutes. *(Your instructor will tell you what the percentage and time limits will be before you begin.)*

KEY: 4 = Satisfactory 0 = Unsatisfactory NA = This step is not counted

PROCEDURE STEPS	SELF	PARTNER	INSTRUCTOR
1. Wash your hands, put on gloves, and obtain the Ishihara color plate book.	❑	❑	❑
2. Prepare the examination area (adequate lighting).	❑	❑	❑
3. Greet and identify the patient and yourself including your title. Explain the procedure.	❑	❑	❑
4. AFF Explain how to respond to a patient who is developmentally challenged.	❑	❑	❑
____ ____ ____ ____			
5. Hold the first bookplate about 30 inches from the patient.	❑	❑	❑
6. Ask if the patient can see the "number" within the series of dots. **a.** Record results of test by noting the number or figure the patient reports. **b.** If patient cannot distinguish a pattern, record plate number–x (e.g., 4–x).	❑	❑	❑
7. The patient should not take more than 3 seconds when reading the plates. **a.** The patient should not squint nor guess. These indicate that the patient is unsure. **b.** Record as plate number–x.	❑	❑	❑
8. Record the results for plates 1 through 10. **a.** Plate number 11 requires patient to trace a winding line between x's. **b.** Patients with a color deficit will not be able to trace the line.	❑	❑	❑

PSY PROCEDURE 30-2 Measuring Color Perception (continued)

9. Store the book in a closed, protected area to protect the integrity of the colors.	❑	❑	❑
10. Remove your gloves and wash your hands.	❑	❑	❑
11. AFF Log into the Electronic Medical Record (EMR) using your username and secure password OR obtain the paper medical record from a secure location and assure it is kept away from public access.	❑	❑	❑
12. Record the procedure in the medical record.	❑	❑	❑
13. When finished, log out of the EMR and/or replace the paper medical record in an appropriate and secure location.	❑	❑	❑

CALCULATION

Total Possible Points: __________

Total Points Earned: __________ Multiplied by 100 = __________ Divided by Total Possible Points = __________ %

PASS ❑ **FAIL** ❑ **COMMENTS:**

Student's signature ____________________ Date __________

Partner's signature ____________________ Date __________

Instructor's signature ____________________ Date __________

PSY PROCEDURE 30-3 Instilling Eye Medication

Name: ______________________ **Date:** __________ **Time:** __________ **Grade:** __________

EQUIPMENT/SUPPLIES: Physician's order and patient record, ophthalmic medications, 2 × 2 gauze pad, tissues, gloves

STANDARDS: Given the needed equipment and a place to work, the student will perform this skill with _____ % accuracy in a total of _____ minutes. *(Your instructor will tell you what the percentage and time limits will be before you begin.)*

KEY: 4 = Satisfactory 0 = Unsatisfactory NA = This step is not counted

PROCEDURE STEPS	SELF	PARTNER	INSTRUCTOR
1. Wash your hands.	❑	❑	❑
2. Obtain the physician order, the correct medication, sterile gauze, and tissues.	❑	❑	❑
3. Greet and identify the patient. Identify yourself including your title. Explain the procedure.	❑	❑	❑
4. Ask the patient about any allergies not recorded in the chart.	❑	❑	❑
5. AFF Explain how to respond to a patient who does not speak English.	❑	❑	❑

____

____

____

____

PROCEDURE STEPS	SELF	PARTNER	INSTRUCTOR
6. Position the patient comfortably. Position the patient comfortably.	❑	❑	❑
7. Put on gloves. Ask the patient to look upward.	❑	❑	❑
8. Use gauze to gently pull lower lid down. Instill the medication: **a.** Ointment **b.** Drops	❑	❑	❑
9. Release the lower lid. Have the patient gently close the eyelid and roll the eye.	❑	❑	❑
10. Wipe off any excess medication with tissue.	❑	❑	❑
11. Instruct patient to apply light pressure on the puncta lacrimalia for several minutes.	❑	❑	❑

PSY PROCEDURE 30-3 Instilling Eye Medication (continued)

12. Properly care for or dispose of equipment and supplies. Clean the work area.	❑	❑	❑
13. Wash your hands.	❑	❑	❑
14. AFF Log into the Electronic Medical Record (EMR) using your username and secure password OR obtain the paper medical record from a secure location and assure it is kept away from public access.	❑	❑	❑
15. Record the procedure.	❑	❑	❑
16. When finished, log out of the EMR and/or replace the paper medical record in an appropriate and secure location.	❑	❑	❑

CALCULATION

Total Possible Points: __________

Total Points Earned: __________ Multiplied by 100 = __________ Divided by Total Possible Points = __________ %

PASS ❑ **FAIL** ❑ **COMMENTS:**

Student's signature ____________________ Date __________

Partner's signature ____________________ Date __________

Instructor's signature ____________________ Date __________

PSY PROCEDURE 30-4 Irrigating the Eye

Name: ______________________ **Date:** __________ **Time:** __________ **Grade:** __________

EQUIPMENT/SUPPLIES: Physician's order and patient record, small basin, irrigating solution and medication if ordered, protective barrier or towels, emesis basin, sterile bulb syringe or 15- to 20-mL syringe, tissues, gloves

STANDARDS: Given the needed equipment and a place to work, the student will perform this skill with _____ % accuracy in a total of _____ minutes. *(Your instructor will tell you what the percentage and time limits will be before you begin.)*

KEY: 4 = Satisfactory 0 = Unsatisfactory NA = This step is not counted

PROCEDURE STEPS	SELF	PARTNER	INSTRUCTOR
1. Wash your hands and put on your gloves.	❑	❑	❑
2. Assemble the equipment, supplies, and medication if ordered by the physician. **a.** Check solution label three times. **b.** Make sure that the label indicates for ophthalmic use.	❑	❑	❑
3. Greet and identify the patient. Identify yourself and your title. Explain the procedure.	❑	❑	❑
4. AFF Explain how to respond to a patient who is hard of hearing. ____ ____ ____ ____	❑	❑	❑
5. Position the patient comfortably. **a.** Sitting with head tilted with the affected eye lower. **b.** Lying with the affected eye downward.	❑	❑	❑
6. Drape patient with the protective barrier or towel to avoid wetting the clothing.	❑	❑	❑
7. Place basin against upper cheek near eye with the towel under the basin. **a.** Wipe the eye from the inner canthus outward with gauze to remove debris. **b.** Separate the eyelids with your thumb and forefinger. **c.** Lightly support your hand, holding the syringe, on the bridge of the patient's nose.	❑	❑	❑

PSY PROCEDURE 30-4 · Irrigating the Eye (continued)

8. Holding syringe 1 inch above the eye, gently irrigate from inner to outer canthus. **a.** Use gentle pressure and do not touch the eye. **b.** The physician will order the period of time or amount of solution required.	❑	❑	❑
9. Use tissues to wipe any excess solution from the patient's face.	❑	❑	❑
10. Properly dispose of equipment or sanitize as recommended.	❑	❑	❑
11. Remove your gloves. Wash your hands.	❑	❑	❑
12. AFF Log into the Electronic Medical Record (EMR) using your username and secure password OR obtain the paper medical record from a secure location and assure it is kept away from public access.	❑	❑	❑
13. Record procedure, including amount, type, and strength of solution; which eye was irrigated; and any observations.	❑	❑	❑
14. When finished, log out of the EMR and/or replace the paper medical record in an appropriate and secure location.	❑	❑	❑

CALCULATION

Total Possible Points: __________

Total Points Earned: __________ Multiplied by 100 = __________ Divided by Total Possible Points = __________ %

PASS **FAIL** **COMMENTS:**

❑ ❑

Student's signature ____________________ Date __________

Partner's signature ____________________ Date __________

Instructor's signature ____________________ Date __________

PSY PROCEDURE 30-5 Irrigating the Ear

Name: ______________________ **Date:** __________ **Time:** __________ **Grade:** __________

EQUIPMENT/SUPPLIES: Physician's order and patient record, emesis basin or ear basin, waterproof barrier or towels, otoscope, irrigation solution, bowl for solution, gauze

STANDARDS: Given the needed equipment and a place to work, the student will perform this skill with _____ % accuracy in a total of _____ minutes. *(Your instructor will tell you what the percentage and time limits will be before you begin.)*

KEY: 4 = Satisfactory 0 = Unsatisfactory NA = This step is not counted

PROCEDURE STEPS	SELF	PARTNER	INSTRUCTOR
1. Wash your hands.	❑	❑	❑
2. Assemble the equipment and supplies.	❑	❑	❑
3. Greet and identify the patient. Identify yourself including your title. Explain the procedure.	❑	❑	❑
4. AFF Explain how to respond to a patient who has dementia.	❑	❑	❑
____________________ ____________________ ____________________ ____________________			
5. Position the patient comfortably in an erect position.	❑	❑	❑
6. View the affected ear with an otoscope to locate the foreign matter or cerumen. **a.** *Adults:* Gently pull up and back to straighten the auditory canal. **b.** *Children:* Gently pull slightly down and back to straighten the auditory canal.	❑	❑	❑
7. Drape the patient with a waterproof barrier or towel.	❑	❑	❑
8. Tilt the patient's head toward the affected side.	❑	❑	❑
9. Place the drainage basin under the affected ear.	❑	❑	❑
10. Fill the irrigating syringe or turn on the irrigating device	❑	❑	❑
11. Gently position the auricle as described above using your non-dominant hand.	❑	❑	❑

PSY PROCEDURE 30-5 Irrigating the Ear (continued)

12. With dominant hand, place the tip of the syringe into the auditory meatus.	❑	❑	❑
13. Direct the flow of the solution gently upward toward the roof of the canal.	❑	❑	❑
14. Irrigate for the prescribed period of time or until the desired results are obtained.	❑	❑	❑
15. Dry the patient's external ear with gauze.	❑	❑	❑
16. Inspect the ear with the otoscope to determine the results.	❑	❑	❑
17. Properly care for or dispose of equipment and supplies. Clean the work area.	❑	❑	❑
18. Wash your hands.	❑	❑	❑
19. AFF Log into the Electronic Medical Record (EMR) using your username and secure password OR obtain the paper medical record from a secure location and assure it is kept away from public access.	❑	❑	❑
20. Record the procedure in the patient's chart.	❑	❑	❑
21. When finished, log out of the EMR and/or replace the paper medical record in an appropriate and secure location.	❑	❑	❑

CALCULATION

Total Possible Points: __________

Total Points Earned: __________ Multiplied by 100 = __________ Divided by Total Possible Points = __________ %

PASS **FAIL** **COMMENTS:**

❑ ❑

Student's signature ____________________ Date __________

Partner's signature ____________________ Date __________

Instructor's signature ____________________ Date __________

PSY PROCEDURE 30-6 Perform an Audiometric Hearing Test

Name: ______________________ **Date:** __________ **Time:** __________ **Grade:** __________

EQUIPMENT/SUPPLIES: Audiometer, otoscope

STANDARDS: Given the needed equipment and a place to work, the student will perform this skill with _____ % accuracy in a total of _____ minutes. *(Your instructor will tell you what the percentage and time limits will be before you begin.)*

KEY: 4 = Satisfactory 0 = Unsatisfactory NA = This step is not counted

PROCEDURE STEPS	SELF	PARTNER	INSTRUCTOR
1. Wash your hands.	❑	❑	❑
2. Greet and identify the patient. Identify yourself and your title. Explain the procedure.	❑	❑	❑
3. AFF Explain how to respond to a patient who is visually impaired.	❑	❑	❑

____

____

____

____

PROCEDURE STEPS	SELF	PARTNER	INSTRUCTOR
4. Take patient to a quiet area or room for testing.	❑	❑	❑
5. Visually inspect the ear canal and tympanic membrane before the examination.	❑	❑	❑
6. Choose the correct size tip for the end of the audiometer.	❑	❑	❑
7. Attach a speculum to fit the patient's external auditory meatus.	❑	❑	❑
8. With the speculum in the ear canal, retract the pinna: **a.** *Adults:* Gently pull up and back to straighten the auditory canal. **b.** *Children:* Gently pull slightly down and back to straighten the auditory canal.	❑	❑	❑
9. Follow audiometer instrument directions for use: **a.** Screen right ear. **b.** Screen left ear.	❑	❑	❑
10. If the patient fails to respond at any frequency, rescreening is required.	❑	❑	❑
11. If the patient fails rescreening, notify the physician.	❑	❑	❑

PSY PROCEDURE 30-6 Perform an Audiometric Hearing Test
(continued)

12. AFF Log into the Electronic Medical Record (EMR) using your username and secure password OR obtain the paper medical record from a secure location and assure it is kept away from public access.	❏	❏	❏
13. Record the results in the medical record	❏	❏	❏
14. When finished, log out of the EMR and/or replace the paper medical record in an appropriate and secure location.	❏	❏	❏

CALCULATION

Total Possible Points: __________

Total Points Earned: __________ Multiplied by 100 = __________ Divided by Total Possible Points = __________ %

PASS ❏ **FAIL** ❏ **COMMENTS:**

Student's signature ____________________ Date __________

Partner's signature ____________________ Date __________

Instructor's signature ____________________ Date __________

PSY PROCEDURE 30-7 Instilling Ear Medication

Name: ______________________ **Date:** __________ **Time:** __________ **Grade:** __________

EQUIPMENT/SUPPLIES: Physician's order and patient record, otic medication with dropper, cotton balls

STANDARDS: Given the needed equipment and a place to work, the student will perform this skill with _____ % accuracy in a total of _____ minutes. *(Your instructor will tell you what the percentage and time limits will be before you begin.)*

KEY: 4 = Satisfactory 0 = Unsatisfactory NA = This step is not counted

PROCEDURE STEPS	SELF	PARTNER	INSTRUCTOR
1. Wash your hands.	❑	❑	❑
2. Assemble the equipment, supplies, and medication if ordered by the physician. **a.** Check solution label three times. **b.** Make sure that the label indicates for otic use.	❑	❑	❑
3. Greet and identify the patient. Identify yourself including your title. Explain the procedure.	❑	❑	❑
4. Ask patient about any allergies not documented.	❑	❑	❑
5. AFF Explain how to respond to a patient who does not speak English.	❑	❑	❑

____

____

____

____

PROCEDURE STEPS	SELF	PARTNER	INSTRUCTOR
6. Have the patient seated with the affected ear tilted upward.	❑	❑	❑
7. Draw up the ordered amount of medication. **a.** Adults: Pull the auricle slightly up and back to straighten the S-shaped canal. **b.** Children: Pull the auricle slightly down and back to straighten the S-shaped canal.	❑	❑	❑
8. Insert the tip of dropper without touching the patient's skin. **a.** Let the medication flow along the side of the canal. **b.** Have the patient sit or lie with affected ear upward for about 5 minutes.	❑	❑	❑
9. To keep medication in the canal, gently insert a moist cotton ball into the external auditory meatus.	❑	❑	❑

PSY PROCEDURE 30-7 Instilling Ear Medication (continued)

10. Properly care for or dispose of equipment and supplies. Clean the work area.	❑	❑	❑
11. Wash your hands.	❑	❑	❑
12. AFF Log into the Electronic Medical Record (EMR) using your username and secure password OR obtain the paper medical record from a secure location and assure it is kept away from public access.	❑	❑	❑
13. Record the procedure in the patient record.	❑	❑	❑
14. When finished, log out of the EMR and/or replace the paper medical record in an appropriate and secure location.	❑	❑	❑

CALCULATION

Total Possible Points: __________

Total Points Earned: __________ Multiplied by 100 = __________ Divided by Total Possible Points = __________ %

PASS ❑ **FAIL** ❑ **COMMENTS:**

Student's signature ____________________ Date __________

Partner's signature ____________________ Date __________

Instructor's signature ____________________ Date __________

PSY PROCEDURE 30-8 Instilling Nasal Medication

Name: ______________________ **Date:** __________ **Time:** __________ **Grade:** __________

EQUIPMENT/SUPPLIES: Physician's order and patient record; nasal medication, drops, or spray; tissues; gloves

STANDARDS: Given the needed equipment and a place to work, the student will perform this skill with _____ % accuracy in a total of _____ minutes. *(Your instructor will tell you what the percentage and time limits will be before you begin.)*

KEY: 4 = Satisfactory 0 = Unsatisfactory NA = This step is not counted

PROCEDURE STEPS	SELF	PARTNER	INSTRUCTOR
1. Wash your hands and put on gloves.	❑	❑	❑
2. Assemble the equipment and supplies. Check the medication label three times.	❑	❑	❑
3. Greet and identify the patient. Identify yourself including your title. Explain the procedure.	❑	❑	❑
4. Ask patient about any allergies not documented.	❑	❑	❑
5. AFF Explain how to respond to a patient who has dementia. ______________________________ ______________________________ ______________________________ ______________________________	❑	❑	❑
6. Position the patient in a comfortable recumbent position. **a.** Extend patient's head beyond edge of examination table. **b.** Or place a pillow under the patient's shoulders. **c.** Support the patient's neck to avoid strain as the head is tilted back.	❑	❑	❑
7. Administering nasal medication: **a.** Nasal drops **(1)** Hold the dropper upright just above each nostril. **(2)** Drop the medication one drop at a time without touching the nares. **(3)** Keep the patient in a recumbent position for 5 minutes. **b.** Nasal spray **(1)** Place tip of the bottle at the naris opening without touching the patient. **(2)** Spray as the patient takes a deep breath.	❑	❑	❑
8. Wipe any excess medication from the patient's skin with tissues.	❑	❑	❑

PSY PROCEDURE 30-8 Instilling Nasal Medication (continued)

9. Properly care for or dispose of equipment and supplies. Clean the work area.	❑	❑	❑
10. Remove your gloves and wash your hands.	❑	❑	❑
11. AFF Log into the Electronic Medical Record (EMR) using your username and secure password OR obtain the paper medical record from a secure location and assure it is kept away from public access.	❑	❑	❑
12. Record the procedure in the patient's chart.	❑	❑	❑
13. When finished, log out of the EMR and/or replace the paper medical record in an appropriate and secure location.	❑	❑	❑

CALCULATION

Total Possible Points: __________

Total Points Earned: __________ Multiplied by 100 = __________ Divided by Total Possible Points = __________ %

PASS ❑ **FAIL** ❑ **COMMENTS:**

Student's signature ____________________ Date __________

Partner's signature ____________________ Date __________

Instructor's signature ____________________ Date __________

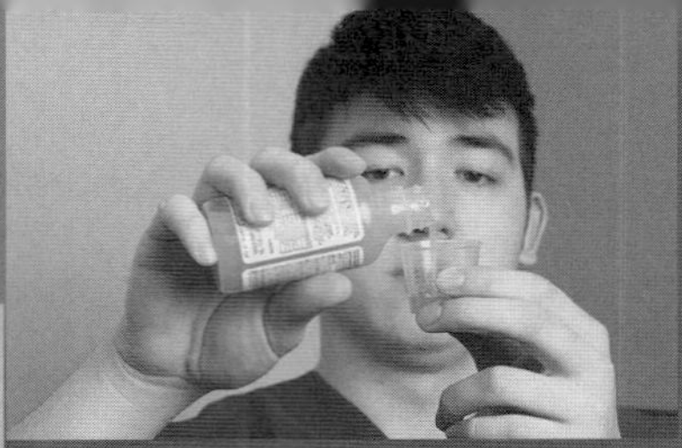

CHAPTER

31 Pulmonary Medicine

Learning Outcomes

COG Cognitive Domain

1. Spell key terms
2. Define medical terms and abbreviations related to all body systems
3. Describe structural organization of the human body
4. List major organs in each body system
5. Identify the anatomical location of major organs in each body system
6. Describe the normal function of each body system
7. Identify common pathology related to each body system including signs, symptoms, and etiology
   a. Identify the primary defense mechanisms of the respiratory system
   b. Identify and explain diagnostic procedures of the respiratory system
   c. Describe the physician's examination of the respiratory system
8. Discuss the role of the medical assistant with regard to various diagnostic and therapeutic procedures

PSY Psychomotor Domain

1. Instruct a patient in the use of the peak flow meter (Procedure 31-1)
2. Administer a nebulized breathing treatment (Procedure 31-2)
3. Collecting a Sputum Specimen (Procedure 31-3)
4. Perform a pulmonary function test (Procedure 31-4)

AFF Affective Domain

1. Incorporate critical thinking skills when performing patient assessment
2. Incorporate critical thinking skills when performing patient care
3. Show awareness of a patient's concerns related to the procedure being performed
4. Demonstrate empathy, active listening, nonverbal communication
5. Demonstrate respect for individual diversity including gender, race, religion, age, economic status, appearance
6. Explain to a patient the rationale for performance of a procedure
7. Demonstrate sensitivity to patient rights
8. Protect the integrity of the medical record

ABHES Competencies

1. Assist the physician with the regimen of diagnostic and treatment modalities as they relate to each body system
2. Comply with federal, state, and local health laws and regulations
3. Communicate on the recipient's level of comprehension
4. Serve as a liaison between the physician and others
5. Show empathy and impartiality when dealing with patients
6. Document accurately

4. Your patient has just been diagnosed with tuberculosis. Explain to him ways in which he should act to protect others while he undergoes treatment.

____

____

____

5. A healthy patient worries that his exposure to secondhand smoke of his coworkers might cause his health to deteriorate. You are aware of research suggesting that this is so; however, much of the research is controversial. How would you advise the patient?

____

____

____

6. A patient has just been diagnosed with lung cancer that the physician described as "not terribly aggressive and potentially curable." The patient asks you if this means that he will be okay. How do you respond?

____

____

____

PSY PROCEDURE 31-1 Instruct a Patient on Using the Peak Flow Meter

Name: ________________ **Date:** ________ **Time:** ________ **Grade:** ________

EQUIPMENT/SUPPLIES: Peak flow meter, recording documentation form

STANDARDS: Given the needed equipment and a place to work, the student will perform this skill with _____ % accuracy in a total of _____ minutes. *(Your instructor will tell you what the percentage and time limits will be before you begin.)*

KEY: 4 = Satisfactory 0 = Unsatisfactory NA = This step is not counted

PROCEDURE STEPS	SELF	PARTNER	INSTRUCTOR
1. Wash your hands.	❑	❑	❑
2. Assemble the peak flow meter, disposable mouthpiece, and patient documentation form.	❑	❑	❑
3. Greet and identify the patient. Identify yourself including your title and explain the procedure.	❑	❑	❑
4. Holding the peak flow meter upright, explain how to read and reset the gauge after each reading.	❑	❑	❑
5. AFF Explain how to respond to a patient who is visually impaired.	❑	❑	❑
____			
____			
____			
____			
6. Instruct the patient to place the peak flow meter mouthpiece into the mouth, forming a tight seal with the lips. After taking a deep breath, the patient should blow hard into the mouthpiece without blocking the back of the flow meter.	❑	❑	❑
7. Note the number on the flow meter denoting the level at which the sliding gauge stopped after the hard blowing into the mouthpiece. Reset the gauge to zero.	❑	❑	❑
8. Instruct the patient to perform this procedure a total of three times consecutively, in both the morning and at night, and to record the highest reading on the form.	❑	❑	❑
9. Explain to the patient the procedure for cleaning the mouthpiece of the flow meter by washing with soapy water and rinsing without immersing the flow meter in water.	❑	❑	❑

PSY PROCEDURE 31-1 Instruct a Patient on Using the Peak Flow Meter (continued)

10. AFF Log into the Electronic Medical Record (EMR) using your username and secure password OR obtain the paper medical record from a secure location and assure it is kept away from public access.	❑	❑	❑
11. Record the procedure including the name of the medication and the patient's response.	❑	❑	❑
12. When finished, log out of the EMR and/or replace the paper medical record in an appropriate and secure location.	❑	❑	❑

CALCULATION

Total Possible Points: __________

Total Points Earned: __________ Multiplied by 100 = __________ Divided by Total Possible Points = __________ %

PASS ❑ **FAIL** ❑ **COMMENTS:**

Student's signature ____________________ Date __________

Partner's signature ____________________ Date __________

Instructor's signature ____________________ Date __________

PSY PROCEDURE 31-2 Perform a Nebulized Breathing Treatment

Name: ______________________ **Date:** __________ **Time:** __________ **Grade:** __________

EQUIPMENT/SUPPLIES: Physician's order and patient's medical record, inhalation medication, nebulizer disposable setup, nebulizer machine

STANDARDS: Given the needed equipment and a place to work, the student will perform this skill with _____ % accuracy in a total of _____ minutes. *(Your instructor will tell you what the percentage and time limits will be before you begin.)*

KEY: 4 = Satisfactory 0 = Unsatisfactory NA = This step is not counted

PROCEDURE STEPS	SELF	PARTNER	INSTRUCTOR
1. Wash your hands.	❑	❑	❑
2. Assemble the equipment and medication, checking the medication label three times as indicated when administering any medications.	❑	❑	❑
3. Greet and identify the patient. Identify yourself including your title and explain the procedure.	❑	❑	❑
4. AFF Explain how you would respond to a patient who is deaf.	❑	❑	❑
____			
____			
____			
____			
5. Remove the nebulizer treatment cup from the setup and add the medication ordered by the physician.	❑	❑	❑
6. Place the top on the cup securely, attach the "T" piece to the top of the cup, and position the mouthpiece firmly on one end of the "T" piece.	❑	❑	❑
7. Attach one end of the tubing securely to the connector on the cup and the other end to the connector on the nebulizer machine.	❑	❑	❑
8. Ask the patient to place the mouthpiece into the mouth and make a seal with the lips, without biting the mouthpiece. Instruct the patient to breathe normally during the treatment, occasionally taking a deep breath.	❑	❑	❑
9. Turn the machine on using the on/off switch. The medication in the reservoir cup will become a fine mist that is inhaled by the patient breathing through the mouthpiece.	❑	❑	❑

PSY PROCEDURE 31-2 Perform a Nebulized Breathing Treatment (continued)

10. Before, during, and after the breathing treatment, take and record the patient's pulse.	❑	❑	❑
11. When the treatment is over and the medication is gone from the cup, turn the machine off and have the patient remove the mouthpiece.	❑	❑	❑
12. Disconnect the disposable treatment setup and dispose of all parts into a biohazard container. Properly put away the machine.	❑	❑	❑
13. Wash your hands.	❑	❑	❑
14. AFF Log into the Electronic Medical Record (EMR) using your username and secure password OR obtain the paper medical record from a secure location and assure it is kept away from public access.	❑	❑	❑
15. Record the procedure including the name of the medication and the patient's pulse before, during, and after the treatment.	❑	❑	❑
16. When finished, log out of the EMR and/or replace the paper medical record in an appropriate and secure location.	❑	❑	❑

CALCULATION

Total Possible Points: __________

Total Points Earned: __________ Multiplied by 100 = __________ Divided by Total Possible Points = __________ %

PASS ❑ **FAIL** ❑ **COMMENTS:**

Student's signature ____________________ Date __________

Partner's signature ____________________ Date __________

Instructor's signature ____________________ Date __________

PSY PROCEDURE 31-3 Collect a Sputum Specimen

Name: ______________________ **Date:** __________ **Time:** __________ **Grade:** __________

EQUIPMENT/SUPPLIES: Physician order, patient's medical record, sterile specimen container, gloves, biohazard transport bag, laboratory request

STANDARDS: Given the needed equipment and a place to work, the student will perform this skill with _____ % accuracy in a total of _____ minutes. *(Your instructor will tell you what the percentage and time limits will be before you begin.)*

KEY: 4 = Satisfactory 0 = Unsatisfactory NA = This step is not counted

PROCEDURE STEPS	SELF	PARTNER	INSTRUCTOR
1. Wash your hands.	❑	❑	❑
2. Assemble the equipment.	❑	❑	❑
3. Greet and identify the patient. Identify yourself including your title and explain the procedure.	❑	❑	❑
4. AFF Explain how to respond to a patient whose first language is not English.	❑	❑	❑
____ ____ ____ ____			
5. Provide the patient with a cup of water and instruct him or her to rinse the mouth with water.	❑	❑	❑
6. Ask the patient to cough deeply, using the abdominal muscles as well as the accessory muscles to bring secretions from the lungs and not just the upper airway.	❑	❑	❑
7. Instruct the patient to expectorate the specimen directly into the container without touching the inside of the container with the lips or tongue and without getting the specimen on the outside of the container.	❑	❑	❑
8. When the specimen is in the container, apply gloves and after taking the container from the patient, cap the container immediately and place into a biohazard bag for transport to the laboratory with a laboratory requisition.	❑	❑	❑
9. Once the specimen has been routed to the laboratory, remove your gloves and wash your hands.	❑	❑	❑

PSY PROCEDURE 31-3 Collect a Sputum Specimen (continued)

10. AFF Log into the Electronic Medical Record (EMR) using your username and secure password OR obtain the paper medical record from a secure location and assure it is kept away from public access.	❑	❑	❑
11. Record the procedure including the name of the medication and the patient's pulse before, during, and after the treatment.	❑	❑	❑
12. When finished, log out of the EMR and/or replace the paper medical record in an appropriate and secure location.	❑	❑	❑

CALCULATION

Total Possible Points: __________

Total Points Earned: __________ Multiplied by 100 = __________ Divided by Total Possible Points = __________ %

PASS ❑ **FAIL** ❑ **COMMENTS:**

Student's signature ____________________ Date __________

Partner's signature ____________________ Date __________

Instructor's signature ____________________ Date __________

PSY PROCEDURE 31-4 Perform a Pulmonary Function Test

Name: ______________________ **Date:** __________ **Time:** __________ **Grade:** __________

EQUIPMENT/SUPPLIES: Physician's order and patient's medical record, spirometer and appropriate cables, calibration syringe and log book, disposable mouthpiece, printer, nose clip

STANDARDS: Given the needed equipment and a place to work, the student will perform this skill with _____ % accuracy in a total of _____ minutes. *(Your instructor will tell you what the percentage and time limits will be before you begin.)*

KEY: 4 = Satisfactory 0 = Unsatisfactory NA = This step is not counted

PROCEDURE STEPS	SELF	PARTNER	INSTRUCTOR
1. Wash your hands.	❑	❑	❑
2. Assemble the equipment.	❑	❑	❑
3. Greet and identify the patient. Identify yourself including your title and explain the procedure.	❑	❑	❑
4. AFF Explain how to respond to a patient who has dementia.	❑	❑	❑
5. Turn the PFT machine on, and if the spirometer has not been calibrated according to the office policy, calibrate the machine using the calibration syringe according to the manufacturer's instructions, and record the calibration in the appropriate logbook.	❑	❑	❑
6. With the machine on and calibrated, attach the appropriate cable, tubing, and mouthpiece for the type of machine being used.	❑	❑	❑
7. Using the keyboard on the machine, input patient data into the machine including the patient's name or identification number, age, weight, height, sex, race, and smoking history.	❑	❑	❑
8. Ask the patient to remove any restrictive clothing, such as a necktie, and instruct the patient in applying the nose clip.	❑	❑	❑
9. Ask the patient to stand, breathe in deeply, and blow into the mouthpiece as hard as possible. He or she should continue to blow into the mouthpiece until the machine indicates that it is appropriate to stop blowing. A chair should be available in case the patient becomes dizzy or lightheaded.	❑	❑	❑
10. Continue the procedure until three adequate readings or maneuvers are performed.	❑	❑	❑
11. Properly care for the equipment and dispose of the mouthpiece into the biohazard container.	❑	❑	❑
12. Wash your hands.	❑	❑	❑

PSY PROCEDURE 31-4 Perform a Pulmonary Function Test
(continued)

13. AFF Log into the Electronic Medical Record (EMR) using your username and secure password OR obtain the paper medical record from a secure location and assure it is kept away from public access.	❑	❑	❑
14. Record the procedure including the patient's response.	❑	❑	❑
15. Print and/or scan the results and place into the medical record.	❑	❑	❑
16. When finished, log out of the EMR and/or replace the paper medical record in an appropriate and a secure location.	❑	❑	❑

CALCULATION

Total Possible Points: __________

Total Points Earned: __________ Multiplied by 100 = __________ Divided by Total Possible Points = __________ %

PASS ❑ **FAIL** ❑ **COMMENTS:**

Student's signature ____________________ Date __________

Partner's signature ____________________ Date __________

Instructor's signature ____________________ Date __________

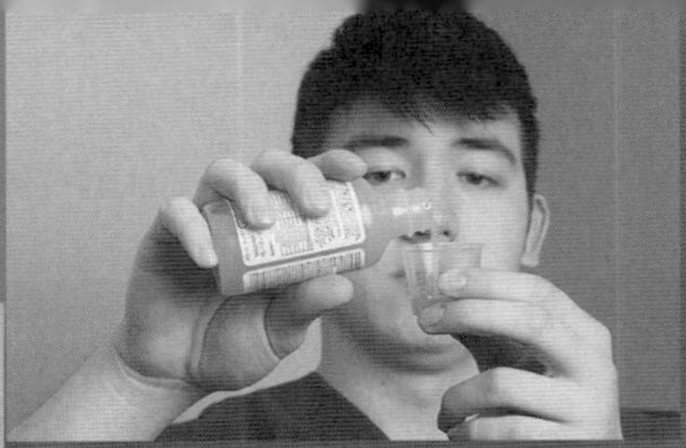

CHAPTER

32 Cardiology

Learning Outcomes

COG Cognitive Domain

1. Spell key terms
2. Define medical terms and abbreviations related to all body systems
3. Describe structural organization of the human body
4. List major organs in each body system
5. Identify the anatomical location of major organs in each body system
6. Describe the normal function of each body system
7. Identify common pathology related to each body system including signs, symptoms, and etiology
   a. List and describe common cardiovascular disorders
   b. Identify and explain common cardiovascular procedures and tests
8. Describe the roles and responsibilities of the medical assistant during cardiovascular examinations and procedures
9. Discuss the information recorded on a basic 12-lead electrocardiogram
10. Explain the purpose of a Holter monitor

PSY Psychomotor Domain

1. Perform electrocardiography (Procedure 32-1)
2. Apply a Holter monitor for a 24-hour test (Procedure 32-2)

AFF Affective Domain

1. Incorporate critical thinking skills when performing patient assessment
2. Incorporate critical thinking skills when performing patient care
3. Show awareness of a patient's concerns related to the procedure being performed
4. Demonstrate empathy, active listening, nonverbal communication
5. Demonstrate respect for individual diversity including gender, race, religion, age, economic status, appearance
6. Explain to a patient the rationale for performance of a procedure
7. Demonstrate sensitivity to patient rights
8. Protect the integrity of the medical record

ABHES Competencies

1. Assist the physician with the regimen of diagnostic and treatment modalities as they relate to each body system
2. Perform electrocardiograms
3. Comply with federal, state, and local health laws and regulations
4. Communicate on the recipient's level of comprehension
5. Serve as a liaison between the physician and others
6. Show empathy and impartiality when dealing with patients
7. Document accurately

55. Which of the following is a question you should ask the patient before a cardiovascular examination?

a. Are you currently pregnant?

b. How long have you had the pain/discomfort?

c. How often do you exercise?

d. What do you like to do in your free time?

56. A Holter monitor is used for:

a. the diagnosis of intermittent cardiac arrhythmias and dysfunctions.

b. obtaining a good-quality ECG without avoidable artifacts.

c. obtaining basic information about the anatomical location and gross structures of the heart, great vessels, and lungs.

d. measuring the response of the cardiac muscle to increased demands for oxygen.

57. Read the risk factors for developing thrombi below and indicate whether the risk factor is primary (P), or inherited, versus secondary (S), or acquired.

a. ______________ hemolytic anemia

b. ______________ long-term immobility

c. ______________ chronic pulmonary disease

d. ______________ thrombophlebitis

e. ______________ sickle cell disease

f. ______________ varicosities

g. ______________ defibrillation after cardiac arrest

58. Identify whether each description describes lead I, lead II, or lead III:

a. ______________ measures the difference in electrical potential between the right arm (RA) and the left leg (LL).

b. ______________ measures the difference in electrical potential between the right arm (RA) and the left arm (LA).

c. ______________ measures the difference in electrical potential between the left arm (LA) and the left leg (LL).

COG SHORT ANSWER

Grade: ____________

59. List five symptoms of the various heart disorders.

____

____

____

____

60. List the four causes of congestive heart failure.

61. Explain how a pacemaker helps the heart maintain normal sinus rhythm.

62. List six potential causes of anemia.

63. Explain angiography, one of the procedures used to diagnose atherosclerosis.

64. Explain why a physician often requires several blood pressure readings before making the diagnosis of hypertension.

65. List the six elements that are taken into consideration during the ECG.

66. Explain the role of the medical assistant during an ECG.

COG TRUE OR FALSE?

Grade: __________

Indicate whether the statements are true or false by placing the letter T (true) or F (false) on the line preceding the statement.

67. ____________ Congestive heart failure (CHF) is a condition in which the heart cannot pump effectively.

68. ____________ Ventricular fibrillation is a medical emergency that occurs when the heart is contracting rather than quivering in an organized fashion.

69. ____________ Diagnosis of atherosclerosis is often made by electrocardiography.

70. ____________ Patients who have cerebrovascular accidents usually have varying degrees of weakness or paralysis of one side of the body.

COG AFF CASE STUDY FOR CRITICAL THINKING

Grade: __________

1. You are interviewing a patient prior to a physical examination of the cardiovascular system. This is his first time in a medical office after many years' absence, and he is considerably anxious. What do you say to him to calm him down? How would you explain the procedure?

____

____

____

____

2. A patient comes into the office complaining of chest pain, nausea, and vomiting. Will he likely be admitted to the hospital right away? Why or why not?

____

____

____

____

3. A patient is given an artificial pacemaker. She would like to know how the device works and what changes she can expect from it. What do you tell her?

____

____

____

____

4. Why is it important that a patient continue taking her prescribed antihypertensive medication, even if her blood pressure has reached a manageable level?

____

____

____

____

5. Many cardiac conditions are preventable with proper diet and exercise. It's important to stress prevention over cure, because in most instances, there is no quick "cure." How will you send this message to patients? What kinds of tools will you use?

____

____

____

____

PSY PROCEDURE 32-1 Perform a 12-Lead Electrocardiogram

Name: ______________________________ **Date:** __________ **Time:** __________ **Grade:** __________

EQUIPMENT/SUPPLIES: Physician order, ECG machine with cable and lead wires, ECG paper, disposable electrodes that contain coupling gel, patient gown and drape, skin preparation materials including a razor and antiseptic wipes

STANDARDS: Given the needed equipment and a place to work, the student will perform this skill with _____ % accuracy in a total of _____ minutes. *(Your instructor will tell you what the percentage and time limits will be before you begin.)*

KEY: 4 = Satisfactory 0 = Unsatisfactory NA = This step is not counted

PROCEDURE STEPS	SELF	PARTNER	INSTRUCTOR
1. Wash your hands.	❑	❑	❑
2. Assemble the equipment.	❑	❑	❑
3. Greet and identify the patient. Identify yourself including your title and explain the procedure.	❑	❑	❑
4. Turn the ECG machine on and enter appropriate data into it. Include the patient's name and/or identification number, age, sex, height, weight, blood pressure, and medications.	❑	❑	❑
5. Instruct the patient to disrobe above the waist. **a.** Provide a gown for privacy. **b.** Female patients should also be instructed to remove any nylons or tights.	❑	❑	❑
6. Position patient comfortably in a supine position. **a.** Provide pillows as needed for comfort. **b.** Drape the patient for warmth and privacy.	❑	❑	❑
7. Prepare the skin as needed. **a.** Wipe away skin oil and lotions with the antiseptic wipes. **b.** Shave hair that will interfere with good contact between skin and electrodes.	❑	❑	❑
8. Apply the electrodes: **a.** Arms and legs: snugly against the fleshy, muscular parts of upper arms and lower legs according to the manufacturer's directions. **b.** Chest: V_1 through V_6.	❑	❑	❑
9. Connect the lead wires securely according to the color codes. **a.** Untangle the wires before applying them to prevent electrical artifacts. **b.** Each lead must lie unencumbered along the contours of the patient's body to decrease the incidence of artifacts. **c.** Double check the placement.	❑	❑	❑
10. Determine the sensitivity and paper speed settings on the ECG machine.	❑	❑	❑
11. Depress the automatic button on the ECG machine to obtain the 12-lead ECG.	❑	❑	❑
12. When the tracing is printed, check the ECG for artifacts and standardization mark.	❑	❑	❑

PSY PROCEDURE 32-1 Perform a 12-Lead Electrocardiogram (continued)

13. If the tracing is adequate, turn off the machine. **a.** Remove the electrodes from the patient's skin. **b.** Assist the patient to a sitting position and help him or her with dressing if needed.	❑	❑	❑
14. AFF Explain how to respond to a patient who has dementia. ________________ ________________ ________________ ________________	❑	❑	❑
15. For a single-channel machine, roll the ECG strip. **a.** Do not secure the roll with clips. **b.** This ECG will need to be mounted on an 8 × 11-inch paper or form.	❑	❑	❑
16. Discard disposable electrodes appropriately and put away the EKG machine. Wash your hands.	❑	❑	❑
17. AFF Log into the Electronic Medical Record (EMR) using your username and secure password OR obtain the paper medical record from a secure location and assure it is kept away from public access.	❑	❑	❑
18. Record the procedure.	❑	❑	❑
19. Place the printed results in the medical record or scan into the electronic medical record if appropriate.	❑	❑	❑
20. Let the physician know that the ECG has been completed and is ready for review.	❑	❑	❑
21. When finished, log out of the EMR and/or replace the paper medical record in an appropriate and secure location.	❑	❑	❑

CALCULATION

Total Possible Points: __________

Total Points Earned: __________ Multiplied by 100 = __________ Divided by Total Possible Points = __________ %

PASS ❑ **FAIL** ❑ **COMMENTS:**

Student's signature ____________________ Date __________

Partner's signature ____________________ Date __________

Instructor's signature ____________________ Date __________

PSY PROCEDURE 32-2 Apply a Holter Monitor for a 24-Hour Test

Name: ______________________ **Date:** __________ **Time:** __________ **Grade:** __________

EQUIPMENT/SUPPLIES: Physician's order, Holter monitor with appropriate lead wires, fresh batteries, carrying case with strap, disposable electrodes that contain coupling gel, adhesive tape, patient gown and drape, skin preparation materials including a razor and antiseptic wipes, patient diary

STANDARDS: Given the needed equipment and a place to work, the student will perform this skill with _____ % accuracy in a total of _____ minutes. *(Your instructor will tell you what the percentage and time limits will be before you begin.)*

KEY: 4 = Satisfactory 0 = Unsatisfactory NA = This step is not counted

PROCEDURE STEPS	SELF	PARTNER	INSTRUCTOR
1. Wash your hands.	❑	❑	❑
2. Assemble the equipment.	❑	❑	❑
3. Greet and identify the patient. Identify yourself including your title and explain the procedure.	❑	❑	❑
4. Explain the importance of carrying out all normal activities during the monitoring and the reason for the incident diary. Emphasize the need to use the diary at all times during the test.	❑	❑	❑
5. Ask the patient to remove all clothing from the waist up; gown and drape appropriately for privacy.	❑	❑	❑
6. Prepare the patient's skin for electrode attachment. **a.** Provide privacy and have the patient in a sitting position. **b.** Shave the skin if necessary and cleanse with antiseptic wipes.	❑	❑	❑
7. Apply the Holter electrodes at the specified sites: **a.** The right manubrium border. **b.** The left manubrium border. **c.** The right sternal border at the fifth rib level. **d.** The fifth rib at the anterior axillary line. **e.** The right lower rib cage over the cartilage as a ground lead.	❑	❑	❑
8. To do this, expose the adhesive backing of the electrodes and follow the manufacturer's instructions to attach each firmly. Check the security of the attachments.	❑	❑	❑
9. Position electrode connectors downward toward the patient's feet.	❑	❑	❑
10. Attach the lead wires and secure with adhesive tape.	❑	❑	❑
11. Connect the cable and run a baseline ECG by hooking the Holter monitor to the ECG machine with the cable hookup.	❑	❑	❑
12. Assist the patient to carefully redress with the cable extending through the garment opening. *Note:* Instruct the patient that clothing that buttons down the front is more convenient.	❑	❑	❑

PSY PROCEDURE 32-2 Apply a Holter Monitor for a 24-Hour Test (continued)

13. Plug the cable into the recorder and mark the diary. **a.** If needed, explain the purpose of the diary to the patient again. **b.** Give instructions for a return appointment to evaluate the recording and the diary.	❑	❑	❑
14. Wash your hands.	❑	❑	❑
15. AFF Log into the Electronic Medical Record (EMR) using your user-name and secure password OR obtain the paper medical record from a secure location and assure it is kept away from public access.	❑	❑	❑
16. Record the procedure.	❑	❑	❑
17. When finished, log out of the EMR and/or replace the paper medical record in an appropriate and secure location.	❑	❑	❑

CALCULATION

Total Possible Points: __________

Total Points Earned: __________ Multiplied by 100 = __________ Divided by Total Possible Points = __________ %

PASS ❑ **FAIL** ❑ **COMMENTS:**

Student's signature ____________________ Date __________

Partner's signature ____________________ Date __________

Instructor's signature ____________________ Date __________

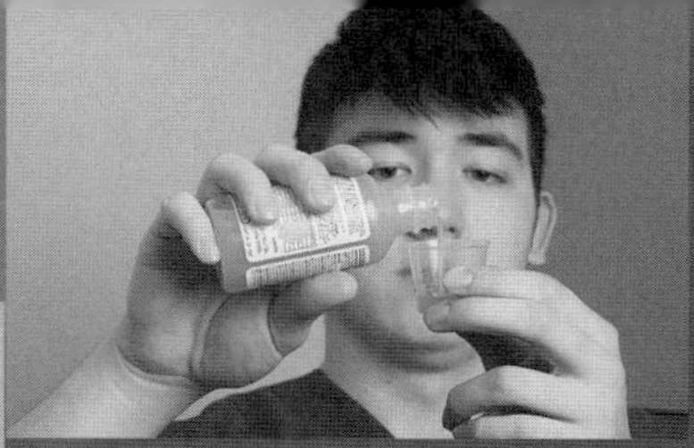

CHAPTER

33 Gastroenterology

Learning Outcomes

COG Cognitive Domain

1. Spell key terms
2. Define medical terms and abbreviations related to all body systems
3. Describe structural organization of the human body
4. List major organs in each body system
5. Identify the anatomical location of major organs in each body system
6. Describe the normal function of each body system
7. Identify common pathology related to each body system including signs, symptoms, and etiology
   a. List and describe common disorders of the alimentary canal and accessory organs
   b. Identify and explain the purpose of common procedures and tests associated with the gastrointestinal system
8. Describe the roles and responsibilities of the medical assistant in diagnosing and treating disorders of the gastrointestinal system

PSY Psychomotor Domain

1. Assist with colon procedures (Procedure 33-1)
2. Test stool specimen for occult blood: Guaiac method (Procedure 33-2)

AFF Affective Domain

1. Incorporate critical thinking skills when performing patient assessment
2. Incorporate critical thinking skills when performing patient care
3. Show awareness of a patient's concerns related to the procedure being performed
4. Demonstrate empathy, active listening, nonverbal communication
5. Demonstrate respect for individual diversity including gender, race, religion, age, economic status, appearance
6. Explain to a patient the rationale for performance of a procedure
7. Demonstrate sensitivity to patient rights
8. Protect the integrity of the medical record

ABHES Competencies

1. Assist the physician with the regimen of diagnostic and treatment modalities as they relate to each body system
2. Prepare the patient for examinations and treatments
3. Recognize and understand various treatment protocols
4. Comply with federal, state, and local health laws and regulations
5. Communicate on the recipient's level of comprehension
6. Serve as a liaison between the physician and others
7. Show empathy and impartiality when dealing with patients
8. Document accurately

Name: ______________________ Date: ____________ Grade: ____________

COG MULTIPLE CHOICE

Circle the letter preceding the correct answer.

1. Which of the following can trigger an outbreak of the herpes simplex virus?
a. Food allergy
b. Illness
c. Lack of sleep
d. Medication
e. Poor diet

2. What commonly causes leukoplakia to develop?
a. Hereditary genes
b. Excessive alcohol intake
c. Lack of exercise
d. Tobacco irritation
e. Obesity

3. Why should a patient complaining of heartburn be assessed immediately?
a. The symptoms of gastroesophageal reflux disease may be similar to the chest pain of a patient with cardiac problems.
b. A patient with heartburn is more likely to develop a serious heart condition.
c. Heartburn is a symptom of a weak lower esophageal sphincter.
d. It is important to assess any gastrointestinal disorder immediately because they are usually serious.
e. Heartburn may be symptomatic of Barrett esophagus, which requires immediate surgery.

4. Abnormal contact between the upper teeth and lower teeth is:
a. malocclusion.
b. dental caries.
c. stomatitis.
d. candidiasis.
e. gingivitis.

5. If a patient is suffering from peptic ulcers, the symptoms will be most severe when the patient:
a. is hungry.
b. has a bowel movement.
c. lies on his back.
d. chews his food.
e. is digesting a meal.

6. Gastroenteritis could become life threatening if a patient:
a. is pregnant.
b. suffers from diabetes mellitus.
c. needs a heart operation.
d. consumes excess alcohol.
e. does not receive treatment immediately.

7. The study of morbid obesity is called:
a. orthodontistry.
b. gerontology.
c. bariatrics.
d. gastroenterology.
e. pediatrics.

8. What is the minimum body mass index that a patient must have to be considered for gastric bypass surgery?
a. 25
b. 30
c. 35
d. 40
e. 45

9. Crohn disease becomes life threatening when:
a. the bowel walls become inflamed and the lymph nodes enlarge.
b. the fluid from the intestinal contents cannot be absorbed.
c. edema of the bowel wall takes place.
d. scarring narrows the colon and obstructs the bowel.
e. patients have periods of constipation, anorexia, and fever.

10. How does irritable bowel syndrome differ from Crohn disease?
a. It does not involve weight loss.
b. It is easily treatable.
c. It is thought to be genetic.
d. It requires a colectomy.
e. It causes scarring.

Scenario for questions 11 and 12: A patient is diagnosed with diverticulitis.

11. Which of the following treatments would the physician most likely recommend?
a. Antibiotics
b. Bed rest
c. Antifungal agent
d. Bland food
e. Drinking less water

12. What advice might the physician have you give to the patient to help maintain good bowel habits in future?
a. Never eat spicy foods.
b. Get some form of daily exercise.
c. Try to force a bowel movement at least once a day.
d. Use laxatives when suffering from constipation.
e. Cut out food products that contain wheat.

13. How can a patient decrease his or her risk of developing a hernia?
a. Avoid lifting heavy objects.
b. Switch from processed to organic foods.
c. Maintain good bowel habits.
d. Have regular medical checkups.
e. Walk at least a mile every day.

14. What is the most effective treatment for appendicitis?
a. Antibiotics
b. Ileostomy
c. Appendectomy
d. Cryosurgery
e. Radiation

15. Which of these factors increases the production of intestinal gas?
a. Excess water
b. Spicy or fatty foods
c. Peristalsis
d. Fast metabolism
e. Lack of exercise

16. The most likely method of contracting hepatitis B is:
a. contaminated food.
b. poor hygiene.
c. contaminated blood.
d. stagnant water.
e. weak immune system.

17. For which of the following procedures would the patient usually be put under anesthesia?
a. Anoscopy
b. Sigmoidoscopy
c. Nuclear imaging
d. Ultrasonography
e. Endoscopic retrograde cholangiopancreatography

18. What is the caustic chemical secreted by the lining of the stomach that may cause erosion if too much of it is secreted?
a. Pepsin
b. Hydrochloric acid
c. Insulin
d. Oral mucosa
e. Melena

19. How does lithotripsy break down gallstones to make them easy to pass?
a. Lasers
b. Sound waves
c. Acidic liquid
d. Heat
e. Air pressure

20. Which piece of advice could best be given to a patient with a malabsorption syndrome by the physician?
a. Drink more water.
b. Eat less processed food.
c. Take vitamin supplements.
d. Cut out spicy foods.
e. Exercise more often.

21. Which of these groups of people are at the highest risk of developing esophageal cancer?
a. Teenagers
b. Pregnant women
c. Young children
d. Elderly women
e. Elderly men

22. A male patient comes to the physician's office complaining of an acute pain in his upper abdomen and back. He also suffers from indigestion and nausea, particularly when he tries to eat foods that have a high fat content. Which of the following gastrointestinal disorders does the patient probably have?
a. Cholelithiasis
b. Peptic ulcers
c. Gastritis
d. Leukoplakia
e. Caries

COG MATCHING

Grade: ______

Place the letter preceding the definition on the line next to the term.

Key Terms

23. ______ anorexia
24. ______ ascites
25. ______ dysphagia
26. ______ guaiac
27. ______ hematemesis
28. ______ hepatomegaly
29. ______ hepatotoxin
30. ______ insufflator
31. ______ leukoplakia
32. ______ malocclusion
33. ______ melena
34. ______ metabolism
35. ______ obturator
36. ______ peristalsis
37. ______ sclerotherapy
38. ______ stomatitis
39. ______ turgor

Definitions

a. an enlarged liver
b. a substance used in a laboratory test for occult blood in the stool
c. a device for blowing air, gas, or powder into a body cavity
d. the sum of chemical processes that result in growth, energy production, elimination of waste, and body functions performed as digested nutrients are distributed
e. black, tarry stools caused by digested blood from the gastrointestinal tract
f. the contraction and relaxation of involuntary muscles of the alimentary canal, producing wavelike movements of products through the digestive system
g. difficulty speaking
h. loss of appetite
i. a substance that can damage the liver
j. an accumulation of serous fluid in the peritoneal cavity
k. the use of chemical agents to treat esophageal varices to produce fibrosis and hardening of the tissue
l. an inflammation of the mucous membranes of the mouth
m. an abnormal contact between the teeth in the upper and lower jaw
n. the normal tension in a cell or the skin
o. vomiting blood or bloody vomitus
p. the smooth, rounded, removable inner portion of a hollow tube, such as an anoscope, that allows for easier insertion
q. white, thickened patches on the oral mucosa or tongue that are often precancerous

COG MATCHING

Grade: ______

Place the letter preceding the description on the line next to the name of the gastrointestinal disorder.

Disorders

40. ______ esophageal varices
41. ______ cholecystitis
42. ______ peptic ulcers
43. ______ stomatitis
44. ______ gastroesophageal reflux disease (GERD)
45. ______ diverticulosis
46. ______ hiatal hernia

Descriptions

a. a chronic disorder characterized by discomfort in the chest due to the backflow of gastric contents into the esophagus
b. a condition that occurs when part of the stomach protrudes up through the diaphragm
c. varicose veins of the esophagus resulting from pressure within the esophageal veins
d. an acute or chronic inflammation of the gall bladder
e. erosions or sores in the GI tract left by sloughed tissue
f. a disorder that usually occurs in the sigmoid colon, attributed to a diet deficient in roughage
g. an inflammation of the oral mucosa, caused by a virus, bacteria, or fungus

COG MATCHING

Grade: ________

Place the letter preceding the description on the line next to the examination method.

Examination Methods

47. _____ endoscopic studies
48. _____ nuclear imaging
49. _____ ultrasonography
50. _____ radiology studies
51. _____ sigmoidoscopy
52. _____ endoscopic retrograde cholangiopancreatography (ERCP)
53. _____ anoscopy

Descriptions

a. instilling barium into the GI tract orally or rectally to outline the organs and identify abnormalities
b. injecting radionuclides into the body and taking images using a nuclear scanning device to detect abnormalities
c. using high-frequency sound waves to diagnose disorders of internal structures
d. passing soft, flexible tubes into the stomach, small intestine, or colon for direct visualization of the organs
e. a method of injecting dye into the ducts of the gallbladder and pancreas; used to visualize the esophagus, stomach, proximal duodenum, and pancreas with a flexible endoscope
f. the insertion of a metal or plastic anoscope into the rectal canal to inspect the anus and rectum and swab for cultures
g. a visual examination of the sigmoid colon

COG IDENTIFICATION

Grade: ________

54. A patient comes into the office with abdominal pain and indigestion. The physician diagnoses the patient with a hiatal hernia. Which of the following diet modifications and treatments would the physician most likely suggest to the patient? Circle the correct answers. There may be more than one.

a. Eat small, frequent meals.

b. Exercise vigorously three times a week.

c. Elevate the head of the bed when sleeping.

d. Do not eat for 2 hours before bedtime.

e. Drink less water.

f. Lose weight.

55. As a medical assistant, you may be called on to assist with colon procedures in the medical office. Place a check mark on the line next to the task(s) that the medical assistant would be responsible for performing in the medical office.

a. ______________ Instruct the patient in the procedure of stool sample collection.

b. ______________ Help to educate the patient about diet and the prevention of gastric disorders.

c. ______________ Prescribe pain medication and antibiotics.

d. ______________ Schedule radiographic and ultrasound procedures in an outpatient facility.

e. ______________ Test the stool specimen when it is returned to the office.

f. ______________ Compile detailed dietary regimens for obese patients.

g. ______________ Assist the physician in performing colon examinations.

h. ______________ Diagnose minor gastrointestinal disorders.

56. Which of the following factors increase a person's risk of developing pancreatic cancer? Circle all that apply.

a. Being female

b. Drinking alcohol

c. Smoking

d. Being of African American descent

e. Being male

f. Being of Caucasian descent

g. Eating high-fat foods

h. A history of working with industrial chemicals

57. Some gastrointestinal disorders require specialist knowledge and equipment outside of the physician's office. In the table below, place a check mark in the appropriate box to indicate whether a procedure could be carried out in the physician's office or would likely require an outpatient facility.

Procedure	Physician's Office	Outpatient Facility
a. Ultrasonography		
b. Anoscopy		
c. Endoscopic retrograde cholangiopancreatography		
d. Nuclear imaging		
e. Sigmoidoscopy examination		

COG SHORT ANSWER

Grade: ______

58. Identify the part of the digestive system where the following gastrointestinal disorders occur.

a. Appendicitis ______

b. Hepatitis ______

c. Cholelithiasis ______

d. Crohn disease ______

e. Peptic ulcers ______

f. Ulcerative colitis ______

g. Diverticulosis ______

59. List three symptoms that could indicate a patient is suffering from gastric cancer.

60. A 40-year-old woman comes to the physician's office complaining of severe stomach cramps and vomiting. To help the physician assess her condition and make a diagnosis, the medical assistant should obtain some personal information. List four things that the physician will ask the patient before continuing with the exam.

61. A 25-year-old woman comes to the physician's office complaining of fatigue and joint pain. She looks jaundiced, and when the physician asks her for her medical history, she says that she recently returned from a 3-month trip to Ghana. Which two tests will the physician most likely recommend?

62. As a medical assistant, part of your job may be to educate patients about the care of teeth and gums. List three things that you could tell a patient to do that might help to prevent dental caries.

63. Which is the more widely accepted instrument to use during an endoscopic study: a rigid sigmoidoscope or a flexible fiberoptic sigmoidoscope? Explain your answer.

COG TRUE OR FALSE?

Grade: ________

Indicate whether the statements are true or false by placing the letter T (true) or F (false) on the line preceding the statement.

64. ______________ Oral cancers are more common among people who smoke.

65. ______________ Cancer of the esophagus is common and can easily be treated.

66. ______________ A sign that a patient has a problem with malabsorption of fats includes stools that are loose.

67. ______________ Irritable bowel syndrome usually results in chronic weight loss.

COG AFF CASE STUDY FOR CRITICAL THINKING

Grade: ________

1. A 55-year-old woman comes to the physician's office and asks about gastric bypass surgery. She says that she has tried every diet available and is unable to lose weight. She suffers from shortness of breath and an inability to walk for long distances. You take the woman's vital signs and measure her height and weight. She appears to be in good health but is at least 60 pounds over the ideal weight for her height. The physician later confirms these facts. Is the patient likely to be a candidate for gastric bypass surgery? Explain your answer.

____

____

____

____

2. The physician tells a patient that he would like to schedule an endoscopic retrograde cholangiopancreatography in a local outpatient facility. After the physician leaves the room, you notice that the patient looks confused and worried. How would you explain the procedure to the patient to reassure him?

____

____

____

____

3. Mr. Thompson, a 50-year-old patient, is scheduled to have an endoscopic examination on Wednesday morning. You have given him all the necessary information to prepare for the examination, including taking a laxative the night before and eating only a light meal on Tuesday evening, with no breakfast Wednesday morning. Mr. Thompson calls you an hour before his appointment to tell you that he forgot to take the laxative the previous evening and has eaten breakfast. Explain what you would do.

____

____

____

____

4. A 15-year-old female patient comes into the physician's office with severe abdominal pains. She is extremely underweight for her height, and you suspect she might be anorexic. When the physician leaves the room, she confesses that she has been using laxatives every day to keep her weight down. Explain what you would do next.

____

____

____

____

5. A 50-year-old male patient has been diagnosed with pancreatic cancer. The patient is clearly devastated and tells you he has heard that people who develop pancreatic cancer have little chance of survival. What do you say to the patient?

____

____

____

____

PSY PROCEDURE 33-1 Assisting with Colon Procedures

Name: ______________________ **Date:** __________ **Time:** __________ **Grade:** __________

EQUIPMENT/SUPPLIES: Appropriate instrument (flexible or rigid sigmoidoscope, anoscope, or proctoscope); water-soluble lubricant; patient gown and drape; cotton swabs; suction (if not part of the scope); biopsy forceps; specimen container with preservative; completed laboratory requisition form; personal wipes or tissues; equipment for assessing vital signs; examination gloves

STANDARDS: Given the needed equipment and a place to work, the student will perform this skill with _____ % accuracy in a total of _____ minutes. *(Your instructor will tell you what the percentage and time limits will be before you begin.)*

KEY: 4 = Satisfactory 0 = Unsatisfactory NA = This step is not counted

PROCEDURE STEPS	SELF	PARTNER	INSTRUCTOR
1. Wash your hands.	❑	❑	❑
2. Assemble the equipment and supplies. **a.** Place the name of the patient on label on outside of specimen container. **b.** Complete the laboratory requisition.	❑	❑	❑
3. Check the illumination of the light source if a flexible sigmoidoscope. Turn off the power after checking for working order.	❑	❑	❑
4. Greet and identify the patient and explain the procedure. Identify yourself including your title. **a.** Inform patient that a sensation of pressure may be felt. **b.** Tell the patient that the pressure is from the instrument. **c.** Gas pressure may be felt when air is insufflated during the sigmoidoscopy.	❑	❑	❑
5. Instruct the patient to empty his or her urinary bladder.	❑	❑	❑
6. Assess the vital signs and record in the medical record.	❑	❑	❑
7. Have the patient undress from the waist down and gown and drape appropriately.	❑	❑	❑
8. Assist the patient onto the examination table. **a.** If the instrument is an anoscope or a fiberoptic device, the Sims position or a side-lying position is most comfortable. **b.** If a rigid instrument is used, position patient when doctor is ready: knee-chest position or on a proctological table. **c.** Drape the patient.	❑	❑	❑
9. Assist the physician with lubricant, instruments, power, swabs, suction, etc.	❑	❑	❑
10. Monitor the patient's response and offer reassurance. **a.** Instruct the patient to breathe slowly through pursed lips. **b.** Encourage relaxing as much as possible.	❑	❑	❑

PSY PROCEDURE 33-1 Assisting with Colon Procedures (continued)

11. When the physician is finished: **a.** Assist the patient into a comfortable position and allow a rest period. **b.** Offer personal cleaning wipes or tissues. **c.** Take the patient's vital signs before allowing him or her to stand. **d.** Assist the patient from the table and with dressing as needed. **e.** Give the patient any instructions regarding postprocedure care.	❑	❑	❑
12. Clean the room and route the specimen to the laboratory with the requisition.	❑	❑	❑
13. Disinfect or dispose of the supplies and equipment as appropriate.	❑	❑	❑
14. Wash your hands.	❑	❑	❑
15. AFF Log into the Electronic Medical Record (EMR) using your username and secure password OR obtain the paper medical record from a secure location and assure it is kept away from public access. Document your part in preparing specimens obtained and patient instructions after the procedure.	❑	❑	❑
16. When finished, log out of the EMR and/or replace the paper medical record in an appropriate and secure location.	❑	❑	❑

CALCULATION

Total Possible Points: __________

Total Points Earned: __________ Multiplied by 100 = __________ Divided by Total Possible Points = __________ %

PASS ❑ **FAIL** ❑ **COMMENTS:**

Student's signature ____________________ Date __________

Partner's signature ____________________ Date __________

Instructor's signature ____________________ Date __________

PSY PROCEDURE 33-2 Test Stool Specimen for Occult Blood: Guaiac Method

Name: ______________________ **Date:** __________ **Time:** __________ **Grade:** __________

EQUIPMENT/SUPPLIES: Gloves, labeled specimen pack or packs (the patient may bring in up to three samples per the office policy), test developer or reagent drops, biohazardous waste container.

STANDARDS: Given the needed equipment and a place to work, the student will perform this skill with _____ % accuracy in a total of _____ minutes. *(Your instructor will tell you what the percentage and time limits will be before you begin.)*

KEY: 4 = Satisfactory 0 = Unsatisfactory NA = This step is not counted

PROCEDURE STEPS	SELF	PARTNER	INSTRUCTOR
1. Wash your hands.	❑	❑	❑
2. Assemble the equipment and supplies and put on gloves.	❑	❑	❑
3. Verify the stool sample collected by the patient appropriately labeled and that the physician has ordered a stool for occult blood.	❑	❑	❑
4. Check the expiration date on the developer or reagent solution.	❑	❑	❑
5. Open the test window on the back of each test pack. Apply one drop of the developer solution to each window according to the manufacturer's instructions.	❑	❑	❑
6. Read the color change within the specified time period, usually 60 seconds.	❑	❑	❑
7. Apply one drop of developer as directed on the control section or window of each test pack. Note whether the control results are positive or negative.	❑	❑	❑
8. Explain the procedure to follow if the control is positive or negative.	❑	❑	❑
9. Properly dispose of the test pack or packs and your gloves in a biohazardous waste container.	❑	❑	❑
10. Wash your hands.	❑	❑	❑
11. AFF Log into the Electronic Medical Record (EMR) using your username and secure password OR obtain the paper medical record from a secure location and assure it is kept away from public access. Document your part in preparing specimens obtained and patient instructions after the procedure.	❑	❑	❑
12. When finished, log out of the EMR and/or replace the paper medical record in an appropriate and secure location.	❑	❑	❑

PSY PROCEDURE 33-2 Test Stool Specimen for Occult Blood: Guaiac Method (continued)

CALCULATION

Total Possible Points: __________

Total Points Earned: __________ Multiplied by 100 = __________ Divided by Total Possible Points = __________ %

PASS ❑ **FAIL** ❑ **COMMENTS:**

Student's signature ____________________ Date __________

Partner's signature ____________________ Date __________

Instructor's signature ____________________ Date __________

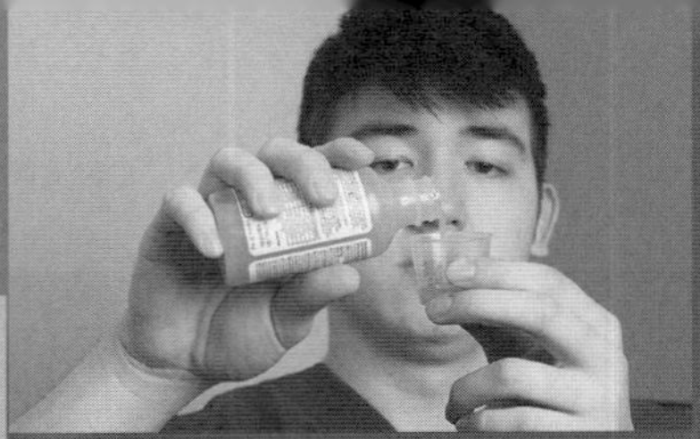

CHAPTER

34 Neurology

Learning Outcomes

COG Cognitive Domain

1. Spell key terms
2. Define medical terms and abbreviations related to all body systems
3. Describe structural organization of the human body
4. List major organs in each body system
5. Identify the anatomical location of major organs in each body system
6. Describe the normal function of each body system
7. Identify common pathology related to each body system including signs, symptoms, and etiology
   a. List and describe common diseases of the nervous system
   b. Describe the physical and emotional effects of degenerative nervous system disorders
   c. List potential complications of a spinal cord injury
   d. Name and describe the common procedures for diagnosing nervous system disorders

PSY Psychomotor Domain

1. Assist with a lumbar puncture (Procedure 34-1)

AFF Affective Domain

1. Incorporate critical thinking skills when performing patient assessment
2. Incorporate critical thinking skills when performing patient care
3. Show awareness of a patient's concerns related to the procedure being performed
4. Demonstrate empathy, active listening, nonverbal communication
5. Demonstrate respect for individual diversity including gender, race, religion, age, economic status, appearance
6. Explain to a patient the rationale for performance of a procedure
7. Demonstrate sensitivity to patient rights
8. Protect the integrity of the medical record

ABHES Competencies

1. Assist the physician with the regimen of diagnostic and treatment modalities as they relate to each body system
2. Comply with federal, state, and local health laws and regulations
3. Communicate on the recipient's level of comprehension
4. Serve as a liaison between the physician and others
5. Show empathy and impartiality when dealing with patients
6. Document accurately

Name: ______________________ Date: __________ Grade: __________

COG MULTIPLE CHOICE

Circle the letter preceding the correct answer.

1. Initial symptoms of tetanus include:
a. muscle spasms and stiff neck.
b. paralysis and stiff neck.
c. drooling and thick saliva.
d. seizures and dysphagia.
e. muscle spasms and clenched teeth.

2. What is another name for grand mal seizures?
a. Absence seizures
b. Tonic–clonic seizures
c. Partial seizures
d. Nervous seizures
e. Flashing seizures

3. Febrile seizures occur in:
a. teenagers.
b. middle-aged men.
c. young children.
d. older adult women.
e. people of all ages.

4. There may be no signs of external deformity with:
a. meningocele.
b. myelomeningocele.
c. spina bifida occulta.
d. amyotrophic lateral sclerosis.
e. poliomyelitis.

5. To diagnose meningitis, the physician may order a(n):
a. urine sample.
b. x-ray.
c. MRI.
d. throat culture.
e. complete blood count.

6. Hydrophobia often occurs after the onset of:
a. rabies.
b. tetanus.
c. encephalitis.
d. cerebral palsy.
e. meningitis.

7. A herpes zoster breakout typically develops on:
a. the legs and arms.
b. the genitals and mouth.
c. the stomach and chest.
d. the face, back, and chest.
e. the face and neck.

8. A disease closely related to poliomyelitis is:
a. encephalitis.
b. meningitis.
c. Parkinson disease.
d. PPMA syndrome.
e. chicken pox.

9. Treatment for brain tumors may include:
a. physical therapy and drug therapy.
b. surgery and radiation therapy.
c. surgery only.
d. radiation therapy only.
e. physical therapy and occupational therapy.

10. CSF removed and sent to the laboratory for a suspected diagnosis of meningitis may be tested for:
a. glucose and white blood cells.
b. cholesterol and white blood cell count.
c. red blood cells and viruses
d. glucose and bacteria.
e. glucose and fatty acids.

11. You should encourage slow, deep breathing for:
a. electrical tests.
b. a lumbar puncture.
c. radiological tests.
d. physical tests.
e. the Romberg test.

12. Contrast medium helps distinguish between the soft tissues of the nervous system and:
a. bones.
b. tendons.
c. tumors.
d. muscles.
e. arteries.

13. When assisting with a Queckenstedt test, you will be directed to:
a. assist the patient into a side-curled position.
b. support a forward-bending sitting position.
c. maintain sterility of instruments.
d. press against the patient's jugular vein.
e. encourage the patient in slow, deep breathing.

14. AFP is generally performed:
a. during the second trimester of pregnancy.
b. during the first trimester of pregnancy.
c. during the third trimester of pregnancy.
d. before a woman gets pregnant.
e. after the baby is born.

15. Which of the following is true of Lou Gehrig disease?
a. It is officially known as multiple sclerosis.
b. It is highly contagious.
c. It is caused by a spinal cord injury.
d. It is found most often in children.
e. It is a terminal disease.

16. During the second phase of a grand mal seizure, the patient experiences:
a. a tingling in extremities.
b. a sensitivity to light.
c. a complete loss of consciousness.
d. an increased awareness of smell.
e. a sense of drowsiness.

17. Which of the following is a cause of febrile seizures?
a. Spinal cord damage
b. Elevated body temperature
c. Hypothermia
d. Reye syndrome
e. Neural tube defects

18. Paraplegia is:
a. paralysis of all limbs.
b. paralysis of the high thoracic vertebrae.
c. paralysis on one side of the body, opposite the side of spinal cord involvement.
d. paralysis of any part of the body above the point of spinal cord involvement.
e. paralysis of any part of the body below the point of spinal cord involvement.

19. Which of the following is an infectious disorder of the nervous system?
a. Tumors
b. ALS
c. Multiple sclerosis
d. Encephalitis
e. Febrile seizures

20. Parkinson disease is a:
a. convulsive disorder.
b. degenerative disorder.
c. developmental disorder.
d. neoplastic disorder.
e. traumatic disorder.

COG MATCHING

Grade: ________

Place the letter preceding the definition on the line next to the term.

Key Terms

21. _____ cephalalgia
22. _____ concussion
23. _____ contusion
24. _____ convulsion
25. _____ dysphagia
26. _____ dysphasia
27. _____ electroencephalogram (EEG)
28. _____ herpes zoster
29. _____ meningocele
30. _____ migraine
31. _____ myelogram
32. _____ myelomeningocele
33. _____ Queckenstedt test
34. _____ Romberg test
35. _____ seizure
36. _____ spina bifida occulta

Definitions

a. tracing of the electrical activity of the brain
b. a headache
c. meninges protruding through the spinal column
d. the protrusion of the spinal cord through the spinal defect
e. an invasive radiological test in which dye is injected into the spinal fluid
f. a test to determine presence of obstruction in the CSF flow performed during a lumbar puncture
g. an injury to the brain due to trauma
h. difficulty speaking
i. sudden, involuntary muscle contraction of a voluntary muscle group
j. an infection caused by reactivation of varicella zoster virus, which causes chicken pox
k. a collection of blood tissues after an injury; a bruise
l. a type of severe headache, usually unilateral; may appear in clusters
m. a congenital defect in the spinal column caused by lack of union of the vertebrae
n. an abnormal discharge of electrical activity in the brain, resulting in involuntary contractions of voluntary muscles
o. a test for the inability to maintain body balance when eyes are closed and feet are together; indication of spinal cord disease
p. inability to swallow or difficulty in swallowing

COG MATCHING

Grade: ________

Place the letter preceding the examination method on the line next to the cranial nerve.

Cranial Nerves

37. ______ Olfactory (I)
38. ______ Trochlear (IV)
39. ______ Facial (VII)
40. ______ Glossopharyngeal (IX)
41. ______ Vagus (X)

Examination Methods

a. Ask patient to raise eyebrows, smile, show teeth, puff out cheeks.
b. Test for downward, inward eye movement.
c. Test each nostril for smell reception, interpretation.
d. Ask patient to say "ah," yawn to observe upward movement of palate; elicit gag response, note ability to swallow.
e. Ask patient to swallow and speak; note hoarseness.

COG MATCHING

Grade: ________

Place the letter preceding the response on the line next to the reflex. Responses may be used more than once.

Reflexes

42. ______ Brachioradialis
43. ______ Biceps
44. ______ Triceps
45. ______ Patellar
46. ______ Achilles
47. ______ Corneal

Responses

a. Closure of eyelid
b. Extension of elbow
c. Flexion of elbow
d. Plantar flexion of foot
e. Extension of leg

COG IDENTIFICATION

Grade: ________

Indicate whether the following disorders are infectious (I), degenerative (DG), convulsive (C), developmental (DV), traumatic (T), neoplastic (N), or a type of headache (H) by placing the identifying letter(s) on the line preceding the disorder.

48. ______________ Amyotrophic lateral sclerosis
49. ______________ Focal or Jacksonian
50. ______________ Hydrocephalus
51. ______________ Meningitis
52. ______________ Neural tube defects
53. ______________ Poliomyelitis
54. ______________ Brain astrocytoma
55. ______________ Herpes zoster
56. ______________ Cerebral palsy
57. ______________ Tetanus

58. ______________ Febrile seizures

59. ______________ Multiple sclerosis

60. ______________ Spinal cord injury

61. Identify whether the disorders listed below affect children, women, men, or older adults. Place a check mark on the line under the appropriate groups.

Disorder	Children	Women	Men	Older Adults
a. Parkinson disease				
b. Amyotrophic lateral sclerosis				
c. Multiple sclerosis				
d. Reye syndrome				
e. Febrile seizures				

62. Indicate whether the following symptoms occur at the onset of a migraine or after the migraine begins. Place a check mark on the line under the word "onset" or "after."

Symptoms	Onset	After Migraine Begins
a. experience of flashing lights		
b. photophobia		
c. nausea		
d. experience of wavy lines		
e. diplopia		

COG SHORT ANSWER

Grade: ______________

63. Explain the difference between dysphagia and dysphasia.

____

____

____

____

64. Name three viral infections that lead to encephalitis.

____

____

____

____

65. What kind of outbreak might be caused by a varicella infection? What generally triggers this outbreak?

66. Which age group is most susceptible to traumatic brain injuries? Why? Which age group is most susceptible to spinal cord injuries? Why?

67. Name seven common diagnostic tests for the nervous system.

68. Explain the difference between the Romberg test and the Queckenstedt test and how or if you would assist the physician in each procedure.

69. List three responsibilities that you may have when working with patients with neurological disorders.

70. Below are some of the steps involved in assisting the physician with a lumbar puncture. Explain the reasons for performing each task listed.

a. Check that the consent form is signed and in the chart. Warn the patient not to move during the procedure. Tell the patient that the area will be numb but pressure may still be felt after the local anesthetic is administered.

b. Throughout the procedure, observe the patient closely for signs such as dyspnea or cyanosis. Monitor the pulse at intervals and record the vital signs after the procedure. Note the patient's mental alertness and any leakage at the site, nausea, or vomiting. Assess lower limb mobility. Assist the physician as necessary.

____

____

____

____

c. If the Queckenstedt test is to be performed, you may be required to press against the patient's jugular veins in the neck (right, left, or both) while the physician monitors the pressure of CSF.

____

____

____

____

COG TRUE OR FALSE?

Grade: __________

Indicate whether the statements are true or false by placing the letter T (true) or F (false) on the line preceding the statement.

71. __________ Ice and alcohol and sponge baths are preferable to cool compresses in returning a child's body temperature to normal.

72. __________ If a patient is bitten by an animal, a copy of the animal's rabies tag and certificate should be placed in the patient's chart.

73. __________ Multiple sclerosis is a contagious disease.

74. __________ A lumbar puncture is more commonly performed in outpatient clinics than in the medical office.

75. __________ Herpes zoster may develop in patients who had a previous varicella infection.

COG AFF CASE STUDIES FOR CRITICAL THINKING

Grade: __________

1. A patient comes in for treatment because of a severe dog bite. The patient has already cleaned the wound himself and the physician attends to the wound immediately. Your patient then receives antibiotic and vaccine therapy. What is the next course of action and what may you be responsible for?

____

____

____

____

2. A patient in your clinic has been treated for epilepsy and is now seizure free. This patient has decided that she is going to stop her medication regimen. She has also expressed her excitement about being able to drive again soon. How might you advise this patient before she makes her decisions?

____

____

____

____

3. There is a patient who has recently started coming to your clinic for treatment for herpes zoster. She doesn't understand why she has shingles. She is a single mom who has been supporting her children and taking care of one child with severe Down syndrome. What would you explain as the likely cause for the herpes zoster outbreak? What kind of advice might you offer this patient toward improving her health?

____

____

____

____

4. A 40-year-old patient has been suffering from severe migraines for the last year. He is concerned about his condition because he is a truck driver. He is worried that it is just a matter time before a migraine sets in while he is driving. Taking rests while he is on the road is a near impossibility. He is usually very tired, and he drinks a lot of coffee to keep himself awake on his long rides. How might you advise and educate this patient?

____

____

____

____

5. A patient comes in to the office and complains of headaches, blurred vision, and memory loss. What would your immediate concern be? What type of tests may need to be performed to learn more about this patient's symptoms?

____

____

____

____

PSY PROCEDURE 34-1 Assist with a Lumbar Puncture

Name: ________________ **Date:** __________ **Time:** __________ **Grade:** __________

EQUIPMENT/SUPPLIES: Sterile gloves, examination gloves, 3- to 5-inch lumbar needle with a stylet (physician will specify gauge and length), sterile gauze sponges, specimen containers, local anesthetic and syringe, needle, adhesive bandages, fenestrated drape, sterile drape, antiseptic, skin preparation supplies (razor), biohazard sharps container, biohazard waste container

STANDARDS: Given the needed equipment and a place to work, the student will perform this skill with _____ % accuracy in a total of _____ minutes. *(Your instructor will tell you what the percentage and time limits will be before you begin.)*

KEY: 4 = Satisfactory 0 = Unsatisfactory NA = This step is not counted

PROCEDURE STEPS	SELF	PARTNER	INSTRUCTOR
1. Wash your hands.	❑	❑	❑
2. Assemble the equipment.	❑	❑	❑
3. Identify yourself including your title.	❑	❑	❑
4. Identify the patient, and explain the procedure.	❑	❑	❑
5. Check that the consent form is signed and available in the chart.	❑	❑	❑
6. Explain the importance of not moving during the procedure and explain that the area will be numbed but pressure may still be felt.	❑	❑	❑
7. Have the patient void.	❑	❑	❑
8. Direct the patient to disrobe and put on a gown with the opening in the back.	❑	❑	❑
9. Prepare the skin unless this is to be done as part of the sterile preparation.	❑	❑	❑
10. Assist as needed with administration of the anesthetic.	❑	❑	❑
11. Assist the patient into the appropriate position. **a.** For the side-lying position: **(1)** Stand in front of the patient and help by holding the patient's knees and top shoulder. **(2)** Ask the patient to move, so the back is close to the edge of the table. **b.** For the forward leaning, supported position: **(1)** Stand in front of the patient and rest your hands on the patient's shoulders. **(2)** Ask the patient to breathe slowly and deeply.	❑	❑	❑
12. Throughout the procedure, observe the patient closely for signs such as dyspnea or cyanosis. **a.** Monitor the pulse at intervals and record the vital signs after the procedure. **b.** Assess lower limb mobility.	❑	❑	❑

PSY PROCEDURE 34-1 Assist with a Lumbar Puncture (continued)

13. When the physician has the needle securely in place, if specimens are to be taken: **a.** Put on gloves to receive the potentially hazardous body fluid. **b.** Label the tubes in sequence as you receive them. **c.** Label with the patient's identification and place them in biohazard bags.	❑	❑	❑
14. If the Queckenstedt test is to be performed, you may be required to press against the patient's jugular veins in the neck, either right, left, or both, while the physician monitors the CSF pressure.	❑	❑	❑
15. At the completion of the procedure: **a.** Cover the site with an adhesive bandage and assist the patient to a flat position. **b.** The physician will determine when the patient is ready to leave.	❑	❑	❑
16. Route the specimens as required.	❑	❑	❑
17. Clean the examination room and care for or dispose of the equipment as needed.	❑	❑	❑
18. Wash your hands.	❑	❑	❑
19. AFF Log into the Electronic Medical Record (EMR) using your username and secure password OR obtain the paper medical record from a secure location and assure it is kept away from public access.	❑	❑	❑
20. Document your part in preparing specimens obtained and patient instructions after the procedure.	❑	❑	❑
21. When finished, log out of the EMR and/or replace the paper medical record in an appropriate and secure location.	❑	❑	❑

CALCULATION

Total Possible Points: __________

Total Points Earned: __________ Multiplied by 100 = __________ Divided by Total Possible Points = __________ %

PASS ❑ **FAIL** ❑ **COMMENTS:**

Student's signature ____________________ Date __________

Partner's signature ____________________ Date __________

Instructor's signature ____________________ Date __________

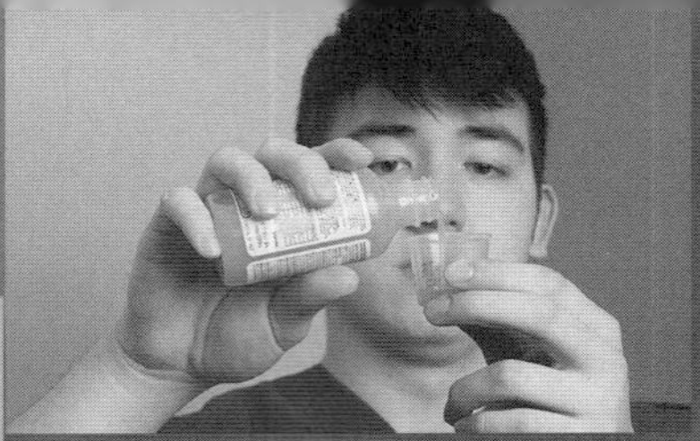

CHAPTER 35 Urology

Learning Outcomes

COG Cognitive Domain

1. Spell key terms
2. Define medical terms and abbreviations related to all body systems
3. Describe structural organization of the human body
4. List major organs in each body system
5. Identify the anatomical location of major organs in each body system
6. Describe the normal function of each body system
7. Identify common pathology related to each body system including signs, symptoms, and etiology
   a. List and describe common diseases of the urinary system and the male reproductive system
   b. Describe and explain the purpose of various diagnostic procedures associated with the urinary system
   c. Name and describe the common procedures for diagnosing urinary system disorders
8. Discuss the role of the medical assistant in diagnosing and treating disorders of the urinary system and the male reproductive system

PSY Psychomotor Domain

1. Perform a female urinary catheterization (Procedure 35-1)
2. Perform a male urinary catheterization (Procedure 35-2)
3. Instruct a male patient on the testicular self-examination (Procedure 35-3)

AFF Affective Domain

1. Incorporate critical thinking skills when performing patient assessment
2. Incorporate critical thinking skills when performing patient care
3. Show awareness of a patient's concerns related to the procedure being performed
4. Demonstrate empathy, active listening, nonverbal communication
5. Demonstrate respect for individual diversity including gender, race, religion, age, economic status, appearance
6. Explain to a patient the rationale for performance of a procedure
7. Demonstrate sensitivity to patient rights
8. Protect the integrity of the medical record

ABHES Competencies

1. Assist the physician with the regimen of diagnostic and treatment modalities as they relate to each body system
2. Comply with federal, state, and local health laws and regulations
3. Communicate on the recipient's level of comprehension
4. Serve as a liaison between the physician and others
5. Show empathy and impartiality when dealing with patients
6. Document accurately

PSY PROCEDURE 35-1 Perform a Female Urinary Catheterization

Name: ______________________ **Date:** __________ **Time:** __________ **Grade:** __________

EQUIPMENT/SUPPLIES: Straight catheterization tray that includes a No. 14 or No. 16 French catheter, a sterile tray, sterile gloves, antiseptic, a specimen cup with a lid, lubricant, and a sterile drape; an examination light; an anatomically correct female torso model for performing the catheterization; a biohazard container

STANDARDS: Given the needed equipment and a place to work, the student will perform this skill with _____ % accuracy in a total of _____ minutes. *(Your instructor will tell you what the percentage and time limits will be before you begin.)*

KEY: 4 = Satisfactory 0 = Unsatisfactory NA = This step is not counted

PROCEDURE STEPS	SELF	PARTNER	INSTRUCTOR
1. Wash your hands.	❑	❑	❑
2. Greet the patient and identify yourself, including your title.	❑	❑	❑
3. Identify the patient and explain the procedure. **a.** Have the patient disrobe from the waist down. **b.** Provide adequate gowning and draping materials.	❑	❑	❑
4. Place the patient in the dorsal recumbent or lithotomy position. **a.** Drape carefully to prevent unnecessary exposure. **b.** Open the tray and place it between the patient's legs. **c.** Adjust examination light to allow adequate visualization of the perineum.	❑	❑	❑
5. Remove the sterile glove package and put on the sterile gloves.	❑	❑	❑
6. Remove sterile drape and place it under the patient's buttocks.	❑	❑	❑
7. Open the antiseptic swabs and place them upright inside the catheter tray.	❑	❑	❑
8. Open the lubricant and squeeze a generous amount onto the tip of the catheter.	❑	❑	❑
9. Remove the sterile urine specimen cup and lid and place them to the side of the tray.	❑	❑	❑
10. Using your nondominant hand, carefully expose the urinary meatus.	❑	❑	❑
11. Using your sterile dominant hand, use antiseptic swabs to cleanse the urinary meatus by starting at the top and moving the swab down each side of the urinary meatus and down the middle, using a new swab for each side and the middle. Do not contaminate the glove on this hand.	❑	❑	❑
12. Pick up the catheter with the sterile, dominant hand and: **a.** Carefully insert the lubricated tip into the urinary meatus approximately 3 inches. **b.** Leave the other end of the catheter in the tray.	❑	❑	❑

PSY PROCEDURE 35-1 Perform a Female Urinary Catheterization (continued)

13. Once the urine begins to flow into the catheter tray, hold the catheter in position with your nondominant hand.	❑	❑	❑
14. Use your dominant hand to direct the flow of urine into the specimen cup.	❑	❑	❑
15. Remove catheter when urine flow slows or stops or 1,000 mL has been obtained.	❑	❑	❑
16. Wipe the perineum carefully with the drape that was placed under the buttocks.	❑	❑	❑
17. Dispose of urine appropriately and discard supplies in a biohazard container. **a.** Label the specimen container and complete the necessary laboratory requisition. **b.** Process the specimen according to the guidelines of the laboratory.	❑	❑	❑
18. Remove your gloves and wash your hands.	❑	❑	❑
19. Instruct patient to dress and give any follow-up information.	❑	❑	❑
20. AFF Log into the Electronic Medical Record (EMR) using your username and secure password OR obtain the paper medical record from a secure location and assure it is kept away from public access.	❑	❑	❑
21. Document the procedure in the patient's medical record.	❑	❑	❑
22. When finished, log out of the EMR and/or replace the paper medical record in an appropriate and secure location.	❑	❑	❑

CALCULATION

Total Possible Points: __________

Total Points Earned: __________ Multiplied by 100 = __________ Divided by Total Possible Points = __________ %

PASS ❑ **FAIL** ❑ **COMMENTS:**

Student's signature ____________________ Date __________

Partner's signature ____________________ Date __________

Instructor's signature ____________________ Date __________

PSY PROCEDURE 35-2 Perform a Male Urinary Catheterization

Name: ______________________ **Date:** __________ **Time:** __________ **Grade:** __________

EQUIPMENT/SUPPLIES: Straight catheterization tray that includes a No. 14 or No. 16 French catheter, a sterile tray, sterile gloves, antiseptic, a specimen cup with a lid, lubricant, and a sterile drape; an examination light; an anatomically correct male torso model for performing the catheterization; a biohazard container

STANDARDS: Given the needed equipment and a place to work, the student will perform this skill with _____ % accuracy in a total of _____ minutes. *(Your instructor will tell you what the percentage and time limits will be before you begin.)*

KEY: 4 = Satisfactory 0 = Unsatisfactory NA = This step is not counted

PROCEDURE STEPS	SELF	PARTNER	INSTRUCTOR
1. Wash your hands.	❑	❑	❑
2. Greet the patient and identify yourself, including your title.	❑	❑	❑
3. Identify the patient. **a.** Explain the procedure and have the patient disrobe from the waist down. **b.** Provide adequate gowning and draping materials.	❑	❑	❑
4. Place the patient in the supine position. **a.** Drape carefully to prevent unnecessary exposure. **b.** Open the tray and place it to the side or on the patient's thighs. **c.** Adjust examination light to allow adequate visualization of the perineum.	❑	❑	❑
5. Remove the sterile glove package and put on the sterile gloves.	❑	❑	❑
6. Carefully remove the sterile drape and place it under the glans penis.	❑	❑	❑
7. Open the antiseptic swabs and place them upright inside the catheter tray.	❑	❑	❑
8. Open lubricant and squeeze a generous amount onto the tip of the catheter.	❑	❑	❑
9. Remove sterile urine specimen cup and lid and place them to the side of the tray.	❑	❑	❑
10. Using your nondominant hand, pick up the penis to expose the urinary meatus.	❑	❑	❑
11. Using your sterile dominant hand, use antiseptic swabs to cleanse the urinary meatus by starting at the top and moving the swab around each side of the urinary meatus and down the middle, using a new swab for each side and the middle. Do not contaminate the glove on this hand.	❑	❑	❑

PSY PROCEDURE 35-2 Perform a Male Urinary Catheterization (continued)

12. Using your sterile dominant hand, pick up the catheter. **a.** Carefully insert the lubricated tip into the meatus approximately 4 to 6 inches. **b.** The other end of the catheter should be left in the tray.	❑	❑	❑
13. Once the urine begins to flow into the catheter tray, hold the catheter in position.	❑	❑	❑
14. Use your dominant hand to direct the flow of urine into the specimen cup.	❑	❑	❑
15. Remove the catheter when urine flow slows or stops or 1,000 mL has been obtained.	❑	❑	❑
16. Wipe the glans penis carefully with the drape that was placed under the buttocks.	❑	❑	❑
17. Dispose of urine appropriately and discard supplies in a biohazard container.	❑	❑	❑
18. Label the specimen container and complete the necessary laboratory requisition.	❑	❑	❑
19. Process specimen according to the guidelines of the laboratory.	❑	❑	❑
20. Remove your gloves and wash your hands.	❑	❑	❑
21. Instruct patient to dress and give any follow-up information.	❑	❑	❑
22. AFF Log into the Electronic Medical Record (EMR) using your username and secure password OR obtain the paper medical record from a secure location and assure it is kept away from public access.	❑	❑	❑
23. Document the procedure in the patient's medical record.	❑	❑	❑
24. When finished, log out of the EMR and/or replace the paper medical record in an appropriate and secure location.	❑	❑	❑

CALCULATION

Total Possible Points: __________

Total Points Earned: __________ Multiplied by 100 = __________ Divided by Total Possible Points = __________ %

PASS ❑ **FAIL** ❑ **COMMENTS:**

Student's signature ____________________ Date __________

Partner's signature ____________________ Date __________

Instructor's signature ____________________ Date __________

PSY PROCEDURE 35-3 **Instruct a Male Patient on the Self-Testicular Examination**

Name: ____________________ **Date:** __________ **Time:** __________ **Grade:** __________

EQUIPMENT/SUPPLIES: A patient instruction sheet if available; a testicular examination model or pictures

STANDARDS: Given the needed equipment and a place to work, the student will perform this skill with _____ % accuracy in a total of _____ minutes. *(Your instructor will tell you what the percentage and time limits will be before you begin.)*

KEY: 4 = Satisfactory 0 = Unsatisfactory NA =This step is not counted

PROCEDURE STEPS	SELF	PARTNER	INSTRUCTOR
1. Wash your hands.	❑	❑	❑
2. Greet the patient and identify yourself, including your title.	❑	❑	❑
3. Identify the patient and explain the procedure.	❑	❑	❑
4. Using the testicular model or pictures, explain the procedure. **a.** Tell the patient to examine each testicle by gently rolling between the fingers and the thumb with both hands. **b.** Check for lumps or thickenings.	❑	❑	❑
5. Explain that the epididymis is located on top of each testicle. **a.** Palpate to avoid incorrectly identifying it as an abnormal growth or lump. **b.** Instruct patient to report abnormal lumps or thickenings to the physician.	❑	❑	❑
6. Allow the patient to ask questions related to the testicular self-examination.	❑	❑	❑
7. AFF Log into the Electronic Medical Record (EMR) using your username and secure password OR obtain the paper medical record from a secure location and assure it is kept away from public access.	❑	❑	❑
8. Document the procedure in the patient's medical record.	❑	❑	❑
9. When finished, log out of the EMR and/or replace the paper medical record in an appropriate and secure location.	❑	❑	❑

CALCULATION

Total Possible Points: __________

Total Points Earned: __________ Multiplied by 100 = __________ Divided by Total Possible Points = __________ %

PASS ❑ **FAIL** ❑ **COMMENTS:**

Student's signature ____________________ Date __________

Partner's signature ____________________ Date __________

Instructor's signature ____________________ Date __________

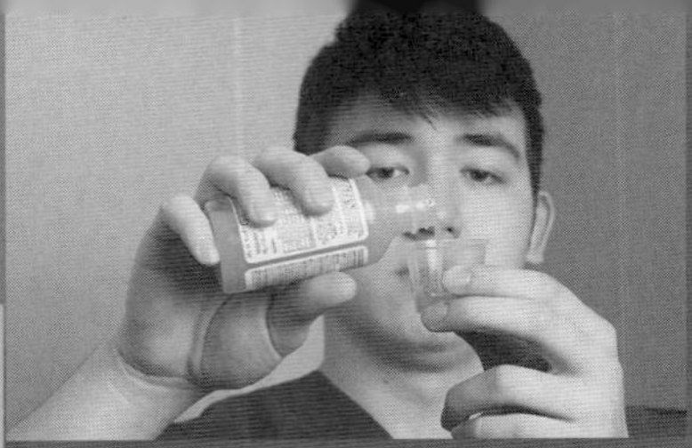

CHAPTER

36 Obstetrics and Gynecology

Learning Outcomes

COG Cognitive Domain

1. Spell key terms
2. Define medical terms and abbreviations related to all body systems
3. Describe structural organization of the human body
4. List major organs in each body system
5. Identify the anatomical location of major organs in each body system
6. Describe the normal function of each body system
7. Identify common pathology related to each body system including signs, symptoms, and etiology
8. List and describe common gynecological and obstetric disorders
9. Identify your role in the care of gynecologic and obstetric patients
10. Describe the components of prenatal and postpartum patient care
11. Explain the diagnostic and therapeutic procedures associated with the female reproductive system
12. Identify the various methods of contraception
13. Describe menopause

PSY Psychomotor Domain

1. Instruct the patient on the breast self-examination (Procedure 36-1)
2. Assist with the pelvic examination and Pap smear (Procedure 36-2)
3. Assist with colposcopy and cervical biopsy (Procedure 36-3)

AFF Affective Domain

1. Incorporate critical thinking skills when performing patient assessment
2. Incorporate critical thinking skills when performing patient care
3. Show awareness of a patient's concerns related to the procedure being performed
4. Demonstrate empathy, active listening, nonverbal communication
5. Demonstrate respect for individual diversity including gender, race, religion, age, economic status, appearance
6. Explain to a patient the rationale for performance of a procedure
7. Demonstrate sensitivity to patient rights
8. Protect the integrity of the medical record

ABHES Competencies

1. Assist the physician with the regimen of diagnostic and treatment modalities as they relate to each body system
2. Comply with federal, state, and local health laws and regulations
3. Communicate on the recipient's level of comprehension
4. Serve as a liaison between the physician and others
5. Show empathy and impartiality when dealing with patients
6. Document accurately

4. A 20-year-old female patient has made an appointment with the physician because she believes that she has PMDD, which she blames for her failing grades and damaged personal relationships. When you meet with the patient to assess her medical history, she asks you to write a note to her professors excusing her from any missed assignments. What should you do next?

____

____

____

____

PSY PROCEDURE 36-1 Instruct the Patient on the Breast Self-Examination

Name: ______________________ **Date:** __________ **Time:** __________ **Grade:** __________

EQUIPMENT/SUPPLIES: Patient education instruction sheet, if available; breast examination model, if available

STANDARDS: Given the needed equipment and a place to work, the student will perform this skill with _____ % accuracy in a total of _____ minutes. *(Your instructor will tell you what the percentage and time limits will be before you begin.)*

KEY: 4 = Satisfactory 0 = Unsatisfactory NA = This step is not counted

PROCEDURE STEPS	SELF	PARTNER	INSTRUCTOR
1. Wash your hands.	❑	❑	❑
2. Greet the patient and identify yourself including your title. Identify the patient.	❑	❑	❑
3. Explain the purpose and frequency of examining the breasts.	❑	❑	❑
4. Describe three positions necessary for the patient to examine the breasts: in front of a mirror, in the shower, and while lying down.	❑	❑	❑
5. In front of a mirror: **a.** Disrobe and inspect the breasts with her arms at sides and with arms raised above her head. **b.** Look for any changes in contour, swelling, dimpling of the skin, or changes in the nipple.	❑	❑	❑
6. In the shower: **a.** Feel each breast with hands over wet skin using the flat part of the first three fingers. **b.** Check for any lumps, hard knots, or thickenings. **c.** Use right hand to lightly press over all areas of left breast. **d.** Use left hand to examine right breast.	❑	❑	❑
7. Lying down: **a.** Place a pillow or folded towel under the right shoulder, and place the right hand behind head to examine the right breast. **b.** With left hand, use flat part of the fingers to palpate the breast tissue. **c.** Begin at the outermost top of the right breast. **d.** Work in a small circular motion around the breast in a clockwise rotation.	❑	❑	❑
8. Encourage patient to palpate the breast carefully moving her fingers inward toward the nipple and palpating every part of the breast including the nipple.	❑	❑	❑
9. Repeat the procedure for the left breast. Place a pillow or folded towel under the left shoulder with the left hand behind the head.	❑	❑	❑

PSY PROCEDURE 36-1 Instruct the Patient on the Breast Self-Examination (continued)

10. Gently squeeze each nipple between the thumb and index finger. **a.** Report any clear or bloody discharge to the physician. **b.** Promptly report any abnormalities found in the breast self-examination to the physician.	❑	❑	❑
11. AFF Explain how to respond to a patient who is visually impaired.	❑	❑	❑
____________________ ____________________ ____________________ ____________________			
12. AFF Log into the Electronic Medical Record (EMR) using your username and secure password OR obtain the paper medical record from a secure location and assure it is kept away from public access.	❑	❑	❑
13. Document the patient education.	❑	❑	❑
14. When finished, log out of the EMR and/or replace the paper medical record in an appropriate and secure location.	❑	❑	❑

CALCULATION

Total Possible Points: __________

Total Points Earned: __________ Multiplied by 100 = __________ Divided by Total Possible Points = __________ %

PASS **FAIL** **COMMENTS:**
❑ ❑

Student's signature ____________________ Date __________

Partner's signature ____________________ Date __________

Instructor's signature ____________________ Date __________

PSY PROCEDURE 36-2 Assist with the Pelvic Examination and Pap Smear

Name: ______________________ **Date:** __________ **Time:** __________ **Grade:** __________

EQUIPMENT/SUPPLIES: Gown and drape; appropriate size vaginal speculum; cotton-tipped applicators; water-soluble lubricant; examination gloves; examination light; tissues; materials for Pap smear: cervical brush, liquid-based preservative (SurePath® or ThinPrep®), laboratory request form, identification labels, and other materials that may be required by laboratory; biohazard transport bag, and biohazard waste container.

STANDARDS: Given the needed equipment and a place to work, the student will perform this skill with _____ % accuracy in a total of _____ minutes. *(Your instructor will tell you what the percentage and time limits will be before you begin.)*

KEY: 4 = Satisfactory 0 = Unsatisfactory NA = This step is not counted

PROCEDURE STEPS	SELF	PARTNER	INSTRUCTOR
1. Wash your hands.	❑	❑	❑
2. Assemble the equipment and supplies. **a.** Warm vaginal speculum by running under warm water. **b.** Do not use lubricant on the vaginal speculum before insertion.	❑	❑	❑
3. Label the outside of the liquid-based preservative container.	❑	❑	❑
4. Greet and identify yourself including your title.	❑	❑	❑
5. Identify the patient and explain the procedure.	❑	❑	❑
6. Ask the patient to empty her bladder and, if necessary, collect a urine specimen.	❑	❑	❑
7. Provide a gown and drape, and ask the patient to disrobe from the waist down.	❑	❑	❑
8. Position patient in the dorsal lithotomy position—buttocks at bottom edge of table.	❑	❑	❑
9. Adjust drape to cover patient's abdomen and knees but expose the genitalia.	❑	❑	❑
10. Adjust light over the genitalia for maximum visibility.	❑	❑	❑
11. Assist physician with the examination as needed.	❑	❑	❑
12. Put on examination gloves. Hold cytology liquid container for physician or insert brush as directed and mix with cytology liquid.	❑	❑	❑
13. Have a basin or other container ready to receive the now-contaminated speculum.	❑	❑	❑
14. Apply lubricant across the physician's two fingers.	❑	❑	❑
15. Encourage the patient to relax during the bimanual examination as needed.	❑	❑	❑

PSY PROCEDURE 36-2 Assist with the Pelvic Examination and Pap Smear (continued)

16. After the examination, assist the patient in sliding up to the top of the examination table and remove both feet at the same time from the stirrups.	❑	❑	❑
17. Offer the patient tissues to remove excess lubricant. **a.** Assist her to a sitting position if necessary. **b.** Watch for signs of vertigo. **c.** Ask the patient to get dressed and assist as needed. **d.** Provide for privacy as the patient dresses.	❑	❑	❑
18. Reinforce any physician instructions regarding follow-up appointments needed. **a.** Advise patient on the procedure for obtaining results from the Pap smear.	❑	❑	❑
19. AFF Explain how to respond to a patient who has dementia.	❑	❑	❑

____

____

____

____

20. Properly care for or dispose of equipment and clean the examination room. Prepare the specimen for transport to the laboratory.	❑	❑	❑
21. Remove your gloves and wash your hands.	❑	❑	❑
22. AFF Log into the Electronic Medical Record (EMR) using your username and secure password OR obtain the paper medical record from a secure location and assure it is kept away from public access.	❑	❑	❑
23. Document your responsibilities during the procedure.	❑	❑	❑
24. When finished, log out of the EMR and/or replace the paper medical record in an appropriate and secure location.	❑	❑	❑

CALCULATION

Total Possible Points: __________

Total Points Earned: __________ Multiplied by 100 = __________ Divided by Total Possible Points = __________ %

PASS **FAIL** **COMMENTS:**

❑ ❑

Student's signature ____________________ Date __________

Partner's signature ____________________ Date __________

Instructor's signature ____________________ Date __________

PSY PROCEDURE 36-3 Assist with Colposcopy and Cervical Biopsy

Name: ______________________ **Date:** __________ **Time:** __________ **Grade:** __________

EQUIPMENT/SUPPLIES: Patient gown and drape, vaginal speculum, colposcope, specimen container with preservative (10% formalin), sterile gloves, appropriate size sterile cotton-tipped applicators, sterile normal saline solution, sterile 3% acetic acid, sterile povidone–iodine (Betadine), silver nitrate sticks or ferric subsulfate (Monsel solution), sterile biopsy forceps or punch biopsy instrument, sterile uterine curette, sterile uterine dressing forceps, sterile 4 × 4 gauze pad, sterile towel, sterile endocervical curette, sterile uterine tenaculum, sanitary napkin, examination gloves, examination light, tissues, biohazard container

STANDARDS: Given the needed equipment and a place to work, the student will perform this skill with _____ % accuracy in a total of _____ minutes. *(Your instructor will tell you what the percentage and time limits will be before you begin.)*

KEY: 4 = Satisfactory 0 = Unsatisfactory NA = This step is not counted

PROCEDURE STEPS	SELF	PARTNER	INSTRUCTOR
1. Wash your hands.	❑	❑	❑
2. Verify that the patient has signed the consent form.	❑	❑	❑
3. Assemble the equipment and supplies.	❑	❑	❑
4. Check the light on the colposcope.	❑	❑	❑
5. Set up the sterile field without contaminating it.	❑	❑	❑
6. Pour sterile normal saline and acetic acid into their respective sterile containers.	❑	❑	❑
7. Cover the field with a sterile drape.	❑	❑	❑
8. Greet and identify yourself including your title.	❑	❑	❑
9. Identify the patient and explain the procedure.	❑	❑	❑
10. When the physician is ready to proceed with the procedure: **a.** Assist the patient into the dorsal lithotomy position. **b.** Put on sterile gloves after positioning the patient if necessary.	❑	❑	❑
11. Hand the physician: **a.** The applicator immersed in normal saline. **b.** Followed by the applicator immersed in acetic acid. **c.** The applicator with the antiseptic solution (Betadine).	❑	❑	❑
12. If you did not apply sterile gloves to assist the physician: **a.** Apply clean examination gloves. **b.** Accept the biopsy specimen into a container of 10% formalin preservative.	❑	❑	❑
13. Provide the physician with Monsel solution or silver nitrate sticks.	❑	❑	❑

PSY PROCEDURE 36-3 Assist with Colposcopy and Cervical Biopsy (continued)

14. When the physician is finished with the procedure: **a.** Assist the patient from the stirrups and into a sitting position. **b.** Explain to the patient that a small amount of bleeding may occur. **c.** Have a sanitary napkin available for the patient. **d.** Ask the patient to get dressed and assist as needed. **e.** Provide for privacy as the patient dresses. **f.** Reinforce any physician instructions regarding follow-up appointments. **g.** Advise the patient on how to obtain the biopsy results.	❑	❑	❑
15. AFF Explain how to respond to a patient who does not speak English or speaks English as a second language.	❑	❑	❑
16. Label the specimen container with the patient's name and date. **a.** Prepare the laboratory request. **b.** Transport the specimen and form to the laboratory.	❑	❑	❑
17. Properly care for, or dispose of, equipment and clean the examination room.	❑	❑	❑
18. Wash your hands.	❑	❑	❑
19. AFF Log into the Electronic Medical Record (EMR) using your username and secure password OR obtain the paper medical record from a secure location and assure it is kept away from public access.	❑	❑	❑
20. Document your responsibilities during the procedure.	❑	❑	❑
21. When finished, log out of the EMR and/or replace the paper medical record in an appropriate and secure location.	❑	❑	❑

CALCULATION

Total Possible Points: __________

Total Points Earned: __________ Multiplied by 100 = __________ Divided by Total Possible Points = __________ %

PASS ❑ **FAIL** ❑ **COMMENTS:**

Student's signature ____________________ Date __________

Partner's signature ____________________ Date __________

Instructor's signature ____________________ Date __________

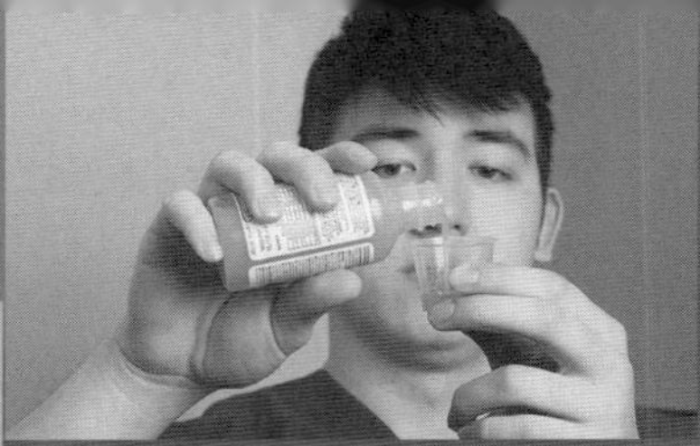

CHAPTER

37 Endocrinology

Learning Outcomes

COG Cognitive Domain

1. Spell key terms
2. Define medical terms and abbreviations related to all body systems
3. Describe structural organization of the human body
4. List major organs in each body system
5. Identify the anatomical location of major organs in each body system
6. Describe the normal function of each body system
7. Identify common pathology related to each body system including signs, symptoms, and etiology
8. Identify abnormal conditions of the thyroid, pancreas, adrenal, and pituitary glands
9. Describe the tests commonly used to diagnose disorders of these endocrine system glands
10. Explain your role in working with patients with endocrine system disorders

PSY Psychomotor Domain

1. Manage a patient with a diabetic emergency (Procedure 37-1)

AFF Affective Domain

1. Incorporate critical thinking skills when performing patient assessment
2. Incorporate critical thinking skills when performing patient care
3. Show awareness of a patient's concerns related to the procedure being performed
4. Demonstrate empathy, active listening, nonverbal communication
5. Demonstrate respect for individual diversity including gender, race, religion, age, economic status, appearance
6. Explain to a patient the rationale for performance of a procedure
7. Demonstrate sensitivity to patient rights
8. Protect the integrity of the medical record

ABHES Competencies

1. Assist the physician with the regimen of diagnostic and treatment modalities as they relate to each body system
2. Comply with federal, state, and local health laws and regulations
3. Communicate on the recipient's level of comprehension
4. Serve as a liaison between the physician and others
5. Show empathy and impartiality when dealing with patients
6. Document accurately

Name: ______________________ Date: __________ Grade: __________

COG MULTIPLE CHOICE

Circle the letter preceding the correct answer:

1. A patient with hypothyroidism must take hormone replacements:
a. for as many years as he has had the disease.
b. until the conclusion of puberty.
c. for his entire life.
d. until middle age.
e. for 10 years.

2. Diabetics may need supplemental insulin to:
a. test blood glucose levels.
b. reverse vascular changes.
c. reduce the presence of ketones.
d. restore pancreatic function.
e. control blood glucose levels.

3. One symptom of ketoacidosis is:
a. shallow respirations.
b. low blood glucose levels.
c. overhydration.
d. abdominal pain.
e. pale, moist skin.

4. Diabetes mellitus affects metabolism of which type of molecule?
a. Neurotransmitters
b. Carbohydrates
c. Hormones
d. Vitamins
e. Lipids

5. One symptom of type 1 diabetes mellitus is:
a. polyuria.
b. exophthalmia.
c. anorexia.
d. weight gain.
e. a goiter.

6. Hyperpigmentation of the skin might be an indication of:
a. Cushing syndrome.
b. Hashimoto thyroiditis.
c. Graves disease.
d. Addison disease.
e. diabetes insipidus.

7. To control gestational diabetes, a blood glucose specimen should be taken from a pregnant woman between:
a. 28 and 32 weeks of gestation.
b. 24 and 28 weeks of gestation.
c. 20 and 24 weeks of gestation.
d. 16 and 20 weeks of gestation.
e. 12 and 16 weeks of gestation.

8. Cushing syndrome sufferers may experience accelerated:
a. Addison disease.
b. endocarditis.
c. osteoporosis.
d. arthritis.
e. dementia.

9. Acromegaly results primarily in:
a. an increase in bone width.
b. muscular atrophy.
c. an increase in bone length.
d. muscular hypertrophy.
e. an increase in bone density.

10. Growth can be stimulated for children with dwarfism by:
a. repairs in the pituitary gland.
b. administration of growth hormone.
c. psychotherapy.
d. increased physical activity.
e. a high-protein diet.

11. Diabetes insipidus results from a deficiency of:
a. adrenocorticotropic hormone.
b. anterior pituitary hormones.
c. human growth hormone.
d. antidiuretic hormone.
e. thyroid hormones.

12. Insulin shock is a result of:
a. Cushing syndrome.
b. Addison disease.
c. Graves disease.
d. hyperglycemia.
e. hypoglycemia.

13. Diabetes mellitus patients need to care for their feet because:
a. they regularly develop ingrown toenails.
b. their peripheral circulation may be poor.
c. they suffer severe joint pain.
d. they have weak calves.
e. foot pain occurs.

14. Exophthalmia is a protrusion of the:
a. thyroid gland.
b. pancreas.
c. gall bladder.
d. eyes.
e. liver.

15. Patients taking corticosteroids may be at risk for:
a. Cushing disease.
b. Addison disease.
c. type 2 diabetes mellitus.
d. Graves disease.
e. Hashimoto thyroiditis.

16. The A1C test determines how well blood glucose has been controlled during the previous:
a. 2 to 3 hours.
b. 2 to 3 days.
c. 2 to 3 weeks.
d. 2 to 3 months.
e. 2 to 3 years.

17. Gigantism is a disorder of the:
a. adrenal glands.
b. pancreas.
c. liver.
d. thyroid.
e. pituitary gland.

18. A thyroid scan relies on a radioactive isotope of what element?
a. Iodine
b. Barium
c. Indium
d. Bismuth
e. Iridium

19. Addison disease is a disorder of the:
a. pituitary gland.
b. pancreas.
c. thyroid.
d. adrenal gland.
e. salivary glands.

20. Both Graves disease and goiters are examples of:
a. hypothyroidism.
b. hypoglycemia.
c. hyperthyroidism.
d. hyperglycemia.
e. hypertension.

COG MATCHING

Grade: ______

Place the letter preceding the definition on the line next to the term.

Key Terms

21. ______ acromegaly
22. ______ Addison disease
23. ______ Cushing syndrome
24. ______ diabetes insipidus
25. ______ dwarfism
26. ______ endocrinologist
27. ______ exophthalmia
28. ______ gigantism
29. ______ glycosuria
30. ______ goiter
31. ______ Graves disease
32. ______ Hashimoto thyroiditis
33. ______ hormones
34. ______ hyperglycemia
35. ______ hyperplasia
36. ______ hypoglycemia
37. ______ insulin-dependent diabetes mellitus

Definitions

a. an enlargement of the thyroid gland
b. a substance that is produced by an endocrine gland and travels through the blood to a distant organ or gland where it acts to modify the structure or function of that gland or organ
c. an adrenal gland disorder that results in an increased production of ACTH from the pituitary glands
d. excess quantities of thyroid hormone in tissues
e. excessive proliferation of normal cells in the normal tissue arrangement of an organism
f. the end products of fat metabolism
g. itching
h. pronounced hyperthyroidism with signs of enlarged thyroid and exophthalmos
i. a type of diabetes in which patients do not require insulin to control blood sugar
j. a deficiency in insulin production that leads to an inability to metabolize carbohydrates

Key Terms	Definitions
38. ______ ketoacidosis	k. partial or complete failure of the adrenal cortex functions, causing general physical deterioration
39. ______ ketones	l. the presence of glucose in the urine
40. ______ non–insulin-dependent diabetes mellitus	m. a disease of the immune system in which the tissue of the thyroid gland is replaced with fibrous tissue
41. ______ polydipsia	n. excessive thirst
42. ______ polyphagia	o. abnormal underdevelopment of the body with extreme shortness but normal proportion; achondroplastic dwarfism is an inherited growth disorder characterized by shortened limbs and a large head but almost normal trunk proportions
43. ______ polyuria	p. acidosis accompanied by an accumulation of ketones in the body
44. ______ pruritus	q. excessive size and stature caused most frequently by hypersecretion of the human growth hormone
45. ______ radioimmunoassay	r. deficiency of sugar in the blood
46. ______ thyrotoxicosis	s. an unusual protrusion of the eyeballs as a result of a thyroid disorder
	t. a disorder of metabolism characterized by polyuria and polydipsia; caused by a deficiency in ADH or an inability of the kidneys to respond to ADH
	u. excessive excretion and elimination of urine
	v. hyperfunction of the anterior pituitary gland near the end of puberty that results in increased bone width.
	w. the introduction of radioactive substances in the body to determine the concentration of a substance in the serum, usually the concentration of antigens, antibodies, or proteins
	x. a doctor who diagnoses and treats disorders of the endocrine system and its hormone-secreting glands
	y. abnormal hunger
	z. an increase in blood sugar, as in diabetes mellitus

COG IDENTIFICATION

Grade: ______

47. Read the following list of symptoms. Are these symptoms representative of hyperglycemia or hypoglycemia? Place the prefix "hyper" on the line preceding the symptoms for hyperglycemia and "hypo" for hypoglycemia.

a. ______________ Pale complexion

b. ______________ Deep respirations

c. ______________ Moist skin

d. ______________ Shallow respirations

e. ______________ Abdominal pain

f. ______________ Rapid, bounding pulse

g. ______________ Fruity breath

h. ______________ Subnormal blood glucose levels

COG SHORT ANSWER

Grade: ___________

48. When does ketoacidosis occur?

____

____

____

____

49. A patient is stunned to learn that she has been diagnosed with type 2 diabetes mellitus. She is 43 years old and in excellent health. As a personal trainer and nutritionist, she has always taken good care of her body. What potential cause of type 2 diabetes mellitus might she be overlooking?

____

____

____

____

50. A patient complains that, lately, his appetite has been ferocious, but he is actually losing weight. He does not understand why this is happening. What do you tell him?

____

____

____

____

51. Why is it difficult for many sufferers of endocrine disorders to comply with physicians' orders?

____

____

____

____

52. A patient who has been diagnosed with type 2 diabetes mellitus explains that a friend told him the disease is sometimes called *non–insulin-dependent diabetes mellitus*. He asks if this means that he will not need to take insulin. Is he correct? Why, or why not?

____

____

____

____

53. Who might be at risk for gestational diabetes mellitus?

____

____

____

____

54. What is the cause of hypoglycemia?

____

____

____

____

55. How is Addison disease treated?

____

____

____

____

56. A patient is diagnosed with dwarfism, and the patient's mother is extremely distressed, wondering if certain body parts will grow normally while others will not. She also wonders if her daughter could ever grow normally. What could you tell the mother?

____

____

____

____

57. What do the fasting glucose test and glucose tolerance test for diabetes mellitus have in common?

____

____

____

____

58. What is the purpose of the A1C blood test?

____

____

____

____

59. Cushing syndrome and Addison disease are both disorders of which gland?

____

____

____

____

60. Why is it important that patients with diseases of the endocrine system wear a medical alert bracelet or necklace?

____

____

____

____

COG TRUE OR FALSE?

Grade: ____________

Indicate whether the statements are true or false by placing the letter T (true) or F (false) on the line preceding the statement.

61. ____________ Endocrine glands are unlike other glands in the body because they are ductless.

62. ____________ Hashimoto thyroiditis is a disease of the endocrine system.

63. ____________ Type 1 diabetes mellitus occurs only in children and young adults.

64. ____________ Addison disease has no effect on the pituitary gland.

COG AFF CASE STUDIES FOR CRITICAL THINKING

Grade: ____________

1. A patient is worried that a thyroid function test requires the use of radioactive material. Explain, to the best of your ability, how the test works and why there is no need to be concerned about radiation. If necessary, do additional research on thyroid function tests to prepare your answer.

____

____

____

____

2. After an examination, a pregnant patient asks why the physician performed a test on her blood glucose level. She says she does not have diabetes. Explain why the physician chose to do the test.

____

____

____

____

3. Young children are sometimes afflicted with diabetes mellitus. This can be difficult for both the child and the family. What is your perspective of the medical assistant's role in this situation?

____

____

____

____

4. A patient with hyperthyroidism says she would prefer not to be treated because she has few negative symptoms, and the increased metabolic rate helps keep her thin. How would you respond to this?

____

____

____

____

PSY PROCEDURE 37-1 Manage a Patient with a Diabetic Emergency

Name: ______________________ **Date:** __________ **Time:** __________ **Grade:** __________

EQUIPMENT/SUPPLIES: Gloves, blood glucose monitor and strips, fruit juice or oral glucose tablets

STANDARDS: Given the needed equipment and a place to work, the student will perform this skill with _____ % accuracy in a total of _____ minutes. *(Your instructor will tell you what the percentage and time limits will be before you begin.)*

KEY: 4 = Satisfactory 0 = Unsatisfactory NA = This step is not counted

PROCEDURE STEPS	SELF	PARTNER	INSTRUCTOR
1. Wash your hands.	❑	❑	❑
2. Recognize the signs and symptoms of hyperglycemia and hypoglycemia.	❑	❑	❑
3. Greet the patient and identify yourself including your title. Identify the patient.	❑	❑	❑
4. Escort the patient into the examination room while making the observation that there is a problem.	❑	❑	❑
5. Determine if the patient has been previously diagnosed with diabetes mellitus and acknowledge that the patient is a diabetic.	❑	❑	❑
6. Ask the patient if he or she has eaten today or taken any medication.	❑	❑	❑
7. Notify the physician about the patient and perform a capillary stick for a blood glucose as directed.	❑	❑	❑
8. Notify the physician with the results of the blood glucose and treat the patient as ordered by the physician. **a.** Administer insulin subcutaneously to a patient with hyperglycemia. **b.** Administer a quick-acting sugar, such as an oral glucose tablet or fruit juice, for a patient with hypoglycemia.	❑	❑	❑
9. AFF Explain how to respond to a patient who is developmentally challenged.	❑	❑	❑

____

____

____

____

PSY PROCEDURE 37-1 Manage a Patient with a Diabetic Emergency (continued)

10. Be prepared to notify EMS as directed by the physician if the symptoms do not improve or worsen.	❑	❑	❑
11. AFF Log into the Electronic Medical Record (EMR) using your username and secure password OR obtain the paper medical record from a secure location and assure it is kept away from public access.	❑	❑	❑
12. Document any observations and treatments given.	❑	❑	❑
13. Document any observations and treatments given.	❑	❑	❑

CALCULATION

Total Possible Points: __________

Total Points Earned: __________ Multiplied by 100 = __________ Divided by Total Possible Points = __________ %

PASS ❑ **FAIL** ❑ **COMMENTS:**

Student's signature ____________________ Date __________

Partner's signature ____________________ Date __________

Instructor's signature ____________________ Date __________

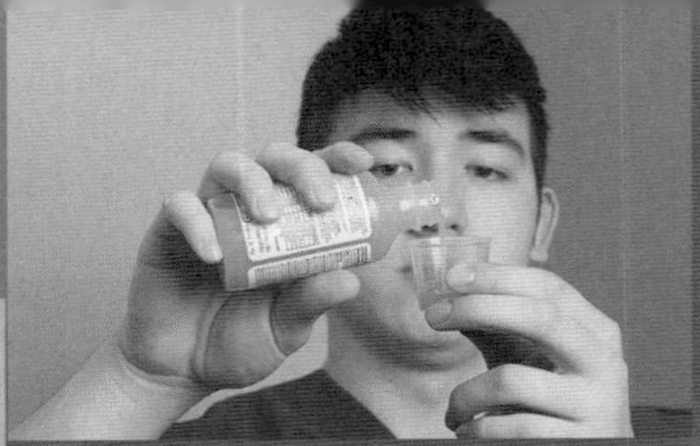

CHAPTER 38 Pediatrics

Learning Outcomes

COG Cognitive Domain

1. Spell key terms
2. Define medical terms and abbreviations related to all body systems
3. Compare structure and function of the human body across the life span
4. Analyze health care results as reported in graphs and tables
5. Identify common pathology related to each body system including signs, symptoms, and etiology
6. List safety precautions for the pediatric office
7. Explain the difference between a well-child and a sick-child visit
8. List types and schedule of immunizations
9. Describe the types of feelings a child might have during an office visit
10. List and explain how to record the anthropometric measurements obtained in a pediatric visit
11. Identify two injection sites to use on an infant and two used on a child
12. Describe the role of the parent during the office visit
13. List the names, symptoms, and treatments for common pediatric illnesses

PSY Psychomotor Domain

1. Obtain an infant's length and weight (Procedure 38-1)
2. Obtain the head and chest circumference (Procedure 38-2)
3. Apply a urinary collection device (Procedure 38-3)

AFF Affective Domain

1. Incorporate critical thinking skills when performing patient assessment
2. Incorporate critical thinking skills when performing patient care
3. Show awareness of a patient's concerns related to the procedure being performed
4. Demonstrate empathy, active listening, nonverbal communication
5. Demonstrate respect for individual diversity including gender, race, religion, age, economic status, appearance
6. Explain to a patient the rationale for performance of a procedure
7. Demonstrate sensitivity to patient rights
8. Protect the integrity of the medical record

ABHES Competencies

1. Assist the physician with the regimen of diagnostic and treatment modalities as they relate to each body system
2. Comply with federal, state, and local health laws and regulations
3. Communicate on the recipient's level of comprehension
4. Serve as a liaison between the physician and others
5. Show empathy and impartiality when dealing with patients
6. Document accurately

Name: ______________________ Date: ___________ Grade: ___________

COG MULTIPLE CHOICE

Circle the letter preceding the correct answer.

1. The top priority in a pediatric office is:
a. organization.
b. safety.
c. efficiency.
d. location.
e. size.

2. In a pediatrician's waiting room, it's most important that the toys are:
a. trendy.
b. interesting to all age groups.
c. large enough to share.
d. washable.
e. educational.

3. Which method of taking a temperature is most readily accepted by children of all ages?
a. Tympanic
b. Oral
c. Rectal
d. Axillary
e. Touch

4. One symptom of meningitis is:
a. dysuria.
b. disorientation.
c. coughing.
d. stiff neck.
e. chills.

5. Which of the following has been associated with Reye syndrome?
a. Pyloric stenosis
b. Aspirin
c. Cerebral palsy
d. Phenylalanine hydroxylase
e. Otitis media

6. Which of the following is something that is routinely done at a child's wellness exam?
a. Blood test
b. Urine test
c. Immunization
d. Radiography
e. Measurements

7. To minimize a child's anxiety during a visit, you should:
a. avoid talking to the child.
b. speak directly to the parent.
c. be gentle but firm.
d. ask the child to be quiet.
e. spend as little time in the room as possible.

8. Which of the following statements is true?
a. The reflexes present in a newborn disappear by age 3 months.
b. A pediatrician is responsible for a child's physical and mental health.
c. Disinfectants should be kept in patient rooms for easy access.
d. Vaccination Information Statements may be provided upon request.
e. The DDST measures all physical and mental aspects of a child.

9. One warning sign of child abuse is a child who:
a. comes in with scraped knees.
b. shrinks away as you approach.
c. has a poor growth pattern.
d. has a bloody nose.
e. screams when you administer a shot.

10. What might make the examination more fun for a 4- or 5-year-old child?
a. Allowing the child to crawl on the floor
b. Answering all the questions he or she asks
c. Showing the child medical pictures
d. Letting the child listen to his or her heartbeat
e. Asking the parent to assist with the exam

Scenario for questions 11 and 12: A child comes in for a well-child visit and begins to panic when she hears she will need to get a vaccination.

11. What should you do?
a. Let another assistant give her the shot.
b. Ask the parent or caregiver to calm her down.
c. Show her the needle ahead of time.
d. Tell her gently that it won't hurt at all.
e. Hide the needle until you give her the shot.

12. After you administer the medication, the girl becomes sullen and withdrawn. What is the best way to address this behavior?
a. Leave and allow her mother to comfort her.
b. Praise and comfort her before you leave.
c. Ask her if the shot was really that bad.
d. Promise it won't hurt so much next time.
e. Laugh and say it was just a little shot.

13. Which of the following disorders has symptoms that may become obvious only with the passage of time?
a. Meningitis
b. Croup
c. Epiglottitis
d. Cerebral palsy
e. Pyloric stenosis

14. Children are more likely to develop ear infections than adults because they have:
a. an immature nervous system.
b. short and straight Eustachian tubes.
c. decreased resistance to diseases.
d. more exposure to bacteria.
e. poor hand-washing skills.

15. Which infant reflex is a result of the cheek being stroked?
a. Rooting
b. Moro
c. Stepping
d. Fencing
e. Babinski

16. Children have lower blood pressure than adults because:
a. they cannot sit still for long periods of time.
b. they require a smaller cuff for measurements.
c. their hearts do not pump as quickly as adults' hearts.
d. their vessels are softer and less resistant.
e. you must use a standard sphygmomanometer.

17. At what age does a child's respiratory rate slow to that of an adult's?
a. 0 to 1 year
b. 1 to 5 years
c. 5 to 10 years
d. 10 to 15 years
e. 15 to 20 years

18. Which of the following can help a physician test an infant for pyloric stenosis?
a. Blood tests
b. Urine tests
c. Parental history
d. Percentile comparisons
e. Weight

19. Which of the following disorders cannot be cured at this time?
a. Meningitis
b. Impetigo
c. Tetanus
d. Syphilis
e. Cerebral palsy

20. A sharp barking cough is a symptom of:
a. meningitis.
b. croup.
c. tetanus.
d. encephalitis.
e. impetigo.

COG MATCHING

Grade: __________

Place the letter preceding the definition on the line next to the term.

Key Terms

21. ______ aspiration
22. ______ autonomous
23. ______ congenital anomaly
24. ______ immunization
25. ______ neonatologist
26. ______ pediatrician

Definitions

a. to control or confine movement
b. a physician who specializes in the care and treatment of newborns
c. a viral infection manifested by the characteristic rash of successive crops of vesicles that scab before resolution; also called chicken pox
d. a physician who specializes in the care of infants, children, and adolescents
e. a visit to the medical office for the administration of immunizations and evaluation of growth and development

Key Terms	Definitions
27. _____ pediatrics	**f.** drawing in or out by suction, as in breathing objects into the respiratory tract or suctioning substances from a site
28. _____ psychosocial	**g.** an abnormality, either structural or functional, present at birth
29. _____ restrain	**h.** a pediatric visit for the treatment of illness or injury
30. _____ sick-child visit	**i.** a specialty of medicine that deals with the care of infants, children, and adolescents
31. _____ varicella zoster	**j.** existing or functioning independently
32. _____ well-child visit	**k.** relating to mental and emotional aspects of social encounters
	l. the act or process of rendering an individual immune to specific disease

COG MATCHING

Grade: _____

Place the letter preceding the pulse rate range on the line preceding the appropriate age.

Ages	Pulse Rate Ranges
33. _____ newborn	**a.** 80 to 150/minute
34. _____ 3 months to 2 years	**b.** 60 to 100/minute
35. _____ 2 years to 10 years	**c.** 100 to 180/minute
36. _____ 10 years and older	**d.** 65 to 130/minute

PSY IDENTIFICATION

Grade: _____

37. Review the most current pediatric immunization schedule on the CDC (Center for Disease Control and Prevention website) to answer the following questions:

a. How many doses of the rotavirus vaccine are given? When?

_____

b. How many immunizations do children receive at 4 months? Which ones?

_____

c. When do children start receiving a yearly influenza vaccination?

_____

d. How many doses of the hepatitis B vaccine are administered?

_____

38. What are five different ways to check a child's temperature?

a. _____

b. _____

c. _____

d. _____

e. _____

39. What are the seven "rights" of drug administration?

a. ______

b. ______

c. ______

d. ______

e. ______

f. ______

g. ______

40. Identify six symptoms of meningitis:

______

COG SHORT ANSWER

Grade: ______

41. What does the Federal Child Abuse Prevention and Treatment Act mandate?

______

42. What is the VIS? Why do you give the parent or caregiver of a child a copy?

______

43. Why do sick-child visits occur frequently during early childhood?

______

44. What is the difference between a well-child and a sick-child visit?

______

45. List five feelings a child might have during an office visit.

46. What role does a parent or caregiver play in the child's exam?

47. How is a child's medication dosage calculated?

48. Why is epiglottitis considered more serious than croup?

49. If a child has been reported as being easily distracted, forgetful, extremely talkative, impulsive, and showing a dislike for school activities, does the child have ADHD?

50. A worried mother calls in because her newborn baby is vomiting. She wants to know if she should bring her baby into the office for examination. What do you tell her?

COG COMPLETION

Grade: ____________

51. Complete the chart below with information about childhood reflexes. Briefly describe each response and note the age it generally disappears.

Reflex	Response	Age When It Generally Disappears
a. Sucking, or rooting		
b. Moro, or startle		
c. Grasp		
d. Tonic neck, or fencing		
e. Placing, or stepping		
f. Babinski		

COG TRUE OR FALSE?

Grade: ____________

Indicate whether the statements are true or false by placing the letter T (true) or F (false) on the line preceding the statement.

52. ____________ Infant scales should always be placed on the floor next to the adult scale.

53. ____________ It is a violation of HIPAA to have two separate waiting rooms for sick children and well children.

54. ____________ There should be no toys in the waiting room because they may help spread germs.

55. ____________ Children outgrow child-sized furniture too quickly, so it is not a worthwhile investment.

56. ____________ Many childhood diseases are highly contagious and can be controlled by stringent hand-washing measures.

57. ____________ Immunization schedules change every 5 years.

58. ____________ A child's heartbeat is much slower than an adult's heart rate.

59. ____________ Asthma is a respiratory problem that usually develops after puberty.

60. ____________ Minors do not need to be informed of what you're going to do.

COG AFF CASE STUDIES FOR CRITICAL THINKING

Grade: ________

1. A mother calls in, saying her 15-month-old daughter has been fussy and tugging at her ear. There is no fever, but the girl has been tired and had a cold a few days before. What do you tell her to do?

2. A young boy, accompanied by his mother, greets you in the examination room and starts asking all kinds of questions about things you do. He enjoys helping you test his reflexes and reading the vision chart, but he firmly refuses to cooperate when you try to give him a shot. What can you or his mother do to get him settled down enough to give him the shot?

3. A 16-year-old boy has been diagnosed as obese, and his parents have come in to find out what they can do to help their son achieve a healthy weight. The physician wants the boy to exercise at a local gym and to return in 6 months to check his progress. What education can you provide that will help the boy and his parents start a healthier lifestyle?

4. A young child has come in with a broken arm. During the examination, you notice the child also has several scrapes and bruises on his legs and feet as well. His mother says he got them from playing outdoors. Do you report this as child abuse to the physician? If not, what do you do?

5. Spanking children for misbehaving is sometimes considered child abuse. However, the parents who spank their children say that they were spanked when they were young, and they believe it is the best way to safely punish bad behavior. They also say that children who are not spanked become spoiled and difficult to control. What do you think? Is it your duty to report spanking as child abuse?

PSY PROCEDURE 38-1 Obtain an Infant's Length and Weight

Name: ______________________ **Date:** __________ **Time:** __________ **Grade:** __________

EQUIPMENT/SUPPLIES: Examining table with clean paper, tape measure, infant scale, protective paper for the scale, appropriate growth chart

STANDARDS: Given the needed equipment and a place to work, the student will perform this skill with _____ % accuracy in a total of _____ minutes. *(Your instructor will tell you what the percentage and time limits will be before you begin.)*

KEY: 4 = Satisfactory 0 = Unsatisfactory NA = This step is not counted

PROCEDURE STEPS	SELF	PARTNER	INSTRUCTOR
1. Wash your hands.	❑	❑	❑
2. Greet the patient and caregiver and identify yourself including your title.	❑	❑	❑
3. Explain the procedure to the parent or caregiver.	❑	❑	❑
4. Ask parent to remove the infant's clothing except for the diaper.	❑	❑	❑
5. Place the child on a firm examination table covered with clean table paper.	❑	❑	❑
6. Fully extend the child's body by holding the head in the midline.	❑	❑	❑
7. Grasp the knees and press flat onto the table gently but firmly.	❑	❑	❑
8. Make a mark on table paper with pen at the top of the head and heel of the feet.	❑	❑	❑
9. Measure between marks in either inches or centimeters.	❑	❑	❑
10. Record the child's length on the growth chart and in the patient's chart.	❑	❑	❑
11. Either carry the infant or have the parent carry the infant to the scale.	❑	❑	❑
12. Place a protective paper on the scale and balance the scale.	❑	❑	❑
13. Remove the diaper just before laying the infant on the scale.	❑	❑	❑
14. Place the child gently on the scale. Keep one of your hands over or near the child on the scale at all times.	❑	❑	❑
15. Balance the scale quickly but carefully.	❑	❑	❑
16. Pick the infant up and instruct the parent to replace the diaper if removed.	❑	❑	❑
17. Wash your hands.	❑	❑	❑

PSY PROCEDURE 38-1 Obtain an Infant's Length and Weight (continued)

18. AFF Log into the Electronic Medical Record (EMR) using your username and secure password OR obtain the paper medical record from a secure location and assure it is kept away from public access.	❑	❑	❑
19. Record the infant's weight on the growth chart and in the patient medical record.	❑	❑	❑
20. When finished, log out of the EMR and/or replace the paper medical record in an appropriate and secure location.	❑	❑	❑

CALCULATION

Total Possible Points: __________

Total Points Earned: __________ Multiplied by 100 = __________ Divided by Total Possible Points = __________ %

PASS **FAIL** **COMMENTS:**

❑ ❑

Student's signature ____________________ Date __________

Partner's signature ____________________ Date __________

Instructor's signature ____________________ Date __________

PSY PROCEDURE 38-2 Obtain the Head and Chest Circumference

Name: ______________________ **Date:** __________ **Time:** __________ **Grade:** __________

EQUIPMENT/SUPPLIES: Paper or cloth measuring tape, growth chart

STANDARDS: Given the needed equipment and a place to work, the student will perform this skill with _____ % accuracy in a total of _____ minutes. *(Your instructor will tell you what the percentage and time limits will be before you begin.)*

KEY: 4 = Satisfactory 0 = Unsatisfactory NA = This step is not counted

PROCEDURE STEPS	SELF	PARTNER	INSTRUCTOR
1. Wash your hands.	❑	❑	❑
2. Place the infant in the supine position on the examination table, or ask the parent to hold the infant.	❑	❑	❑
3. Measure around the head above the eyebrow and posteriorly at the largest part of the occiput.	❑	❑	❑
4. Record the child's head circumference on the growth chart.	❑	❑	❑
5. With the infant's clothing removed from the chest, measure around the chest at the nipple line, keeping the measuring tape at the same level anteriorly and posteriorly.	❑	❑	❑
6. Wash your hands.	❑	❑	❑
7. AFF Log into the Electronic Medical Record (EMR) using your username and secure password OR obtain the paper medical record from a secure location and assure it is kept away from public access.	❑	❑	❑
8. Record the child's chest circumference on the growth chart.	❑	❑	❑
9. When finished, log out of the EMR and/or replace the paper medical record in an appropriate and secure location.	❑	❑	❑

CALCULATION

Total Possible Points: __________

Total Points Earned: __________ Multiplied by 100 = __________ Divided by Total Possible Points = __________ %

PASS ❑ **FAIL** ❑ **COMMENTS:**

Student's signature ____________________ Date __________

Partner's signature ____________________ Date __________

Instructor's signature ____________________ Date __________

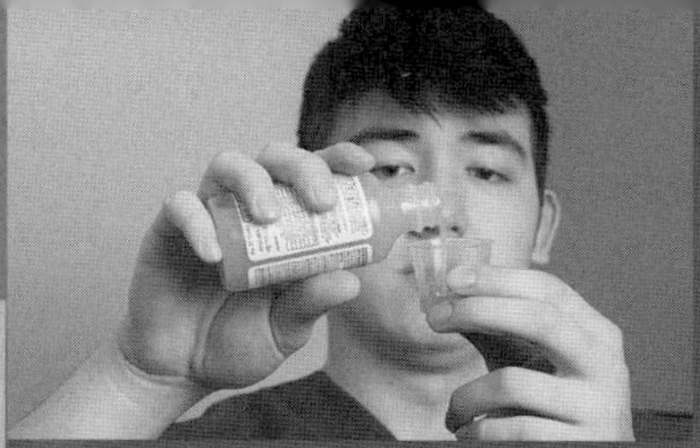

CHAPTER

39 Geriatrics

Learning Objectives

COG Cognitive Domain

1. Spell key terms
2. Define medical terms and abbreviations related to all body systems
3. Compare structure and function of the human body across the life span
4. Identify common pathology related to each body system including signs, symptoms, and etiology
5. Explain how aging affects thought processes
6. Describe methods to increase compliance with health maintenance programs among older adults
7. Discuss communication problems that may occur with the older adult and list steps to maintain open communication
8. Recognize and describe the coping mechanisms used by the older adult to deal with multiple losses
9. Name the risk factors and signs of elder abuse
10. Explain the types of long-term care facilities available
11. Describe the effects of aging on the way the body processes medication
12. Discuss the responsibility of medical assistants with regard to teaching older adult patients
13. List and describe physical changes and diseases common to the aging process

AFF Affective Domain

1. Incorporate critical thinking skills when performing patient assessment
2. Incorporate critical thinking skills when performing patient care
3. Demonstrate empathy, active listening, nonverbal communication
4. Demonstrate respect for individual diversity including gender, race, religion, age, economic status, appearance

ABHES Competencies

1. Assist the physician with the regimen of diagnostic and treatment modalities as they relate to each body system
2. Comply with federal, state, and local health laws and regulations
3. Communicate on the recipient's level of comprehension
4. Serve as a liaison between the physician and others
5. Show empathy and impartiality when dealing with patients
6. Document accurately

Name: ______________________ Date: __________ Grade: __________

COG MULTIPLE CHOICE

Circle the letter preceding the correct answer.

1. Which of the following statements is true about older adult patients who require long-term medication?
   a. If older adult patients take their medication every day, they are unlikely to forget a dosage.
   b. Compliance over a long period of time can become problematic in older adult patients.
   c. With a chronic illness, an older adult patient can neglect to take his or her medication for a few weeks with no side effects.
   d. Patients who take their medications for a long period of time will eventually notice a significant improvement.
   e. Older adult patients will eventually become immune to long-term medication.

2. Which of these conditions can sometimes be improved by taking the herbal supplement gingko?
   a. Arthritis
   b. Parkinson disease
   c. Loss of appetite
   d. Poor concentration
   e. Alzheimer disease

3. The purpose of an advance directive is to:
   a. divide a person's possessions in the event of death.
   b. inform the physician of any allergies that an individual has to specific medications.
   c. outline a person's wishes about end-of-life care.
   d. transfer a patient's medical records between physicians' offices.
   e. order a physician not to resuscitate a patient under any circumstances.

4. Which of these is a task performed by a home health aide?
   a. Light housecleaning
   b. Refilling prescriptions
   c. Reorganizing bulky furniture
   d. Writing daily task lists and reminders
   e. Keeping the older adult occupied

5. Which of these is a good place to find information about respite care for older adult relatives?
   a. Local newspaper
   b. Television advertisement
   c. Community senior citizen program
   d. Local business directory
   e. Library bulletin board

6. What is an example of passive neglect of an older adult patient?
   a. Withholding medication from the patient
   b. Locking the patient in a room
   c. Overmedicating the patient to make him or her easier to care for
   d. Isolating the patient from friends and family
   e. Forgetting to give the patient regular baths

7. Which of the following statements is true about the aging process?
   a. Longevity is based entirely on environmental factors.
   b. People who have dangerous occupations will not live as long as people who do not.
   c. Longevity is hereditary, so it does not make a difference how you live your life.
   d. Longevity is largely hereditary, but environmental factors play a significant role.
   e. An obese, physically inactive smoker will have a shorter lifespan than a healthy nonsmoker.

8. What is the best way to deal with a patient who is hearing impaired?
   a. Raise your voice until the patient can hear you.
   b. Give written instructions whenever possible.
   c. Talk to the patient with your back to the light.
   d. Talk directly into the patient's ear.
   e. Find a coworker who is able to communicate using sign language.

Scenario for questions 9 to 11: A 55-year-old patient comes into the physician's office and tells you that he thinks he is suffering from Parkinson disease.

9. The physician would diagnose the patient by:
   a. taking a blood test.
   b. performing dexterity tasks.
   c. excluding other causes.
   d. performing an MRI scan.
   e. testing his reflexes.

10. How would you explain deep brain stimulation to the patient?
    a. It increases the levels of dopamine in the brain.
    b. It lowers a person's acetylcholine levels.
    c. It blocks the impulses that cause tremors.
    d. It controls a person's stress and anxiety levels.
    e. It acts as a muscle relaxant and prevents rigidity.

11. What would you tell the patient about Levodopa?
a. It has no serious side effects.
b. It remains effective for the entire length of the disease.
c. It can cause headaches and migraines.
d. It should not be taken with alcohol.
e. It may aggravate stomach ulcers.

12. When older adult patients are beginning a new exercise regime, it is a good idea for them to:
a. rest when they get tired.
b. start with a brisk 30-minute jog.
c. keep to the same weekly routine.
d. exercise alone so they are not distracted.
e. work through any initial pain or discomfort.

13. Which of the following statements is true about the nutritional requirements of older adult patients?
a. Older adult patients need less food and water than younger patients because older adults are not as active.
b. It is easier for older adult patients to maintain good nutrition because they have more time to prepare meals.
c. Vitamin and mineral requirements are lower in older adult patients than in younger patients.
d. Older adult patients should eat smaller, more frequent meals to aid digestion.
e. Older adult patients can replace meals with liquid dietary supplements without damaging their health.

14. A caregiver can help increase safety in the home of an older adult patient by:
a. installing handrails in the bathtub and near the commode.
b. placing childproof locks on the kitchen cupboards.
c. encouraging the patient to exercise regularly.
d. covering highly polished floors with scatter rugs.
e. keeping the patient's medicine in a locked bathroom cabinet.

15. What action should you take if you suspect older adult abuse?
a. Try to separate the caregiver from the patient for the examination.
b. Tell the caregiver you will be reporting him or her to the authorities.
c. Question the patient about suspicious injuries until she tells you the truth.
d. Call the police while the patient is in the examination room.
e. Wait to inform the physician of your suspicions until you are sure they are correct.

16. What does the acronym HOH mean in a patient's chart?
a. Has ordinary hearing
b. Head of household
c. Has own home
d. Hard on health
e. Hard of hearing

17. Another name for the herbal supplement gingko is:
a. folic acid.
b. kew tree.
c. aloe vera.
d. green tea.
e. milk thistle.

18. What is the best advice to give a patient who is having difficulty swallowing medication?
a. Grind the medication into powder.
b. Ask the pharmacist for smaller pills.
c. Put the medication on the back of the tongue, and drink water with a straw.
d. Lie down and swallow the medication with a lot of water.
e. Dissolve the medication in a hot drink.

19. A physician who specializes in disorders that affect the aging population is called a(n):
a. gastroenterologist.
b. gerontologist.
c. oncologist.
d. otorhinolaryngologist.
e. rheumatologist.

20. An eye condition that causes increased intraocular pressure and intolerance to light is:
a. cataracts.
b. kyphosis.
c. bradykinesia.
d. osteoporosis.
e. glaucoma.

COG MATCHING

Grade: ______

Place the letter preceding the definition on the line next to the term.

Key Terms

21. ______ activities of daily living (ADL)
22. ______ biotransform
23. ______ bradykinesia
24. ______ cataracts
25. ______ cerebrovascular accident (CVA)
26. ______ compliance
27. ______ degenerative joint disease (DJD)
28. ______ dementia
29. ______ dysphasia
30. ______ gerontologist
31. ______ glaucoma
32. ______ Kegel exercises
33. ______ keratosis (senile)
34. ______ kyphosis (dowager's hump)
35. ______ lentigines
36. ______ osteoporosis
37. ______ potentiation
38. ______ presbycusis
39. ______ presbyopia
40. ______ senility
41. ______ syncope
42. ______ transient ischemic attack (TIA)
43. ______ vertigo

Definitions

a. a specialist who studies aging
b. general mental deterioration associated with old age
c. to convert the molecules of a substance from one form to another, as in medications within the body
d. a sensation of whirling of oneself or the environment, dizziness
e. abnormally slow voluntary movements
f. a sudden fall in blood pressure or cerebral hypoxia resulting in loss of consciousness
g. progressive organic mental deterioration with loss of intellectual function
h. a skin condition characterized by overgrowth and thickening
i. difficulty speaking
j. an abnormal porosity of the bone, most often found in the older adult, predisposing the affected bony tissue to fracture
k. an acute episode of cerebrovascular insufficiency, usually a result of narrowing of an artery by atherosclerotic plaques, emboli, or vasospasm; usually passes quickly but should be considered a warning for predisposition to cerebrovascular accidents
l. a progressive loss of transparency of the lens of the eye, resulting in opacity and loss of sight
m. describes the actions of two drugs taken together in which the combined effects are greater than the sum of the independent effects
n. a vision change (farsightedness) associated with aging
o. isometric exercises in which the muscles of the pelvic floor are voluntarily contracted and relaxed while urinating
p. brown skin macules occurring after prolonged exposure to the sun; freckles
q. a loss of hearing associated with aging
r. an abnormally deep dorsal curvature of the thoracic spine; also known as humpback or hunchback
s. activities usually performed in the course of the day, i.e., bathing, dressing, feeding oneself
t. also known as *osteoarthritis*; arthritis characterized by degeneration of the bony structure of the joints, usually noninflammatory
u. willingness of a patient to follow a prescribed course of treatment
v. ischemia of the brain due to an occlusion of the blood vessels supplying the brain, resulting in varying degrees of debilitation
w. an abnormal increase in the fluid of the eye, usually as a result of obstructed outflow, resulting in degeneration of the intraocular components and blindness

COG MATCHING

Grade: ________

Place the letter preceding the description of the facility on the line preceding the type of facility.

Facilities

44. _____ Group homes or assisted living facilities
45. _____ Long-term care facilities
46. _____ Skilled-nursing facilities

Descriptions

a. Facilities for those who need help with most areas of personal care and moderate medical supervision
b. Facilities for those who are gravely or terminally ill and need constant supervision
c. Facilities for those who can tend to their own activities of daily living but need companionship and light supervision for safety

COG IDENTIFICATION

Grade: ________

47. Some older adult patients suffer from memory loss, which may make it difficult for them to remember to take their medications. As a medical assistant, it is important to give these patients tools to help them remember and maintain their medication regimens. Identify and list five ways you can help older adult patients remember their medication regimens.

____

____

____

____

48. Which of the following are common reasons for older adult patients not taking their medications correctly? Place a check mark on the line next to all that apply.

a. __________ Financial difficulties

b. __________ To attract attention

c. __________ Forgetfulness

d. __________ Tiring of the constraints of taking long-term medication

e. __________ Deliberate defiance

49. Mrs. Kim is 89 years old and suffers from memory lapses. It is apparent that she is both frustrated and lonely. Identify and list three ways that you can maintain good communication with her and help her express her feelings.

____

____

____

____

50. Mrs. Driscoll is 84 years old with poor eyesight who suffers from forgetfulness. She needs to take two different types of medication three times a day. Identify and list four ways that you could help ensure that Mrs. Driscoll adheres to her medication regimen.

____

____

____

____

51. Patients who react negatively to moving to a long-term care facility can show signs of grief. Identify and list five symptoms that could indicate that a patient is suffering from a sense of loss.

____

____

____

____

52. Sometimes an older adult patient will turn to alcohol as a way of coping. The effects of drinking alcohol can often be mistaken for other ailments. Identify and list three conditions that exhibit symptoms similar to the influence of alcohol.

____

____

____

____

53. Suicide is a risk for older adult patients, especially those who have recently lost a spouse to death or divorce. Which of the following warning signs indicate that an older adult patient is contemplating suicide? Place a check mark on the line next to all that apply.

a. ______________ Giving away favored objects

b. ______________ Increased interest in family affairs

c. ______________ Secretive behavior

d. ______________ Increased anger, hostility, or isolation

e. ______________ Increased forgetfulness

f. ______________ Increased alcohol or drug use

g. ______________ Loss of interest in matters of health

54. Which of the following indicate that a patient is suffering from older adult abuse? Place a check mark on the line preceding all that apply.

a. ______________ Disturbed sleep patterns

b. ______________ Signs of restraint on the wrists or ankles

c. ______________ Large, deep pressure ulcers

d. ______________ Incontinence

e. ______________ Poor hygiene or poor nutrition

f. ______________ Untreated injury or condition

g. ______________ Dehydration not caused by disease

55. Which of the following are symptoms of Parkinson disease? Circle the letter preceding all that apply.

a. Muscle rigidity
b. Increased anger
c. Involuntary tremors
d. Difficulty walking
e. Loss of memory
f. Dysphagia and drooling
g. Expressionless face and infrequent blinking

56. Identify and list three reasons why an older adult patient can have difficulty maintaining good nutrition.

a. ____

b. ____

c. ____

COG SHORT ANSWER

Grade: ___________

57. You ask Mr. Walton if he is taking his blood pressure medication and he tells you that he is taking it every day. Later, the physician tells you that Mr. Walton has been taking three pills a day instead of just one. How could this situation be avoided with other older adult patients?

____

____

____

____

58. Mrs. Dawson is a widow who lives in a long-term care facility. Her family is worried that she has recently become withdrawn and uncommunicative. Before her husband died, Mrs. Dawson led an active life and took a large role in running the household. What could you say to Mrs. Dawson's family to help her cope with the loss of her spouse and her independence?

____

____

____

____

59. Mr. Gonzalez is an 85-year-old patient who lives alone. He is still fairly active and is able to carry out most activities of daily living by himself. However, members of his family have expressed some concerns that he is lonely and that they are not able to visit him as often as they would like. What options could you discuss with the family?

____

____

____

____

COG COMPLETION

Grade: _______

60. Older adult patients whose health and economic situation are unstable may experience feelings of grief and loss. These feelings can be about both specific and nonspecific aspects of their lives. Fill in the chart below, listing five specific and nonspecific losses older adult patients may find difficult to cope with.

Specific Losses	Nonspecific Losses
a.	
b.	
c.	
d.	
e.	

61. The passage below describes how medications affect the body of an older adult. However, some of the important terms are missing. Read the passage and fill in the correct words from the list below.

The ______________ system no longer moves medications along as efficiently because ______________ has slowed. The ______________ system does not absorb dissolved medication from the ______________ or the ______________ and deliver it to the target tissue as quickly. The ______________ does not ______________ medication as quickly, causing medications to remain in the body longer than desirable and possibly add to the cumulative effect. Finally, the ______________ receive less blood, so less medication is filtered and removed from the body. These decreases in body system function can result in possible ______________ of medications in the older adult.

circulatory system	*gastrointestinal system*	*intestines*	*biotransform*	*kidneys*
toxic effects		*liver*	*peristalsis*	*injection site*

62. Complete the following table by indicating whether the following suggestions are appropriate for a patient with Parkinson disease or for a patient with Alzheimer disease. Place a checkmark in the appropriate box.

Suggestion	Patient with Parkinson Disease	Patient with Alzheimer Disease
a. Speak calmly and without condescension.		
b. Do not argue with the patient.		
c. Tell the patient to take small bites and chew each mouthful carefully before swallowing.		
d. Encourage the patient to use no-spill cups, plates with high sides, and special utensils.		
e. Free the home from rugs and loose cords that may cause tripping.		
f. Speak in short, simple, direct sentences and explain one action at a time.		
g. Listen to the patient and stimulate his intelligence.		
h. Remind the patient who you are and what you must do.		

COG TRUE OR FALSE?

Grade: ______________

Indicate whether the statements are true or false by placing the letter T (true) or F (false) on the line preceding the statement.

63. ______________ Newspaper word puzzles are just a temporary distraction to help entertain older adults.

64. ______________ Attempts to commit suicide by older adults are usually just a cry for help.

65. ______________ If a patient has an advance directive on file somewhere other than the medical office, it should be noted in her medical record.

66. ______________ Most older adult abuse is committed by workers in long-term care facilities.

COG AFF CASE STUDIES FOR CRITICAL THINKING

Grade: ________

1. Read the following case studies and think about what you know about the causes of older adult abuse. Circle the letter preceding the case study that describes the patient who falls in the highest risk category for abuse.

a. Mr. Simpson is an 89-year-old widower who lives alone. He is still fairly active and is able to carry out most daily activities by himself. He has a daughter and a son, who take turns visiting him every week and doing his shopping and laundry for him. Mr. Simpson takes medication for high blood pressure and angina.

b. Mrs. Lewis is an 83-year-old patient who lives in a long-term care facility. She suffers from mild senile dementia, which her family sometimes finds frustrating, but is learning to cope with. Mrs. Lewis has a home health aide and private nurse to help her carry out activities of daily living. She sleeps for most of the day.

c. Mrs. Beddowes is a 90-year-old widow who lives with her son. She suffers from senile dementia, incontinence, and insomnia. Her family members cannot afford to place her in a long-term care facility, so they share the responsibility of taking care of her. However, most of the responsibility falls onto her son, who helps Mrs. Beddowes carry out most activities of daily living.

d. Mr. Williams is an 81-year-old patient who lives in an assisted living facility. He was recently widowed and is having difficulty coming to terms with his wife's death. Mr. Williams used to be extremely active but has recently become withdrawn and has started drinking heavily. He has two daughters who visit him regularly.

2. Your patient is a 90-year-old man with various age-associated health problems. He has been recently diagnosed with dementia, but during his recent visits to the physician's office, you have smelled alcohol on his breath. How would you handle this situation? What would you do?

____

____

____

____

3. Your patient is an 82-year-old woman who suffers from mild hearing loss. She recently lost her husband and has been making frequent appointments at the physician's office for minor complaints. You suspect that the patient is lonely and is visiting the office for company and human interaction. Explain what you would do.

____

____

____

____

4. Your patient is an 80-year-old woman who has recently lost a noticeable amount of weight. She tells you that she has not been very hungry lately and has not felt like eating very much. The physician has asked you to write a list of nutritional guidelines for her to follow and explain why they are important. What would you put in the guidelines?

____

____

____

____

5. Your patient is a 91-year-old man with Alzheimer disease. After his appointment with the physician, you overhear his family trying to get him into the car. The patient has forgotten where he is and refuses to leave the physician's office. His daughter loses her temper and shouts at her father loudly until he complies. What would you do? Explain your actions.

____

____

____

____

6. You overhear a coworker asking a 77-year-old patient about her medical history. When the patient tells your coworker that she is taking gingko to improve her memory, your coworker tells her that she needs to know only about actual medications. What would you say to your coworker?

____

____

____

____

PART

4

The Clinical Laboratory

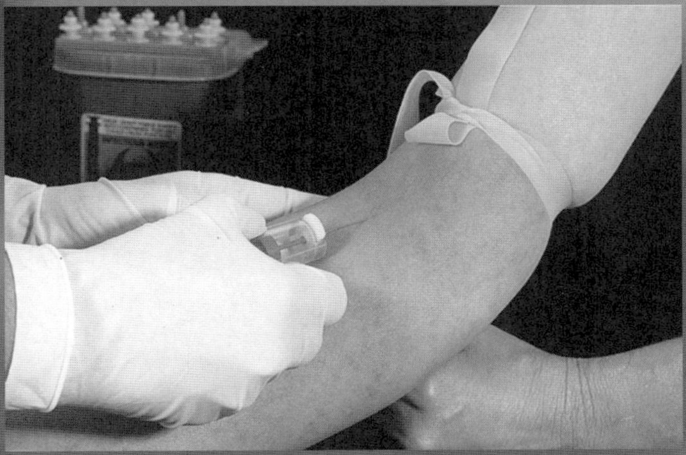

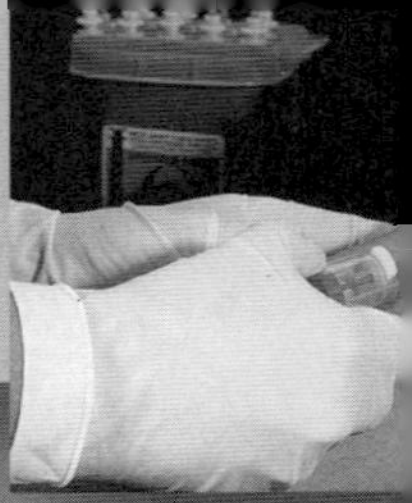

UNIT SIX FUNDAMENTALS OF LABORATORY PROCEDURES

CHAPTER 40

Introduction to the Physician Office Laboratory

Learning Outcomes

COG Cognitive Domain

1. Spell key terms
2. Define medical terms and abbreviations related to all body systems
3. List the various types of clinical laboratories including the physician office laboratory
4. Explain the types of departments found in most large laboratories
5. Describe common laboratory tests ordered to diagnose disease and illness
6. Explain the significance of CLIA and how to maintain compliance in the physician office laboratory
7. Identify disease processes that are indications for CLIA-waived tests
8. Identify equipment found in the physician office laboratory and routine maintenance
9. List and describe the parts of a microscope
10. Discuss the role of the medical assistant in clinical laboratory testing
11. Define critical values
12. Analyze charts, graphs, and/or tables in the interpretation of health care results

PSY Psychomotor Domain

1. Care of the microscope (Procedure 40-1)
2. Screen test results (Procedure 40-2)
3. Maintain laboratory test results using flow sheets (Procedures 40-3 and 40-4)

ABHES Competencies

1. Incorporate critical thinking skills when performing patient assessment
2. Distinguish between normal and abnormal test results

PSY PROCEDURE 40-1 Care of the Microscope (continued)

____

____

____

____

CALCULATION

Total Possible Points: __________

Total Points Earned: __________ Multiplied by 100 = __________ Divided by Total Possible Points = __________ %

PASS ❑ **FAIL** ❑ **COMMENTS:**

Student's signature ____________________ Date __________

Partner's signature ____________________ Date __________

Instructor's signature ____________________ Date __________

PSY PROCEDURE 40-2 Screen and Follow Up Test Results

Name: ____________________ **Date:** __________ **Time:** __________ **Grade:** __________

EQUIPMENT/SUPPLIES: Patient laboratory results, critical values list for office, patient medical record

STANDARDS: Given the needed equipment and a place to work, the student will perform this skill with _____ % accuracy in a total of _____ minutes. *(Your instructor will tell you what the percentage and time limits will be before you begin practicing.)*

KEY: 4 = Satisfactory 0 = Unsatisfactory NA = This step is not counted

PROCEDURE STEPS	SELF	PARTNER	INSTRUCTOR
1. Review laboratory reports received from reference laboratory.	❏	❏	❏
2. Note which reports may be placed directly on the patient's chart and which require immediate notification due to critical results.	❏	❏	❏
3. Notify the physician of the result. Take any immediate instructions from the physician.	❏	❏	❏
4. Follow instructions and document notification and follow-up.	❏	❏	❏
5. Chart remaining reports appropriately.	❏	❏	❏

CALCULATION

Total Possible Points: __________

Total Points Earned: __________ Multiplied by 100 = __________ Divided by Total Possible Points = __________ %

PASS ❏ **FAIL** ❏ **COMMENTS:**

Student's signature ____________________ Date __________

Partner's signature ____________________ Date __________

Instructor's signature ____________________ Date __________

PSY PROCEDURE 40-3 Use a Laboratory Flow Sheet

Name: ______________________ **Date:** __________ **Time:** __________ **Grade:** __________

EQUIPMENT/SUPPLIES: Flow sheet for documenting a patient's anticoagulation therapy and test results; scenarios for patient Jacob Wisliki.

STANDARDS: Patient Jacob Wisliki is on Coumadin (warfarin) therapy following a stroke. Dr. Wilson requests that you maintain a flow sheet on this patient and orders weekly INR (coagulation) testing.

The student will perform this skill with ________% accuracy in a total of ________ minutes. *(Your instructor will tell you what the percentage and time limits will be before you begin practicing.)*

PATIENT SCENARIOS:

- Today is November 1, 2016. Mr. Wisliki's INR is 1.8, which is below Dr. Wilson's target range. Dr. Wilson increases Mr. Wisliki's dose to 2.5 mg qd and requests that Mr. Wisliki return in a week for another INR.
- Mr. Wisliki returns and his INR is 2.1, which is in Dr. Wilson's therapeutic range. Dr. Wilson would like to see the value higher so he increases Mr. Wisliki's Coumadin dose to 3.5 mg qd and have another INR performed in 1 week.
- The following week, Mr. Wisliki returns and his INR result is 3.5, which is higher than Dr. Wilson's therapeutic range. Dr. Wilson decreases Mr. Wisliki's dose to 3.0 mg qd and requests Mr. Wisliki to return in 1 week.
- Mr. Wisliki returns on schedule the following week and his INR is 3.1. Dr. Wilson is concerned that Mr. Wisliki's INR did not respond as usual to the decrease in the dose. Mr. Wisliki is instructed to avoid eating green leafy vegetables while on anticoagulant therapy and his dose is not changed. He is instructed to return in a week as ordered by Dr. Wilson.
- Mr. Wisliki is back for his weekly INR check, and today, it is 2.5. Dr. Wilson is pleased with this INR result and does not change the dose. You instruct Mr. Wisliki to return in a week as Dr. Wilson ordered.
- Mr. Wisliki is back for his INR, which is 2.5. Because his INR is stable, Dr. Wilson does not change his dose.

KEY: 4 = Satisfactory 0 = Unsatisfactory NA = This step is not counted

PROCEDURE STEPS	SELF	PARTNER	INSTRUCTOR
1. Obtain the anticoagulant flow sheet and the scenarios and data for Jacob Wisliki.	❑	❑	❑
2. Record the INR results, medication dosage change (new dose), and your name (first initial, last name) on the first line (date 11/01/2016) of the flow sheet.	❑	❑	❑
3. Record the date, INR results, medication dosage change, and your name for the 2nd week of the scenario.	❑	❑	❑
4. Record the date, INR results, medication dosage change, and your name for each of the following weeks (weeks # 2, 3, 4, 5, and 6).	❑	❑	❑
5. Each weekly entry is complete, legible, and accurate.	❑	❑	❑
6. Explain that the flow sheet is maintained in the patient medical record.	❑	❑	❑

PSY PROCEDURE 40-3 Use a Laboratory Flow Sheet (continued)

CALCULATION

Total Possible Points: __________

Total Points Earned: __________ Multiplied by 100 = __________ Divided by Total Possible Points = __________ %

PASS **FAIL** **COMMENTS:**

❑ ❑

Student's signature ____________________ Date __________

Partner's signature ____________________ Date __________

Instructor's signature ____________________ Date __________

PSY PROCEDURE 40-4 Anticoagulant Flow Sheet

Name: ______________________ **Date:** __________ **Time:** __________ **Grade:** __________

PATIENT'S NAME: Jacob Wisliki

DATE OF BIRTH: 03/20/1940

TARGET INTERNATIONAL NORMALIZED RATIO (INR): √ 2.0–3.0 □ 2.5–3.5 Other: _______

Date	Current Dose	INR	Medication	New Dose	Signature
11/01/2016	2 mg qd				

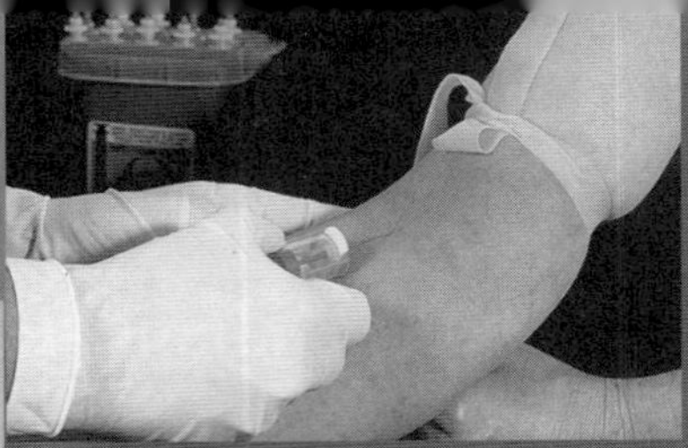

CHAPTER

41 Phlebotomy

Learning Outcomes

COG Cognitive Domain

1. Spell and define the key terms
2. Define medical terms and abbreviations related to all body systems
3. Identify equipment and supplies used to obtain a routine venous specimen and a routine capillary skin puncture
4. Describe proper use of specimen collection equipment
5. List the major anticoagulants, their color codes, and the suggested order in which they are filled during a venipuncture
6. Describe the location and selection of the blood collection sites using capillaries and veins
7. Differentiate between the feel of a vein, tendon, and artery
8. Describe care for a puncture site after blood has been drawn
9. Explain quality assessment issues in specimen collection procedures

PSY Psychomotor Domain

1. Obtain a blood specimen by evacuated tube or winged infusion set (Procedure 41-1)
   a. Perform venipuncture
   b. Instruct and prepare a patient for a procedure or treatment
   c. Coach patients appropriately considering cultural diversity, developmental life stage, communication barriers
   d. Document patient care accurately in the medical record.
2. Obtain a blood specimen by capillary puncture (Procedure 41-2)
   a. Perform capillary puncture
   b. Instruct and prepare a patient for a procedure or treatment
   c. Coach patients appropriately considering cultural diversity, developmental life stage, communication barriers
   d. Document patient care accurately in the medical record.

AFF Affective Domain

1. Incorporate critical thinking skills when performing patient assessment.
2. Incorporate critical thinking skills when performing patient care.
3. Show awareness of a patient's concerns related to the procedure being performed.
4. Demonstrate empathy, active listening, nonverbal communication
5. Demonstrate respect for individual diversity including gender, race, religion, age, economic status, appearance.
6. Explain to a patient the rationale for performance of a procedure
7. Demonstrate sensitivity to patient rights
8. Protect the integrity of the medical record.

ABHES Competencies

1. Define and use entire basic structure of medical words and be able to accurately identify in the correct context, that is, root, prefix, suffix, combinations, spelling, and definitions
2. Build and dissect medical terms from roots/suffixes to understand the word element combinations that create medical terminology
3. Document accurately
4. Comply with federal, state, and local health laws and regulations
5. Identify and respond appropriately when working/caring for patients with special needs
6. Maintain inventory equipment and supplies
7. Communicate on the recipient's level of comprehension
8. Use pertinent medical terminology
9. Recognize and respond to verbal and nonverbal communication
10. Use standard precautions
11. Dispose of biohazardous materials
12. Collect, label, and process specimens
13. Perform venipuncture
14. Perform capillary puncture

COG PLACE IN ORDER

Grade: ______

61. Numbering from 1 to 25, place the steps for performing a venipuncture in the correct order.

______ Greet and identify the patient. Explain the procedure. Ask for and answer any questions.

______ Tap the tubes that contain additives to ensure that the additive is dislodged from the stopper and wall of the tube. Insert the tube into the adaptor until the needle slightly enters the stopper. Do not push the top of the tube stopper beyond the indentation mark. If the tube retracts slightly, leave it in the retracted position.

______ Check the physician order and fill out a laboratory requisition form if necessary.

______ If a fasting specimen is required, ask the patient the last time he or she ate or drank anything other than water.

______ Select a vein by palpating. Use your gloved index finger to trace the path of the vein and judge its depth.

______ Wash your hands.

______ Apply the tourniquet around the patient's arm 3 to 4 inches above the elbow.

______ Cleanse the venipuncture site with an alcohol pad, starting in the center of puncture site and working outward in a circular motion. Allow the site to dry or dry the site with sterile gauze. Do not touch the area after cleansing.

______ With the bevel up, line up the needle with the vein approximately one quarter to half an inch below the site where the vein is to be entered. At a 15- to 30-degree angle, rapidly and smoothly insert the needle through the skin. Place two fingers on the flanges of the adapter, and with the thumb, push the tube onto the needle inside the adapter. Allow the tube to fill to capacity. Release the tourniquet and allow the patient to release the fist. When blood flow ceases, remove the tube from the adapter by gripping the tube with your nondominant hand and placing your thumb against the flange during removal. Twist and gently pull out the tube. Steady the needle in the vein. Avoid pulling up or pressing down on the needle while it is in the vein. Insert any other necessary tubes into adapter and allow each to fill to capacity.

______ Assemble the equipment. Check the expiration date on the tubes.

______ Record the procedure.

______ Put on nonsterile latex or vinyl gloves. Use other personal protective equipment as defined by facility policy.

______ Place a sterile gauze pad over the puncture site at the time of needle withdrawal. Do not apply any pressure to the site until the needle is completely removed. After the needle is removed, immediately activate the safety device and apply pressure or have the patient apply direct pressure for 3 to 5 minutes. Do not bend the arm at the elbow.

______ Instruct the patient to sit with a well-supported arm.

______ Label the tubes with patient information as defined in facility protocol.

______ Release the tourniquet after palpating the vein if it has been left on for more than 1 minute. Have patient release his or her fist.

______ Test, transfer, or store the blood specimen according to the medical office policy.

______ Remove the needle cover. Hold the needle assembly in your dominant hand, thumb on top of the adaptor and fingers under it. Grasp the patient's arm with the other hand, using your thumb to draw the skin taut over the site. This anchors the vein about 1 to 2 inches below the puncture site and helps keep it in place during needle insertion.

______ If the vacuum tubes contain an anticoagulant, they must be mixed immediately by gently inverting the tube 8 to 10 times. Do not shake the tube.

______ If blood being drawn for culture will be used in diagnosing a septic condition, make sure the specimen is sterile. To do this, apply alcohol to the area for 2 full minutes. Then apply a 2% iodine solution in ever widening circles. Never move the wipes back over areas that have been cleaned; use a new wipe for each sweep across the area.

______ Thank the patient. Instruct the patient to leave the bandage in place at least 15 minutes and not to carry a heavy object (such as a purse) or lift heavy objects with that arm for 1 hour.

______ Properly care for or dispose of all equipment and supplies. Clean the work area. Remove personal protective equipment and wash your hands.

______ Reapply the tourniquet if it was removed after palpation. Ask patient to make a fist.

______ Check the puncture site for bleeding. Apply a dressing, a clean 2 × 2 gauze pad folded in quarters, and hold in place by an adhesive bandage or 3-inch strip of tape.

______ With the tourniquet released, remove the tube from the adapter before removing the needle from the arm.

62. Numbering from 1 to 16, place the steps for performing a capillary puncture in the correct order.

______ Thank the patient. Instruct the patient to leave the bandage in place at least 15 minutes.

______ Greet and identify the patient. Explain the procedure. Ask for and answer any questions.

______ Check the physician order and fill out a laboratory requisition form if necessary.

______ Select the puncture site. Use the appropriate puncture device for the site selected.

______ Obtain the first drop of blood. Wipe away the first drop of blood with dry gauze. Apply pressure toward the site but do not milk the site.

______ Wash your hands.

______ Grasp the finger firmly between your nondominant index finger and thumb, or grasp the infant's heel firmly with your index finger wrapped around the foot and your thumb wrapped around the ankle. Cleanse the selected area with 70% isopropyl alcohol and allow to air dry.

______ Record the procedure.

______ Assemble the equipment.

______ Hold the patient's finger or heel firmly and make a swift, firm puncture. Perform the puncture perpendicular to the whorls of the fingerprint or footprint. Dispose of the used puncture device in a sharps container.

______ Test, transfer, or store the specimen according to the medical office policy.

______ Put on gloves.

______ Collect the specimen in the chosen container or slide. Touch only the tip of the collection device to the drop of blood. Blood flow is encouraged if the puncture site is held downward and gentle pressure is applied near the site. Cap microcollection tubes with the caps provided and mix the additives by gently tilting or inverting the tubes 8 to 10 times.

______ Make sure the site chosen is warm and not cyanotic or edematous. Gently massage the finger from the base to the tip or massage the infant's heel.

______ Properly care for or dispose of equipment and supplies. Clean the work area. Remove gloves and wash your hands.

______ When collection is complete, apply clean gauze to the site with pressure. Hold pressure or have the patient hold pressure until bleeding stops. Label the containers with the proper information. Do not apply a dressing to a skin puncture of an infant under age 2 years. Never release a patient until the bleeding has stopped.

2. You are reviewing test results received from the referral laboratory. You notice that the HIV results on your neighbor, Alice Sihotang, are positive. Your friend Kaylene Oyakawa meets you for lunch. She tells you that all of your neighbors are worried about Alice because she looks so ill and has been losing weight. Kaylene says that she knows Alice is a patient at your medical office and asks you what is wrong with Alice. What do you say?

____

____

____

____

3. After drawing blood with a winged set, you inadvertently stick yourself with the needle. How would you handle this situation?

____

____

____

____

4. Your last patient of the day, a young child accompanied by her mother, accidentally knocks over your collection tubes that were within her reach as you were disposing of sharps. How would you handle this situation?

____

____

____

____

5. The medical office has closed and you are completing preparation of specimens for the reference laboratory pick-up. You find you have two requisitions without labeled specimens to accompany them. You have two unlabeled blood tubes. There is no way to identify the two specimens. What do you do?

____

____

____

____

PSY PROCEDURE 41-1 Obtain a Blood Specimen by Evacuated Tube or Winged Infusion Set

Name: ______________________ **Date:** ________ **Time:** ________ **Grade:** ________

EQUIPMENT/SUPPLIES: Multisample needle and adaptor or winged infusion set, evacuated tubes, tourniquet, sterile gauze pads, bandages, sharps container, 70% alcohol pad, permanent marker or pen, appropriate personal protective equipment (e.g., gloves, impervious gown, face shield)

STANDARDS: Given the needed equipment and a place to work, the student will perform this skill with _____ % accuracy in a total of _____ minutes. *(Your instructor will tell you what the percentage and time limits will be before you begin practicing.)*

KEY: 4 = Satisfactory 0 = Unsatisfactory NA =This step is not counted

PROCEDURE STEPS	SELF	PARTNER	INSTRUCTOR
1. Check the physician order and complete the requisition slip if appropriate.	❑	❑	❑
2. Wash your hands and assemble the equipment.	❑	❑	❑
3. Check the expiration date on the tubes. Discard expired supplies according to office policy and procedure.	❑	❑	❑
4. AFF Greet and identify the patient and yourself including your title. Explain the procedure.	❑	❑	❑
5. AFF Demonstrate recognition of the patient's level of understanding communications. Apply active listening skills. Modify communication to the patient's level of understanding, or obtain assistance with language differences.	❑	❑	❑
6. Ask the patient about any dietary restrictions and the use of medications that increase bleeding time. If a fasting or NPO specimen is required, ask the patient for the last time he or she ate or drank anything.	❑	❑	❑
7. Put on nonsterile latex or vinyl gloves. Use other personal protective equipment as defined by office policy.	❑	❑	❑
8. *For evacuated tube collection*: Break the seal of the needle cover and thread the sleeved needle into the adaptor, using the needle cover as a wrench. *For winged infusion set collection*: Extend the tubing. Thread the sleeved needle into the adaptor. *For both methods*: Tap the tubes that contain additives to ensure that the additive is dislodged from the stopper and wall of the tube. Insert the tube into the adaptor until the needle slightly enters the stopper. Do not push the top of the tube stopper beyond the indentation mark. If the tube retracts slightly, leave it in the retracted position.	❑	❑	❑
9. Instruct the patient to sit with a well-supported arm.	❑	❑	❑

PSY PROCEDURE 41-1 Obtain a Blood Specimen by Evacuated Tube or Winged Infusion Set (continued)

10. After reviewing veins in both arms, choose one arm and apply the tourniquet 3 –to 4 inches above the elbow. **a.** Apply the tourniquet snuggly, but not too tightly. **b.** Secure the tourniquet by using the half-bow knot. **c.** Make sure the tails of the tourniquet extend upward to avoid contaminating the venipuncture site. **d.** Ask the patient to make a fist and hold it, but not to pump the fist.	❑	❑	❑
11. Select a vein by palpating. Use your gloved index finger to trace the path of the vein and judge its depth.	❑	❑	❑
12. Release tourniquet after palpating the vein if it has been left on for more than one minute. Have patient release fist.	❑	❑	❑
13. Cleanse the venipuncture site with an alcohol pad, starting in the center of puncture site and working outward in a circular motion. Allow the site to dry or dry the site with sterile gauze. Do not touch the area after cleansing.	❑	❑	❑
14. If blood is being drawn for a blood culture, make sure the area is cleansed using a 2% iodine solution for 2 full minutes.	❑	❑	❑
15. Reapply the tourniquet if it was removed after palpation. Ask patient to make a fist.	❑	❑	❑
16. Remove the needle cover. Hold the needle assembly in your dominant hand, thumb on top of the adaptor and fingers under it. Grasp the patient's arm with the other hand, using your thumb to draw the skin taut over the site. This anchors the vein about 1 –to 2 inches below the puncture site and helps keep it in place during needle insertion.	❑	❑	❑
17. With the bevel up, line up the needle with the vein approximately one quarter to half an inch below the site where the vein is to be entered. At a 15- to 30-degree angle, rapidly and smoothly insert the needle through the skin. Use a lesser angle for winged infusion set collections. Place two fingers on the flanges of the adapter and with the thumb push the tube onto the needle inside the adapter. Allow the tube to fill to capacity. Release the tourniquet and allow the patient to release the fist. When blood flow ceases, remove the tube from the adapter by gripping the tube with your non-dominant hand and placing your thumb against the flange during removal. Twist and gently pull out the tube. Steady the needle in the vein. Avoid pulling up or pressing down on the needle while it is in the vein. Insert any other necessary tubes into adapter and allow each to fill to capacity.	❑	❑	❑

PSY PROCEDURE 41-1 Obtain a Blood Specimen by Evacuated Tube or Winged Infusion Set (continued)

18. With the tourniquet released, remove the tube from the adapter before removing the needle from the arm.	❑	❑	❑
19. Place a sterile gauze pad over the puncture site at the time of needle withdrawal. Do not apply any pressure to the site until the needle is completely removed. **a.** After the needle is removed, immediately activate the safety device and apply pressure or have the patient apply direct pressure for 3 to 5 minutes. Do not bend the arm at the elbow.	❑	❑	❑
20. After the needle is removed, immediately activate the safety device and apply pressure, or have the patient apply direct pressure for 3 to 5 minutes. Do not bend the arm at the elbow.	❑	❑	❑
21. If the vacuum tubes contain an anticoagulant, they must be mixed immediately by gently inverting the tube 8 to 10 times. Do not shake the tube.	❑	❑	❑
22. Label the tubes with patient information as defined by the office or laboratory protocol.	❑	❑	❑
23. Check the puncture site for bleeding. Apply a dressing, a clean 2 × 2 gauze pad folded in quarters, and hold in place by an adhesive bandage or 3-inch strip of tape.	❑	❑	❑
24. AFF Thank the patient. Instruct the patient to leave the bandage in place at least 15 minutes and not to carry a heavy object (such as a purse) or lift heavy objects with that arm for 1 hour.	❑	❑	❑
25. Properly care for or dispose of all equipment and supplies. Clean the work area. Remove personal protective equipment and wash your hands.	❑	❑	❑
26. Test, transfer, or store the blood specimen according to the medical office policy.	❑	❑	❑
27. Log into the Electronic Medical Record (EMR) using your username and secure password OR obtain the paper medical record from a secure location and assure it is kept away from public access. Record the procedure noting the date, time, site of the venipuncture, test results for CLIA-waived POC procedures or the name of the lab where the specimen was sent, and your name.	❑	❑	❑
28. When finished, log out of the EMR and/or replace the paper medical record in an appropriate and secure location.	❑	❑	❑

PSY PROCEDURE 41-1 Obtain a Blood Specimen by Evacuated Tube or Winged Infusion Set (continued)

29. AFF Explain how to respond to a patient who is deaf, hearing impaired, visually impaired, developmentally challenged, or speaks English as a second language (ESL) or who has dementia, cultural or religious concerns, or generational differences.	❑	❑	❑

____

____

____

____

CALCULATION

Total Possible Points: __________

Total Points Earned: __________ Multiplied by 100 = __________ Divided by Total Possible Points = __________ %

PASS **FAIL** **COMMENTS:**

❑ ❑

Student's signature ____________________ Date __________

Partner's signature ____________________ Date __________

Instructor's signature ____________________ Date __________

PSY PROCEDURE 41-2 Obtain a Blood Specimen by Capillary Puncture

Name: ______________________ **Date:** __________ **Time:** __________ **Grade:** __________

EQUIPMENT/SUPPLIES: Skin puncture device, 70% alcohol pads, 2 × 2 gauze pads, microcollection tubes or containers, heel warming device if needed, small band aids, pen or permanent marker and personal protective equipment (e.g., gloves, impervious gown, face shield)

STANDARDS: Given the needed equipment and a place to work the student will perform this skill with _____ % accuracy in a total of _____ minutes. *(Your instructor will tell you what the percentage and time limits will be before you begin.)*

KEY: 4 = Satisfactory 0 = Unsatisfactory NA = This step is not counted

PROCEDURE STEPS	SELF	PARTNER	INSTRUCTOR
1. Check the physician order and complete the requisition slip if appropriate.	❑	❑	❑
2. Wash your hands.	❑	❑	❑
3. Assemble the equipment.	❑	❑	❑
4. AFF Greet and identify the patient and yourself including your title. Explain the procedure.	❑	❑	❑
5. AFF Evaluate your patient for his or her ability to understand your instructions. When indicated, whether the problem is deafness, hearing impairment, visual impairment, a developmental challenge, English as a second language (ESL), dementia, cultural or religious concerns, or generational differences, you are responsible for helping the patient understand the procedure before beginning the phlebotomy. This may include help from the person who brought the patient to the office or from a translator.	❑	❑	❑
6. Put on gloves.	❑	❑	❑
7. Ask the patient or caregiver of an infant or small child about any dietary restrictions and the use of medications that increase bleeding time as appropriate. If a fasting or NPO specimen is required, ask the patient for the last time he or she ate or drank anything.	❑	❑	❑
8. Select the puncture site (the lateral portion of the tip of the middle or ring finger of the non-dominant hand or lateral curved surface of the heel of an infant). The puncture should be made in the fleshy central portion of the second or third finger, slightly to the side of center, and perpendicular to the grooves of the fingerprint. Perform heel puncture only on the plantar surface of the heel, medial to an imaginary line extending from the middle of the great toe to the heel, and lateral to an imaginary line drawn from between the fourth and fifth toes to the heel. Use the appropriate puncture device for the site selected.	❑	❑	❑

PSY PROCEDURE 41-2 Obtain a Blood Specimen by Capillary Puncture (continued)

9. Make sure the site chosen is warm and not cyanotic or edematous. Gently massage the finger from the base to the tip or massage the infant's heel.	❑	❑	❑
10. Grasp the finger firmly between your nondominant index finger and thumb, or grasp the infant's heel firmly with your index finger wrapped around the foot and your thumb wrapped around the ankle. Cleanse the selected area with 70% isopropyl alcohol and allow to air dry.	❑	❑	❑
11. Hold the patient's finger or heel firmly and make a swift, firm puncture. Perform the puncture perpendicular to the whorls of the fingerprint or footprint. Dispose of the used puncture device in a sharps container.	❑	❑	❑
12. Obtain the first drop of blood. **a.** Wipe away the first drop of blood with dry gauze. **b.** Apply pressure toward the site but do not milk the site.	❑	❑	❑
13. Collect the specimen in the chosen container or slide. Touch only the tip of the collection device to the drop of blood. Blood flow is encouraged if the puncture site is held downward, and gentle pressure is applied near the site. Cap micro-collection tubes with the caps provided and mix the additives by gently tilting or inverting the tubes 8 to 10 times.	❑	❑	❑
14. When collection is complete, apply clean gauze to the site with pressure. Hold pressure or have the patient or caregiver hold pressure until bleeding stops. Label the containers with the proper information. Do not apply a dressing to a skin puncture of an infant under age 2 years. Never release a patient until the bleeding has stopped.	❑	❑	❑
15. AFF Thank the patient. Instruct the patient to leave the bandage in place at least 15 minutes if appropriate.	❑	❑	❑
16. Properly care for or dispose of equipment and supplies. Clean the work area. Remove gloves and wash your hands.	❑	❑	❑
17. Test, transfer, or store the specimen according to the medical office policy.	❑	❑	❑
18. Log into the Electronic Medical Record (EMR) using your username and secure password OR obtain the paper medical record from a secure location and assure it is kept away from public access. Record the procedure noting the date, time, site of the capillary puncture, test results for CLIA-waived POC procedures or the name of the lab where the specimen was sent, and your name.	❑	❑	❑
19. When finished, log out of the EMR and/or replace the paper medical record in an appropriate and secure location.	❑	❑	❑

PROCEDURE 41-2 Obtain a Blood Specimen by Capillary Puncture (continued)

____

____

____

____

CALCULATION

Total Possible Points: __________

Total Points Earned: __________ Multiplied by 100 = __________ Divided by Total Possible Points = __________ %

PASS ❑ **FAIL** ❑ **COMMENTS:**

Student's signature ____________________ Date __________

Partner's signature ____________________ Date __________

Instructor's signature ____________________ Date __________

2. A trauma patient arrives in the hospital with extensive bleeding and internal injuries. The next day you are asked to run lab tests on this patient's bloodwork. How do you expect her results to differ from those of a healthy patient?

3. Your patient presents with a persistent headache and nasal congestion. His WBC count is normal, but the eosinophil count is high. What is the probable cause of the patient's complaint?

4. You are performing an erythrocyte sedimentation rate. After 60 minutes, you look at the tube to report the test results. You cannot determine the separation between the cells and the plasma. The separation is not straight, and there are bubbles in the tube. What are the probable causes of your problem?

5. You are preparing to collect a fingerstick specimen from your patient for a PT and INR test. The puncture wound continues to bleed heavily after the specimen is completed. How do you stop the bleeding and reassure the patient?

6. Explain the rationale used when explaining a procedure to the patient within parameters set by the physician.

7. Your patient arrives for a fingerstick hematocrit test. She tells you she is worried because she continues to have anemia and treatment does not seem to be helping. How do you show awareness of the patient's feelings within the scope of practice of a medical assistant?

PSY PROCEDURE 42-1 Performing a Hemoglobin Determination

Name: ______________________________ **Date:** __________ **Time:** __________ **Grade:** __________

EQUIPMENT/SUPPLIES: Hemoglobin meter, applicator sticks, whole blood, hand disinfectant, surface disinfectant, gloves, biohazard container, medical record

STANDARDS: Given the needed equipment and a place to work, the student will perform this skill with _____ % accuracy in a total of _____ minutes. *(Your instructor will tell you what the percentage and time limits will be before you begin practicing.)*

KEY: 4 = Satisfactory 0 = Unsatisfactory NA = This step is not counted

PROCEDURE STEPS	SELF	PARTNER	INSTRUCTOR
1. Check the physician order and wash your hands. Put on personal protective equipment.	❑	❑	❑
2. Assemble the necessary equipment and supplies. Check the expiration dates on supplies that require this and ensure the equipment is in good working order. Perform any calibration or quality control procedures as required per the manufacturer and office policy and procedure.	❑	❑	❑
3. Take the equipment and supplies to the patient examination room or take the patient to the phlebotomy station if available.	❑	❑	❑
4. Greet and identify the patient and yourself including your title. Explain the procedure and put on gloves.	❑	❑	❑
5. Explain how you would respond to an elderly patient.	❑	❑	❑
6. Obtain a blood specimen from the patient by capillary puncture.	❑	❑	❑
7. Place well-mixed whole blood into the hemoglobinometer chamber or place the blood specimen on the reagent strip as described by the manufacturer.	❑	❑	❑
8. Slide the chamber into the hemoglobinometer or process the specimen using the CLIA-waived machine as required by the manufacturer. Slide the chamber into the hemoglobin meter.	❑	❑	❑
9. Record the hemoglobin level from the digital readout.	❑	❑	❑
10. Dispose of the contaminated supplies into a biohazard waste receptacle according to office policy and procedure. Clean the work area with surface disinfectant. Remove gloves and wash your hands. *Note:* This procedure may vary with the instrument.	❑	❑	❑

PSY PROCEDURE 42-1 Performing a Hemoglobin Determination (continued)

11. Log into the Electronic Medical Record (EMR) using your username and secure password OR obtain the paper medical record from a secure location and assure it is kept away from public access. Record the procedure, noting the date, time, site of the venipuncture, test results for CLIA-waived POC procedures or the name of the lab where the specimen was sent, and your name.	❑	❑	❑
12. When finished, log out of the EMR and/or replace the paper medical record in an appropriate and secure location.	❑	❑	❑

____

____

____

____

CALCULATION

Total Possible Points: __________

Total Points Earned: __________ Multiplied by 100 = __________ Divided by Total Possible Points = __________ %

PASS **FAIL** **COMMENTS:**

❑ ❑

Chart Documentation ____________________ Date __________

Student's signature ____________________ Date __________

Partner's signature ____________________ Date __________

Instructor's signature ____________________ Date __________

PSY PROCEDURE 42-2 Performing a Microhematocrit Determination

Name: ____________________ **Date:** __________ **Time:** __________ **Grade:** __________

EQUIPMENT/SUPPLIES: Microcollection tubes, sealing clay, microhematocrit centrifuge, microhematocrit reading device, hand disinfectant, surface disinfectant, gloves, biohazard container, sharps container, medical record

STANDARDS: Given the needed equipment and a place to work, the student will perform this skill with _____ % accuracy in a total of _____ minutes. *(Your instructor will tell you what the percentage and time limits will be before you begin practicing.)*

KEY: 4 = Satisfactory 0 = Unsatisfactory NA = This step is not counted

PROCEDURE STEPS	SELF	PARTNER	INSTRUCTOR
1. Check the physician order and wash your hands.	❑	❑	❑
2. Assemble the equipment and supplies. Check the expiration dates on supplies that require this and ensure the equipment is in good working order. Perform any calibration or quality control procedures as required per the manufacturer and office policy and procedure.	❑	❑	❑
3. Take the equipment and supplies to the patient examination room or take the patient to the phlebotomy station if available.	❑	❑	❑
4. Greet and identify the patient and yourself including your title. Explain the procedure and put on gloves.	❑	❑	❑
5. Explain how you would respond to a patient who does not speak English as their first language.	❑	❑	❑
6. Obtain a blood specimen from the patient by capillary puncture. Draw blood into the capillary tube by holding the capillary microhemaocrit microhematocrit tube horizontally and touching one end of the tube to the blood coming from the capillary puncture. Allow the tube to fill to ¾ or the indicated mark on the capillary tube.	❑	❑	❑
7. With the microhematocrit tube in a horizontal position, place your forefinger over the opposite end of the tube, lift it up, and push the tube into the clay sealant with the blood side in the clay.	❑	❑	❑
8. Draw a second specimen in the same manner using a second microhematocrit tube.	❑	❑	❑
9. Place the tubes, clay-sealed end out, in the radial grooves of the microhematocrit centrifuge opposite each other. Put the lid on the grooved area and tighten by turning the knob clockwise. Close the centrifuge lid. Spin for 5 minutes or as directed by the centrifuge manufacturer.	❑	❑	❑
10. Remove the tubes from the centrifuge and read the results; instructions are printed on the device. Results should be within 5% of each other. Take the average and report as a percentage.	❑	❑	❑

PSY PROCEDURE 42-2 Performing a Microhematocrit Determination (continued)

11. Dispose of the contaminated supplies into a biohazard waste receptacle according to office policy and procedure. Clean the work area with surface disinfectant. Dispose of equipment and supplies appropriately. Remove gloves and wash your hands. *Note:* Some microhematocrit centrifuges have the scale printed in the machine at the radial grooves.	❑	❑	❑
12. Log into the Electronic Medical Record (EMR) using your username and secure password OR obtain the paper medical record from a secure location and assure it is kept away from public access. Record the procedure, noting the date, time, site of the venipuncture, test results for CLIA-waived POC procedures or the name of the lab where the specimen was sent, and your name.	❑	❑	❑
13. When finished, log out of the EMR and/or replace the paper medical record in an appropriate and secure location.	❑	❑	❑

____

____

____

____

CALCULATION

Total Possible Points: __________

Total Points Earned: __________ Multiplied by 100 = __________ Divided by Total Possible Points = __________ %

PASS ❑ **FAIL** ❑ **COMMENTS:**

Chart Documentation ____________________ Date __________

Student's signature ____________________ Date __________

Partner's signature ____________________ Date __________

Instructor's signature ____________________ Date __________

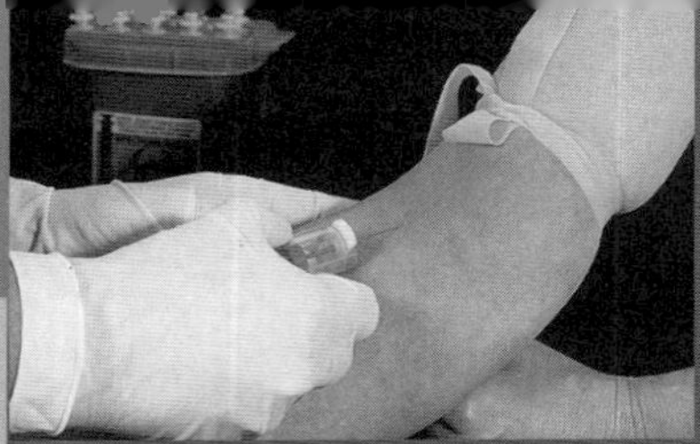

CHAPTER

43 Clinical Chemistry

Learning Outcomes

COG Cognitive Domain

1. Spell key terms
2. Define medical terms and abbreviations related to all body systems
3. List the common electrolytes and explain the relationship of electrolytes to acid–base balance
4. Describe the nonprotein nitrogenous compounds and name conditions with abnormal values
5. Identify CLIA-waived tests associated with common diseases
6. Analyze health care results as reported in graphs and tables
7. List and describe the substances commonly tested in liver function assessment
8. Describe glucose use and regulation and the purpose of the various glucose tests
9. Describe the function of cholesterol and other lipids and their correlation to heart disease

PSY Psychomotor Domain

1. Perform blood glucose testing (Procedure 43-1)
2. Perform blood cholesterol testing (Procedure 43-2)

AFF Affective Domain

1. Distinguish between normal and abnormal test results
2. Incorporate critical thinking skills when performing patient assessment
3. Incorporate critical thinking skills when performing patient care
4. Show awareness of a patient's concerns related to the procedure being performed.
5. Demonstrate empathy, active listening, nonverbal communication
6. Demonstrate respect for individual diversity including gender, race, religion, age, economic status, appearance
7. Explain to a patient the rationale for performance of a procedure
8. Demonstrate sensitivity to patient rights
9. Protect the integrity of the medical record

ABHES Competencies

1. Perform CLIA-waived tests that assist with diagnosis and treatment
2. Perform chemistry testing
3. Perform routine maintenance of clinical equipment safely
4. Screen and follow up patient test results
5. Use standard precautions

Name: ____________________ Date: __________ Grade: __________

COG AFF MULTIPLE CHOICE

Circle the letter preceding the correct answer.

1. Sodium is used to maintain:
a. blood urea nitrogen.
b. TSH stimulation.
c. waste materials.
d. fluid balance.
e. blood oxygen.

2. An enzyme is a(n):
a. cell that speeds up the production of proteins.
b. protein that quickens chemical reactions.
c. chemical reaction that ionizes electrolytes.
d. ion that has an electrical charge.
e. specialized cell that deals with blood levels.

3. Which of the following is formed in the liver?
a. Urea
b. TSH
c. Creatinine
d. Lipase
e. Amylase

4. A patient's blood work shows her amylase level is found to be high. What other substance would indicate pancreatitis?
a. Hemoglobin
b. Triglycerides
c. Potassium
d. Lipase
e. Lipoproteins

5. The function of LDLs is to:
a. transport enzymes to the heart and lungs.
b. assist in the production of lipoproteins.
c. store energy in adipose tissue.
d. move cholesterol from the liver to arteries.
e. carry cholesterol from the cells to the liver.

6. Chloride, bicarbonate, and electrolytes are all a part of:
a. maintaining thyroid function.
b. bile formation.
c. red blood cell maturation.
d. glucose storage.
e. acid-base balance.

7. Women are screened for gestational diabetes:
a. before they conceive.
b. during the first month of pregnancy.
c. during the second trimester.
d. during the third trimester.
e. after the baby is born.

8. When blood sugar levels go below 45 mg/dL, a person may experience:
a. trembling.
b. vomiting.
c. diarrhea.
d. chills.
e. a high temperature.

9. If you are testing for a substance only found in serum, what should you do with a blood specimen?
a. Use reagent strips to check for serum presence.
b. Create a slide and analyze it under a microscope.
c. Put the clotted specimen in the centrifuge to separate.
d. Allow the specimen a few days to sit and separate.
e. Run tests without doing anything to the specimen.

10. What is the body's normal blood pH range?
a. 7.35 to 7.45
b. 6.9 to 7.35
c. 7.0 to 7.5
d. 6.0 to 6.5
e. 7.45 to 8.25

11. Hemoglobin A1C is tested to measure the patient's:
a. fasting glucose.
b. level of anemia.
c. glucose that is attached to hemoglobin molecules.
d. hemoglobin attached to glucose molecules.
e. glucose tolerance.

12. Why is fasting required to accurately measure lipid levels?
a. To evaluate how the body handles fat intake
b. To establish fasting glucose levels
c. To measure how much water is in body fat
d. To limit the action of digestion on increasing lipid levels
e. To lower HDL levels

COG MATCHING

Grade: ________

Match each key term with the correct definition.

Key Terms

13. ______ acidosis
14. ______ alkalosis
15. ______ amylase
16. ______ azotemia
17. ______ bicarbonate
18. ______ buffer systems
19. ______ creatinine
20. ______ electrolyte
21. ______ enzyme
22. ______ ions
23. ______ lipase
24. ______ lipoproteins
25. ______ urea

Definitions

a. electrically charged atoms
b. any substance-containing ions
c. an electrolyte with a negative charge formed when carbon dioxide dissolves in the blood
d. keeps the pH changes balanced
e. blood pH is below 7.4 caused by too much acid or too little base
f. blood pH is above 7.4 caused by too much base or too little acid
g. waste product from the body's metabolism of protein
h. abnormally high levels of nitrogen-containing compounds
i. a protein produced by living cells that speeds up chemical reactions
j. helps in the digestion of fats
k. breaks down starch into sugar
l. substances composed of lipids and proteins
m. a waste product from making the energy muscles use to function

COG IDENTIFICATION

Grade: ________

Identify the electrolyte by the stated relationship to acid–base balance.

Relationship	Electrolyte
26. It causes the most problems when its level is not stable	
27. When the level is extremely low, it becomes difficult for the patient to breathe	
28. Can be made unstable if the patient is suffering diabetic ketoacidosis and metabolic acidosis	
29. Most important electrolyte used in acid–base balance	
30. Low levels are seen in patients experiencing a long-term severe illness	
31. Low levels result from inadequate absorption from the diet, GI losses, electrolyte shifts, and endocrine disorders	
32. A waste product of oxygen metabolism	

COG IDENTIFY

Grade: ________

The following table lists nonprotein nitrogenous compound descriptions and associated abnormal conditions. Identify the nonprotein nitrogenous compound that is described.

Compound	Description	Abnormal Condition
33.	Waste product from the body's metabolism of protein	Dehydration, renal disease, inadequate dialysis, azotemia
34.	Waste product from making the energy muscles use to function	Kidney damage, kidney disease
35.	Waste product from breaking down protein	Gout, kidney stones

COG FILL IN THE BLANK

Grade: ________

36. ________ is elevated in MI.

37. Most of the CK is located in ________ muscle.

38. CK has three parts: ________, ________, and ________.

39. The ________ ________ is present in both cardiac and skeletal muscle.

40. The ________ ________ is much more specific for cardiac muscle.

41. The CKMB fraction increases within ________ following MI.

42. Troponins will begin to rise following MI within ________.

43. ________ levels are the best indicator of MI.

44. Rise in myoglobin can help to determine the ________ of an infarction.

45. Since inflammation is part of MI, ________ ________ is tested to predict the diagnosis of MI.

COG SHORT ANSWER

Grade: ________

46. What is pancreatitis, and what two enzymes are elevated in this condition?

____

____

____

____

47. The pancreas makes two endocrine hormones that are important in diabetes. What are they and what do they do?

____

____

____

____

48. What are the two hormones that regulate the process of storing glucose as glycogen?

a. ______________________________

b. ______________________________

49. What glucose test is used for screening?

____

____

____

____

50. What glucose test is used to monitor insulin therapy?

____

____

____

____

51. How does hemoglobin A1C gives the physician a picture of the patient's glucose levels over the past 3 months?

____

____

____

____

52. What are the four fats measured in a lipid panel?

____

____

____

____

AFF CASE STUDIES

Grade: __________

1. Your patient is a 5-year-old girl. The physician has ordered a fingerstick glucose. The mother of the child accompanied her to the office and gave the child a piece of candy because she thought her sugar might be low. You collect the specimen and run the test. The glucose is 60 mg/dL. You realize that you forgot to help the child wash her hands before the test. How could the result be affected if traces of the candy were on the child's finger? What do you do? What will make it difficult to do the right thing? How do you manage the parent and the child?

____

____

____

____

2. Your patient, Sarah Ingle, had an electrolyte panel ordered by Dr. Willis. The results are back from the reference lab, and your job includes screening test results. What are the reference intervals (normal ranges) you expect to see for these tests: sodium, potassium, chloride, and CO_2? You find that the potassium level is 6.0 mmol/L. What action do you take, and how do you document your action?

____

____

____

____

3. Melissa Woermann had a glucose tolerance test, and her results are noted on the graph is below. Her fasting glucose was 90 mg/dL. Estimate Ms. Woermann's 1/2-, 1-, 2-, and 3-hour glucose levels. What are the criteria proposed by the National Diabetes Data Group and the World Health Organization and endorsed by the ADA for a diagnosis of diabetes? Does it appear from the graph that Ms. Woermann could be diagnosed with diabetes?

____

____

____

____

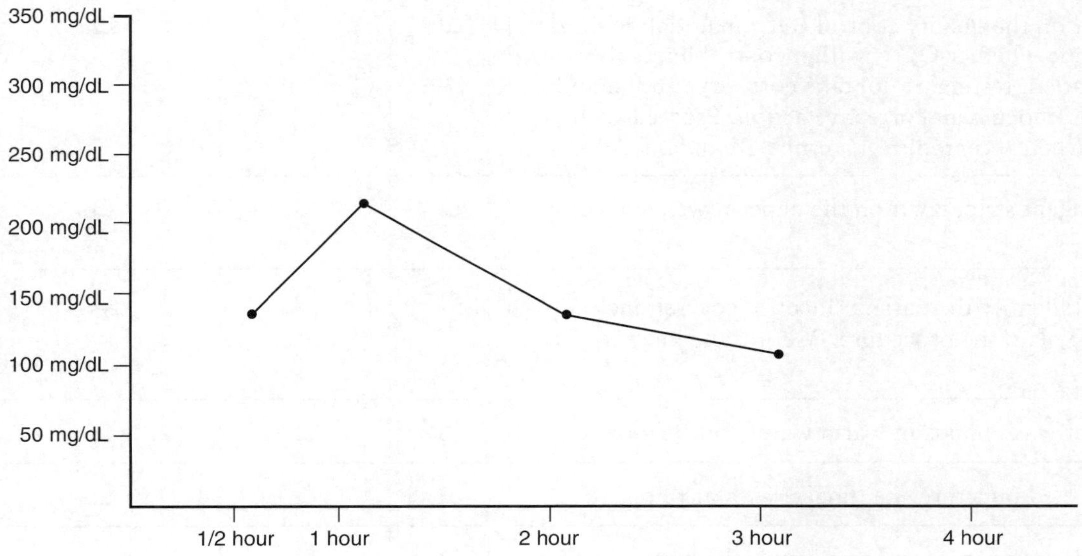

PSY PROCEDURE 43-1 Perform Blood Glucose Testing

Name: ______________________ **Date:** ___________ **Time:** ___________ **Grade:** ___________

EQUIPMENT/SUPPLIES: Glucose meter, glucose reagent strips, control solutions, capillary puncture device, personal protective equipment, gauze, paper towel, adhesive bandage, lancet, alcohol pad, hand sanitizer, surface sanitizer, contaminated waste container.

NOTE: These are generic instructions for using a glucose meter. Refer to the manufacturer's instructions shipped with the meter for instructions specific to the instrument in use.

STANDARDS: Given the needed equipment and a place to work, the student will perform this skill with _____ % accuracy in a total of _____ minutes. *(Your instructor will tell you what the percentage and time limits will be before you begin practicing.)*

KEY: 4 = Satisfactory 0 = Unsatisfactory NA = This step is not counted

PROCEDURE STEPS	SELF	PARTNER	INSTRUCTOR
1. Check the physician order and wash your hands	❑	❑	❑
2. Assemble the equipment and supplies.	❑	❑	❑
3. Review the instrument manual for your glucose meter.	❑	❑	❑
4. Turn on the instrument and verify that it is calibrated.	❑	❑	❑
5. Perform the test on the quality control (QC) material. Record results. Determine whether QC is within control limits. If yes, proceed with patient testing. If no, take corrective action and recheck controls. Document corrective action. Proceed with patient testing when acceptable QC results are obtained.	❑	❑	❑
6. Remove one reagent strip, lay it on the paper towel, and recap the container.	❑	❑	❑
7. AFF Greet and identify the patient. Identify yourself including your title. Explain the procedure. Ask for and answer any questions.	❑	❑	❑
8. Have the patient wash hands in warm water. Put on gloves.	❑	❑	❑
9. Cleanse the selected puncture site (finger) with alcohol.	❑	❑	❑
10. Perform a capillary puncture and wipe away the first drop of blood.	❑	❑	❑
11. Turn the patient's hand palm down and gently squeeze the finger to form a large drop of blood.	❑	❑	❑
12. Bring the reagent strip up to the finger and touch the pad to the blood. **a.** Do not touch the finger. **b.** Completely cover the pad or fill the testing chamber with blood.	❑	❑	❑

PSY PROCEDURE 43-1 Perform Blood Glucose Testing (continued)

13. Insert the reagent strip into the analyzer. **a.** Meanwhile, apply pressure to the puncture wound with gauze. **b.** The meter will continue to incubate the strip and measure the reaction.	❑	❑	❑
14. The instrument reads the reaction strip and displays the result on the screen in mg/dL.	❑	❑	❑
15. Apply a small adhesive bandage to the patient's fingertip.	❑	❑	❑
16. Properly care for or dispose of equipment and supplies.	❑	❑	❑
17. Clean the work area. Remove personal protective equipment and wash your hands.	❑	❑	❑
18. Log into the Electronic Medical Record (EMR) using your username and secure password OR obtain the paper medical record from a secure location and assure it is kept away from public access. Record the procedure noting the date, time, test results for CLIA-waived POC procedure, and your name.	❑	❑	❑
19. When finished, log out of the EMR and/or replace the paper medical record in an appropriate and secure location.	❑	❑	❑

____

____

____

____

CALCULATION

Total Possible Points: __________

Total Points Earned: __________ Multiplied by 100 = __________ Divided by Total Possible Points = __________ %

PASS ❑ **FAIL** ❑ **COMMENTS:**

Student's signature ____________________ Date __________

Partner's signature ____________________ Date __________

Instructor's signature ____________________ Date __________

PSY PROCEDURE 43-2 Perform Blood Cholesterol Testing

Name: ______________________ **Date:** __________ **Time:** __________ **Grade:** __________

EQUIPMENT/SUPPLIES: Cholesterol meter and supplies or test kit, control solutions, capillary puncture equipment or blood specimen as indicated by manufacturer, personal protective equipment, hand sanitizer, surface sanitizer, contaminated waste container

NOTE: These are generic instructions for using a cholesterol meter or test kit. Refer to the manufacturer's instructions shipped with the testing tool for instructions specific for the instrument in use.

STANDARDS: Given the needed equipment and a place to work, the student will perform this skill with _____ % accuracy in a total of _____ minutes. *(Your instructor will tell you what the percentage and time limits will be before you begin practicing.)*

KEY: 4 = Satisfactory 0 = Unsatisfactory NA = This step is not counted

PROCEDURE STEPS	SELF	PARTNER	INSTRUCTOR
1. Check the physician order and wash your hands. Wash your hands.	❑	❑	❑
2. Assemble the equipment and supplies.	❑	❑	❑
3. Review the instrument manual for your cholesterol meter or kit. Put on gloves.	❑	❑	❑
4. Perform the test on the quality control material. Record results. Determine whether QC is within control limits. If yes, proceed with patient testing. If no, take corrective action and recheck controls. Document corrective action. Proceed with patient testing when acceptable QC results are obtained.	❑	❑	❑
5. Follow manufacturer's instructions in using a patient specimen obtained by capillary puncture or from evacuation a tube.	❑	❑	❑
6. Follow manufacturer's instructions for applying the sample to the testing device and inserting the device into the analyzer. Record results.	❑	❑	❑
7. Properly care for or dispose of equipment and supplies.	❑	❑	❑
8. Clean the work area. Remove personal protective equipment and wash your hands.	❑	❑	❑
9. AFF Log into the Electronic Medical Record (EMR) using your username and secure password OR obtain the paper medical record from a secure location and assure it is kept away from public access. Record the procedure noting the date, time, test results for CLIA-waived POC procedure, and your name.	❑	❑	❑
10. When finished, log out of the EMR and/or replace the paper medical record in an appropriate and secure location.	❑	❑	❑

PSY **PROCEDURE 43-2 Perform Blood Cholesterol Testing**
(continued)

____

____

____

____

CALCULATION

Total Possible Points: __________

Total Points Earned: __________ Multiplied by 100 = __________ Divided by Total Possible Points = __________ %

PASS FAIL COMMENTS:

❑ ❑

Student's signature ____________________ Date __________

Partner's signature ____________________ Date __________

Instructor's signature ____________________ Date __________

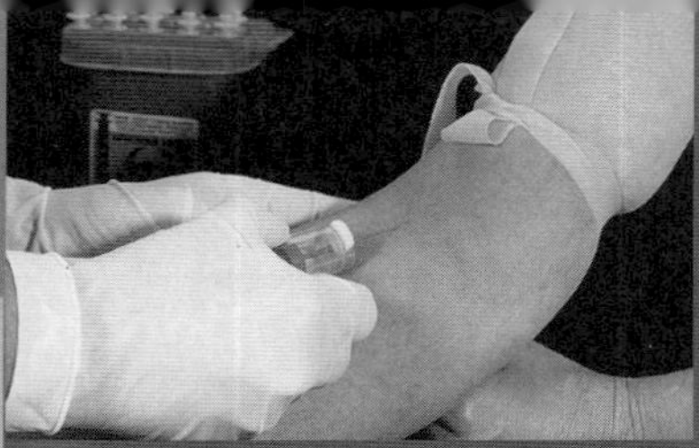

CHAPTER

44 Microbiology and Immunology

Learning Outcomes

COG Cognitive Domain

1. Spell the key terms
2. Define medical terms and abbreviations related to all body systems
3. Identify CLIA-waived tests associated with common diseases
4. Analyze health care results as reported in graphs and tables
5. List major types of infectious agents
6. Discuss quality control issues related to handling microbiological specimens

PSY Psychomotor Domain

1. Collect throat specimens (Procedure 44-1)
2. Collect nasopharyngeal specimens (Procedure 44-2)
3. Collect wound specimens (Procedure 44-3)
4. Collect stool specimen for ova and parasites (Procedure 44-4)
5. Inoculate a culture (Procedure 44-5)
6. Perform mononucleosis testing (Procedure 44-6)
7. Perform HCG pregnancy testing (Procedure 44-7)
8. Perform rapid group A strep testing (Procedure 44-8)

AFF Affective Domain

1. Incorporate critical thinking skills when performing patient assessment.
2. Incorporate critical thinking skills when performing patient care.
3. Show awareness of a patient's concerns related to the procedure being performed.
4. Demonstrate empathy, active listening, nonverbal communication
5. Demonstrate respect for individual diversity including gender, race, religion, age, economic status, appearance.
6. Explain to a patient the rationale for performance of a procedure
7. Demonstrate sensitivity to patient rights
8. Protect the integrity of the medical record.

ABHES Competencies

1. Document patient care
2. Perform quality control measures
3. Screen test results
4. Perform immunology testing
5. Practice standard precautions
6. Perform handwashing
7. Obtain specimens for microbiology testing
8. Perform CLIA-waived microbiology testing
9. Perform pregnancy test
10. Perform strep A test
11. Instruct patients in the collection of fecal specimens

PSY PROCEDURE 44-1 Collect a Throat Specimen

Name: ____________________ **Date:** __________ **Time:** __________ **Grade:** __________

EQUIPMENT/SUPPLIES: Tongue blade, light source, sterile specimen container and swab, personal protective equipment, hand sanitizer, surface sanitizer and biohazard transport bag (if to be sent to the laboratory for analysis)

STANDARDS: Given the needed equipment and a place to work, the student will perform this skill with _____ % accuracy in a total of _____ minutes. *(Your instructor will tell you what the percentage and time limits will be before you begin practicing.)*

KEY: 4 = Satisfactory 0 = Unsatisfactory NA = This step is not counted

PROCEDURE STEPS	SELF	PARTNER	INSTRUCTOR
1. Check the physician order. Wash your hands.	❑	❑	❑
2. Assemble the equipment and supplies.	❑	❑	❑
3. Apply gloves.	❑	❑	❑
4. AFF Greet and identify the patient. Identify yourself including your title. Explain the rationale of the performance of the collection to the patient.	❑	❑	❑
5. AFF If the patient is hearing impaired, you need to speak clearly and distinctly in front of the patient's face.	❑	❑	❑
6. AFF Use active listening to observe patients' body language and detect a lack of understanding of instructions. Obtain assistance when you realize that you are not able to communicate with the patient.	❑	❑	❑
7. AFF Allow time for the adult or patient or caregiver if the patient is a child to ask questions.	❑	❑	❑
8. AFF Display empathy for the patient and family.	❑	❑	❑
9. Have the patient sit with a light source directed the throat.	❑	❑	❑
10. Carefully remove the sterile swab from the container. If performing both the rapid strep and culture or confirming negative results with a culture, swab with two swabs held together.	❑	❑	❑
11. Have the patient say "Ah" as you press down on the midpoint of the tongue with the tongue depressor. If the tongue depressor is placed too far forward, it will not be effective; if it is placed too far back, the patient will gag unnecessarily.	❑	❑	❑
12. Swab the mucous membranes, especially the tonsillar area, the crypts, and the posterior pharynx in a "figure 8" motion. Turn the swab to expose all of its surfaces to the membranes. Avoid touching teeth, sides of mouth, and uvula.	❑	❑	❑

PSY PROCEDURE 44-1 Collect a Throat Specimen (continued)

13. Maintain the tongue depressor position while withdrawing the swab from the patient's mouth.	❑	❑	❑
14. Follow the instructions on the specimen container for transferring the swab or processing the specimen in the office using a commercial kit. Label the specimen with the patient's name, the date and time of collection, and the origin of the material.	❑	❑	❑
15. Properly dispose of the equipment and supplies in a biohazard waste container. Remove PPE and wash your hands.	❑	❑	❑
16. Route the specimen or store it appropriately until routing can be completed.	❑	❑	❑
17. AFF Log into the Electronic Medical Record (EMR) using your username and secure password OR obtain the paper medical record from a secure location and assure it is kept away from public access. Record the procedure noting the date, time, specimen collected, and specimen processing procedure (i.e., sent to lab, tested using CLIA-waived test, etc.). Include your name and title according to office policy and procedure.	❑	❑	❑

____

____

____

____

CALCULATION

Total Possible Points: __________

Total Points Earned: __________ Multiplied by 100 = __________ Divided by Total Possible Points = __________ %

PASS ❑ **FAIL** ❑ **COMMENTS:**

Student's signature ____________________ Date __________

Partner's signature ____________________ Date __________

Instructor's signature ____________________ Date __________

PSY PROCEDURE 44-2 Collect a Nasopharyngeal Specimen

Name: ______________________ **Date:** ________ **Time:** ________ **Grade:** ________

EQUIPMENT/SUPPLIES: Penlight, tongue blade, sterile flexible wire swab, transport media, personal protective equipment, hand sanitizer, surface sanitizer and biohazard transport bag (if to be sent to the laboratory for analysis)

STANDARDS: Given the needed equipment and a place to work, the student will perform this skill with _____ % accuracy in a total of _____ minutes. *(Your instructor will tell you what the percentage and time limits will be before you begin practicing.)*

KEY: 4 = Satisfactory 0 = Unsatisfactory NA =This step is not counted

PROCEDURE STEPS	SELF	PARTNER	INSTRUCTOR
1. Check the physician order. Wash your hands.	❑	❑	❑
2. Assemble the equipment and supplies.	❑	❑	❑
3. Put on gloves.	❑	❑	❑
4. AFF Greet and identify the patient. Greet and identify the patient. Identify yourself including your title. Explain the rationale of the performance of the collection to the patient.	❑	❑	❑
5. AFF If your patient is developmentally challenged, have the individual who transported the patient to the office assist you with communicating with the patient. The developmentally challenged patient may struggle if you have to proceed with something he or she does not understand. Have another medical assistant available to help you should extra support be necessary to support the patient.	❑	❑	❑
6. AFF Leave time for the adult patient or caregiver of a child to ask questions.	❑	❑	❑
7. Position the patient with his head tilted back.	❑	❑	❑
8. Using a penlight, inspect the nasopharyngeal area.	❑	❑	❑
9. Gently pass the swab through the nostril and into the nasopharynx, keeping the swab near the septum and floor of the nose. Rotate the swab quickly and then remove it and place it in the transport media.	❑	❑	❑
10. Label the specimen with the patient's name, the date and time of collection, and the origin of repeated.	❑	❑	❑
11. Properly dispose of the equipment and supplies in a biohazard waste container. Remove gloves and wash your hands.	❑	❑	❑

PSY PROCEDURE 44-2 Collect a Nasopharyngeal Specimen
(continued)

12. Route the specimen or store it appropriately until routing can be completed.	❑	❑	❑
13. AFF Log into the Electronic Medical Record (EMR) using your username and secure password OR obtain the paper medical record from a secure location and assure it is kept away from public access. Record the procedure noting the date, time, specimen collected, and specimen processing procedure (i.e., sent to lab, tested using CLIA-waived test, etc.). Include your name and title according to office policy and procedure.	❑	❑	❑

____

____

____

____

CALCULATION

Total Possible Points: __________

Total Points Earned: __________ Multiplied by 100 = __________ Divided by Total Possible Points = __________ %

PASS **FAIL** **COMMENTS:**

❑ ❑

Student's signature ____________________ Date __________

Partner's signature ____________________ Date __________

Instructor's signature ____________________ Date __________

PSY PROCEDURE 44-3 Collect a Wound Specimen

Name: ______________________________ **Date:** __________ **Time:** __________ **Grade:** __________

EQUIPMENT/SUPPLIES: Sterile swab, transport media, personal protective equipment, hand sanitizer, surface sanitizer, and biohazard transport bag (if to be sent to the laboratory for analysis)

STANDARDS: Given the needed equipment and a place to work, the student will perform this skill with _____ % accuracy in a total of _____ minutes. *(Your instructor will tell you what the percentage and time limits will be before you begin practicing.)*

KEY: 4 = Satisfactory 0 = Unsatisfactory NA = This step is not counted

PROCEDURE STEPS	SELF	PARTNER	INSTRUCTOR
1. Check the physician order. Wash your hands.	❑	❑	❑
2. Assemble the equipment and supplies.	❑	❑	❑
3. Put on gloves.	❑	❑	❑
4. AFF Greet and identify the patient. Identify yourself including your title. Explain the procedure.	❑	❑	❑
5. AFF If your patient is struggling with dementia, be prepared to gently repeat yourself as necessary until you have collected your specimen. You may have to physically adjust your patient as necessary to collect the specimen. Be gentle but remember to speak to the patient as an adult.	❑	❑	❑
6. If dressing is present, remove it and dispose of it in biohazard container. Assess the wound by observing color, odor, and amount of exudate. Remove contaminated gloves and put on clean gloves.	❑	❑	❑
7. Use the sterile swab to sample the exudate. Saturate swab with exudate, avoiding the skin edge around the wound.	❑	❑	❑
8. Place swab back into container and crush the ampule of transport medium.	❑	❑	❑
9. Label the specimen with the patient's name, the date and time of collection, and the origin of specimen.	❑	❑	❑
10. Route the specimen or store it appropriately until routing can be completed.	❑	❑	❑
11. Clean the wound and apply a sterile dressing using sterile technique.	❑	❑	❑
12. Properly dispose of the equipment and supplies in a biohazard waste container. Remove gloves and wash your hands.	❑	❑	❑

PSY PROCEDURE 44-3 Collect a Wound Specimen (continued)

13. AFF Log into the Electronic Medical Record (EMR) using your username and secure password OR obtain the paper medical record from a secure location and assure it is kept away from public access. Record the procedure noting the date, time, specimen collected, and specimen processing procedure (i.e., sent to lab, tested using CLIA-waived test, etc.). Include your name and title according to office policy and procedure.	❑	❑	❑

____

____

____

____

CALCULATION

Total Possible Points: __________

Total Points Earned: __________ Multiplied by 100 = __________ Divided by Total Possible Points = __________ %

PASS ❑ **FAIL** ❑ **COMMENTS:**

Student's signature ____________________ Date __________

Partner's signature ____________________ Date __________

Instructor's signature ____________________ Date __________

PSY PROCEDURE 44-4 Collect a Stool Specimen for Ova and Parasites

Name: ______________________ **Date:** ________ **Time:** ________ **Grade:** ________

EQUIPMENT/SUPPLIES: Specimen container dependent on test ordered (sterile container or Para-Pak collection system for C&S or ova and parasites, tongue blade or wooden spatula, personal protective equipment, hand sanitizer, surface sanitizer, and biohazard transport bag

STANDARDS: Given the needed equipment and a place to work, the student will perform this skill with _____ % accuracy in a total of _____ minutes. *(Your instructor will tell you what the percentage and time limits will be before you begin practicing.)*

KEY: 4 = Satisfactory 0 = Unsatisfactory NA = This step is not counted

PROCEDURE STEPS	SELF	PARTNER	INSTRUCTOR
1. Check the physician order. Wash your hands.	❑	❑	❑
2. Assemble the equipment and supplies.	❑	❑	❑
3. AFF Greet and identify the patient. Identify yourself including your title. Explain the procedure.	❑	❑	❑
4. AFF If you are in a significantly different generation than the patient, you will need to take extra precautions with communication. First, remember that collecting a stool specimen is embarrassing for most patients. Watch the patient's facial expressions to note if he or she is understanding your instructions. This is one of the times you may find that your patient does not understand professional terminology.	❑	❑	❑
5. When obtaining a stool specimen for C&S or ova and parasites, the patient should collect an amount of the first and last portion of the stool after the bowel movement with the wooden spatula or tongue blade and place it in the specimen container without contaminating the outside of the container. Fill Para-Pak until fluid reaches "fill" line, and recap the container.	❑	❑	❑
6. Upon receipt of the specimen, you should put on gloves and place the specimen into the biohazard bag for transport to the reference laboratory. Fill out a laboratory requisition slip to accompany the specimen.	❑	❑	❑
7. Label the specimen with the patient's name, the date and time of collection, and the origin of the specimen.	❑	❑	❑
8. Transport the specimen to the laboratory or store the specimen as directed. Refer to the laboratory procedure manual since some samples require refrigeration, others are kept at room temperature, and some must be placed in an incubator at a laboratory as soon as possible after collecting.	❑	❑	❑

PSY PROCEDURE 44-4 Collect a Stool Specimen for Ova and Parasites (continued)

9. Properly dispose of the equipment and supplies in a biohazard waste container. Remove gloves and wash your hands.	❑	❑	❑
10. AFF Log into the Electronic Medical Record (EMR) using your username and secure password OR obtain the paper medical record from a secure location and assure it is kept away from public access. Record the procedure noting the date, time, specimen collected, and specimen processing procedure (i.e., sent to lab, tested using CLIA-waived test, etc.). Include your name and title according to office policy and procedure.	❑	❑	❑

____

____

____

____

CALCULATION

Total Possible Points: __________

Total Points Earned: __________ Multiplied by 100 = __________ Divided by Total Possible Points = __________ %

PASS ❑ **FAIL** ❑ **COMMENTS:**

Student's signature ____________________ Date __________

Partner's signature ____________________ Date __________

Instructor's signature ____________________ Date __________

PROCEDURE 44-5 Inoculating a Culture

Name: ______________________ **Date:** __________ **Time:** __________ **Grade:** __________

EQUIPMENT/SUPPLIES: Specimen on a swab, permanent laboratory marker, Petri dish, , gloves, hand sanitizer, surface sanitizer, biohazard waste container.

STANDARDS: Given the needed equipment and a place to work, the student will perform this skill with _____ % accuracy in a total of _____ minutes. *(Your instructor will tell you what the percentage and time limits will be before you begin practicing.)*

KEY: 4 = Satisfactory 0 = Unsatisfactory NA =This step is not counted

PROCEDURE STEPS	SELF	PARTNER	INSTRUCTOR
1. Check the physician order. Wash your hands.	❑	❑	❑
2. Assemble the equipment and supplies, checking expiration dates.	❑	❑	❑
3. Put on gloves.	❑	❑	❑
4. Label the medium side of the plate with the permanent marker. Include the patient's name, identification number, source of specimen, time collected, time inoculated, your initials, and date.	❑	❑	❑
5. Remove the Petri plate from the cover (the Petri plate is always stored with the cover down), and place the cover on the work surface with the opening up. Do not open the cover unnecessarily.	❑	❑	❑
6. Using a rolling and sliding motion, streak the specimen swab across one fourth of the plate, starting at the top and working to the center. Dispose of the swab in a biohazard container. The specimen will spread in gradually thinning colonies of bacteria.	❑	❑	❑
7. Use a disposable sterile loop and turn the plate a quarter turn from its previous position. Pass the loop a few times in the original inoculum, and then across the medium approximately a quarter of the surface of the plate. Do not enter the originally streaked area after the first few sweeps.	❑	❑	❑
8. Turn the plate another quarter turn so that now it is 180 degrees to the original smear. Working in the previous manner, draw the loop at right angles through the most recently streaked area. Again, do not enter the originally streaked area after the first few sweeps.	❑	❑	❑
9. Place the prepared culture with the lid on in an incubator per office policy and procedure. Properly dispose of the contaminated supplies in a biohazard waste container. Remove gloves and wash your hands.	❑	❑	❑

PSY PROCEDURE 44-5 Inoculating a Culture (continued)

10. AFF Log into the Electronic Medical Record (EMR) using your username and secure password OR obtain the paper medical record from a secure location and assure it is kept away from public access. Record the procedure noting the date, time, specimen collected, and specimen processing procedure (i.e., sent to lab, tested using CLIA-waived test, etc.). Include your name and title according to office policy and procedure.	❑	❑	❑

____

____

____

____

CALCULATION

Total Possible Points: __________

Total Points Earned: __________ Multiplied by 100 = __________ Divided by Total Possible Points = __________ %

PASS ❑ **FAIL** ❑ **COMMENTS:**

Student's signature ____________________ Date __________

Partner's signature ____________________ Date __________

Instructor's signature ____________________ Date __________

PSY PROCEDURE 44-6 Mononucleosis Testing

Name: ______________________ **Date:** __________ **Time:** __________ **Grade:** __________

EQUIPMENT/SUPPLIES: Patient's labeled specimen (whole blood, plasma, or serum, depending on the kit), CLIA-waived mononucleosis kit (slide or test strip) with instructions, stopwatch or timer, gloves, hand sanitizer, surface sanitizer, biohazard waste container

STANDARDS: Given the needed equipment and a place to work, the student will perform this skill with _____ % accuracy in a total of _____ minutes. *(Your instructor will tell you what the percentage and time limits will be before you begin practicing.)*

KEY: 4 = Satisfactory 0 = Unsatisfactory NA =This step is not counted

PROCEDURE STEPS	SELF	PARTNER	INSTRUCTOR
1. Check the physician order. Wash your hands.	❑	❑	❑
2. Assemble the equipment and ensure that the materials in the kit and the patient specimen are at room temperature.	❑	❑	❑
3. Label the test pack or test strip (depending on type of kit) with the patient's name, positive control, and negative control. Use one test pack or strip per patient and control.	❑	❑	❑
4. Put on gloves. Collect the blood specimen according to the test kit instructions.	❑	❑	❑
5. Perform the test as directed. Also, perform the controls according to the kit instructions.	❑	❑	❑
6. Set timer for the period indicated in package insert.	❑	❑	❑
7. Read reaction results at the end of time period.	❑	❑	❑
8. Verify the results of the controls before documenting the patient's results. Log the QC and patient information on any worksheet required per the office policy and procedure manual.	❑	❑	❑
9. Properly dispose of the equipment and supplies in a biohazard waste container.	❑	❑	❑
10. Remove your gloves and wash your hands	❑	❑	❑
11. AFF Log into the Electronic Medical Record (EMR) using your username and secure password OR obtain the paper medical record from a secure location and assure it is kept away from public access. Record the procedure noting the date, time, specimen collected, and specimen processing procedure (i.e., sent to lab, tested using CLIA-waived test, etc.). Include your name and title according to office policy and procedure.	❑	❑	❑

PSY PROCEDURE 44-6 Mononucleosis Testing (continued)

____
____
____
____

CALCULATION

Total Possible Points: __________

Total Points Earned: __________ Multiplied by 100 = __________ Divided by Total Possible Points = __________ %

PASS FAIL COMMENTS:

❑ ❑

Student's signature ____________________ Date __________

Partner's signature ____________________ Date __________

Instructor's signature ____________________ Date __________

PSY PROCEDURE 44-7 Perform HCG Pregnancy Test

Name: ______________________ **Date:** __________ **Time:** __________ **Grade:** __________

EQUIPMENT/SUPPLIES: Patient's labeled urine specimen, CLIA-waived HCG pregnancy kit, timer, gloves, hand sanitizer, surface sanitizer, biohazard waste container

STANDARDS: Given the needed equipment and a place to work, the student will perform this skill with _____ % accuracy in a total of _____ minutes. *(Your instructor will tell you what the percentage and time limits will be before you begin practicing.)*

KEY: 4 = Satisfactory 0 = Unsatisfactory NA = This step is not counted

PROCEDURE STEPS	SELF	PARTNER	INSTRUCTOR
1. Check the physician order. Wash your hands.	❑	❑	❑
2. Assemble the equipment and supplies.	❑	❑	❑
3. Verify the urine specimen is for the correct patient. Verify the HCG test kit is not expired.	❑	❑	❑
4. Perform the test as indicated on the test kit package insert directions.	❑	❑	❑
5. Sample the positive and negative controls as directed for the test kit.	❑	❑	❑
6. Set the timer for running the test as indicated in package insert.	❑	❑	❑
7. Read reaction results at the end of prescribed period of time.	❑	❑	❑
8. Verify the results of the controls before documenting the patient's results. Log controls and patient information on the worksheet according to office policy and procedure.	❑	❑	❑
9. Properly dispose of the equipment and supplies in a biohazard waste container.	❑	❑	❑
10. Remove gloves and wash your hands.	❑	❑	❑
11. AFF Log into the Electronic Medical Record (EMR) using your username and secure password OR obtain the paper medical record from a secure location and assure it is kept away from public access. Record the procedure noting the date, time, specimen collected, and specimen processing procedure (i.e., sent to lab, tested using CLIA-waived test, etc.). Include your name and title according to office policy and procedure.	❑	❑	❑

PROCEDURE 44-7 Perform HCG Pregnancy Test (continued)

____

____

____

____

CALCULATION

Total Possible Points: __________

Total Points Earned: __________ Multiplied by 100 = __________ Divided by Total Possible Points = __________ %

PASS **FAIL** **COMMENTS:**

❑ ❑

Student's signature ____________________ Date __________

Partner's signature ____________________ Date __________

Instructor's signature ____________________ Date __________

PSY PROCEDURE 44-8 Rapid Group A Strep Testing

Name: ______________________ **Date:** __________ **Time:** __________ **Grade:** __________

EQUIPMENT/SUPPLIES: CLIA-waived Group A strep kit (controls may be included, depending on the kit), timer, gloves, hand sanitizer, surface sanitizer, biohazard waste container

STANDARDS: Given the needed equipment and a place to work, the student will perform this skill with _____ % accuracy in a total of _____ minutes. *(Your instructor will tell you what the percentage and time limits will be before you begin practicing.)*

KEY: 4 = Satisfactory 0 = Unsatisfactory NA = This step is not counted

PROCEDURE STEPS	SELF	PARTNER	INSTRUCTOR
1. Check the physician order. Wash your hands.	❑	❑	❑
2. Assemble the equipment including the test kit. Familiarize yourself with the instructions before obtaining the specimen and performing the procedure.	❑	❑	❑
3. Apply gloves. Obtain the throat specimen from the patient after assuring you have the correct patient. Use the swabs that come with the testing kit.	❑	❑	❑
4. Follow the directions for the kit. Add the appropriate reagents and drops to each of the extraction appropriate test tubes.	❑	❑	❑
5. Insert the patient swab into the labeled extraction tube.	❑	❑	❑
6. Add the appropriate controls to each of the labeled extraction tubes.	❑	❑	❑
7. Set the timer for the appropriate time to ensure accuracy.	❑	❑	❑
8. Add the appropriate reagent and drops to each of the extraction tubes.	❑	❑	❑
9. Use the swab to mix the reagents. Then press out any excess fluid on the swab against the inside of the tube.	❑	❑	❑
10. Add the appropriate number of drops from the well-mixed extraction tube to the sample window of the strep A test unit. Do the same for each control.	❑	❑	❑
11. Set the timer for the time indicated in the kit package insert.	❑	❑	❑
12. Depending on the test kit used, a positive result may appear as a line in the result window within 5 minutes. The strep A test unit or strip has an internal control; if a line appears in the control window, the test is valid.	❑	❑	❑
13. Read a negative result at exactly 5 minutes or as per the test kit instructions to avoid a false negative.	❑	❑	❑
14. Verify results of the controls before recording or reporting test results. Log the controls and the patient's information on the worksheet according to office policy and procedure.	❑	❑	❑

PSY PROCEDURE 44-8 Rapid Group A Strep Testing (continued)

15. Properly dispose of the equipment and supplies in a biohazard waste container.	❑	❑	❑
16. Remove your gloves and wash your hands.	❑	❑	❑
17. AFF Log into the Electronic Medical Record (EMR) using your username and secure password OR obtain the paper medical record from a secure location and assure it is kept away from public access. Record the procedure noting the date, time, specimen collected, and specimen processing procedure (i.e., sent to lab, tested using CLIA-waived test, etc.). Include your name and title according to office policy and procedure.	❑	❑	❑

____

____

____

____

CALCULATION

Total Possible Points: __________

Total Points Earned: __________ Multiplied by 100 = __________ Divided by Total Possible Points = __________ %

PASS **FAIL** **COMMENTS:**

❑ ❑

Student's signature ____________________ Date __________

Partner's signature ____________________ Date __________

Instructor's signature ____________________ Date __________

COG PSY AFF CASE STUDIES

Grade: ________

1. One of your patients needs to provide a 24-hour urine collection. She has never done it before and is unsure how to carry out the procedure. Write the patient a list of instructions, explaining what she should do in order to provide an accurate specimen. Why is it important that the patient thoroughly understands and complies with your instructions?

2. You instruct a patient how to perform a clean-catch midstream urine specimen. When you test the sample, you discover that the urine is cloudy, with a pH level of 7.5, and contains traces of red blood cells, nitrites, and leukocytes. How would you document this information on the patient's chart?

3. A patient asks you what types of drugs can be detected in urine. Two weeks later, the same patient comes into the office to provide a urine specimen. He appears to be acting suspiciously and you think you see him pick up a bottle before entering the bathroom. What should you do next?

4. Your patient, Sharon, has never collected a clean-catch midstream urine specimen before. As you describe the procedure, her facial expressions begin to change, and she becomes aloof. What are the possible reasons for her response? How do you adjust your behavior to support the patient's understanding of the procedure? How do you demonstrate empathy to this patient?

5. The results have come back from the testing laboratory on a drug screen test you collected. The medical assistant working in the front office comes to you asking about this patient's test results. She says the woman babysits her children after school, and she wants to know if the patient is taking drugs. How do you respond?

PSY PROCEDURE 45-1 Obtaining a Clean-Catch Midstream Urine Specimen

Name: ______________________ **Date:** __________ **Time:** __________ **Grade:** __________

EQUIPMENT/SUPPLIES: Sterile urine container labeled with patient's name, cleansing towelettes (two for males, three for females), gloves if you are to assist patient, hand sanitizer

STANDARDS: Given the needed equipment and a place to work, the student will perform this skill with _____ % accuracy in a total of _____ minutes. *(Your instructor will tell you what the percentage and time limits will be before you begin practicing.)*

KEY: 4 = Satisfactory 0 = Unsatisfactory NA = This step is not counted

PROCEDURE STEPS	SELF	PARTNER	INSTRUCTOR
1. Check the physician order. Wash your hands.	❑	❑	❑
2. Assemble the equipment and supplies.	❑	❑	❑
3. AFF Identify the patient and explain the procedure. Identify yourself including your title. Explain the rationale for performance of a procedure to the patient.	❑	❑	❑
4. AFF If the patient is hearing impaired, you may need to face the person and speak clearly, not loudly. You should have an easy-to-read instruction guide for the patient to follow and point out where there are questions. If the patient can sign and you cannot, have someone proficient in sign language assist you in instructing the patient.	❑	❑	❑
5. If the patient is to perform the procedure, provide the necessary supplies.	❑	❑	❑
6. Have the patient perform the procedure properly with the following instructions: **A.** Male patients: **i.** If uncircumcised, expose the glans penis by retracting the foreskin, then clean the meatus with an antiseptic wipe. The glans should be cleaned in a circular motion away from the meatus. A new wipe should be used for each cleaning sweep. **ii.** Keeping the foreskin retracted, initially void a few seconds into the toilet or urinal. **iii.** Bring the sterile container into the urine stream and collect a sufficient amount (about 30 to 60 mL). Instruct the patient to avoid touching the inside of the container with the penis. **iv.** Finish voiding into the toilet or urinal. **B.** Female patients: **i.** Kneel or squat over the toilet bowl. Spread the labia minora widely to expose the meatus. Using an antiseptic wipe, cleanse on either side of the meatus, and then cleanse the meatus itself. Use a wipe only once in a sweep from the anterior to the posterior surfaces, and then discard it. **ii.** Keeping the labia separated, initially void a few seconds into the toilet. **iii.** Bring the sterile container into the urine stream and collect a sufficient amount (about 30 to 60 mL). **iv.** Finish voiding into the toilet.	❑	❑	❑

PSY PROCEDURE 45-1 Obtaining a Clean-Catch Midstream Urine Specimen (continued)

7. Cap the filled container and place it in a designated area.	❑	❑	❑
8. Transport the specimen in a biohazard container for testing or test the urine specimen according to office policy and procedure.	❑	❑	❑
9. Properly care for or dispose of equipment and supplies. Clean the work area. Remove gloves and wash your hands.	❑	❑	❑
10. AFF Log into the Electronic Medical Record (EMR) using your username and secure password OR obtain the paper medical record from a secure location and assure it is kept away from public access. Record the procedure noting the date, time, specimen collected, and specimen processing procedure (i.e., sent to lab, tested using CLIA-waived test, etc.). Include your name and title according to office policy and procedure.	❑	❑	❑

CALCULATION

Total Possible Points: ________

Total Points Earned: ________ Multiplied by 100 = ________ Divided by Total Possible Points = ________ %

PASS ❑ **FAIL** ❑ **COMMENTS:**

Student's signature ________________ Date ________

Partner's signature ________________ Date ________

Instructor's signature ________________ Date ________

PSY PROCEDURE 45-2 Perform a Physical and Chemical Urinalysis

Name: ______________________ **Date:** __________ **Time:** __________ **Grade:** __________

EQUIPMENT/SUPPLIES: Gloves, patient's labeled urine specimen, chemical reagent strips (such as Multistix™ or Chemstrip™), hand disinfectant, biohazard waste container

STANDARDS: Given the needed equipment and a place to work, the student will perform this skill with _____ % accuracy in a total of _____ minutes. *(Your instructor will tell you what the percentage and time limits will be before you begin practicing.)*

KEY: 4 = Satisfactory 0 = Unsatisfactory NA = This step is not counted

PROCEDURE STEPS	SELF	PARTNER	INSTRUCTOR
1. Check the physician order. Wash your hands.	❑	❑	❑
2. Assemble the equipment.	❑	❑	❑
3. Put on gloves.	❑	❑	❑
4. Verify the name on the specimen container and the physician order.	❑	❑	❑
5. In bright light against a white background, examine the color of the specimen. The most common colors are straw (very pale yellow), yellow, dark yellow, and amber (brown–yellow).	❑	❑	❑
6. Determine clarity. Hold the specimen container in front of a surface with print such as blank print. If you see the image or print clearly (not obscured), record as clear. If you see the image or print but they are not well delineated, record as hazy. If you cannot see the image or print at all, record as cloudy.	❑	❑	❑
7. Remove the reagent strip from its container and replace the lid to prevent deterioration of the strips by humidity.	❑	❑	❑
8. Immerse the reagent strip in the urine completely, immediately remove it, sliding the edge of the strip along the lip of the container to remove excess urine. Pooling of excess urine on the dipstick causes cross-contamination among the reactions, possibly obscuring accurate color detection.	❑	❑	❑
9. Start your stopwatch or timer immediately.	❑	❑	❑
10. Compare the reagent pads to the color chart, determining results at the intervals stated by the manufacturer. Example: Glucose is read at 30 seconds. To determine results, examine that pad 30 seconds after dipping and compare with color chart for glucose.	❑	❑	❑
11. Read all reactions at the times indicated and record the results.	❑	❑	❑

PSY PROCEDURE 45-2 Perform a Physical and Chemical Urinalysis (continued)

12. Discard the reagent strips in the biohazard receptacle. Discard urine.	❑	❑	❑
13. Remove your gloves and wash your hands.	❑	❑	❑
14. AFF Log into the Electronic Medical Record (EMR) using your username and secure password OR obtain the paper medical record from a secure location and assure it is kept away from public access. Record the procedure noting the date, time, specimen collected, and specimen processing procedure (i.e., sent to lab, tested using CLIA-waived test, etc.). Include your name and title according to office policy and procedure.	❑	❑	❑

____

____

____

____

CALCULATION

Total Possible Points: __________

Total Points Earned: __________ Multiplied by 100 = __________ Divided by Total Possible Points = __________ %

PASS ❑ **FAIL** ❑ **COMMENTS:**

Student's signature ____________________ Date __________

Partner's signature ____________________ Date __________

Instructor's signature ____________________ Date __________

PART

5

Career Strategies

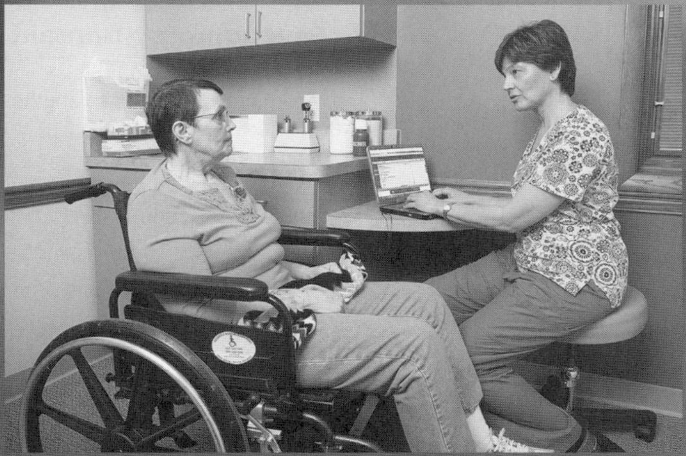

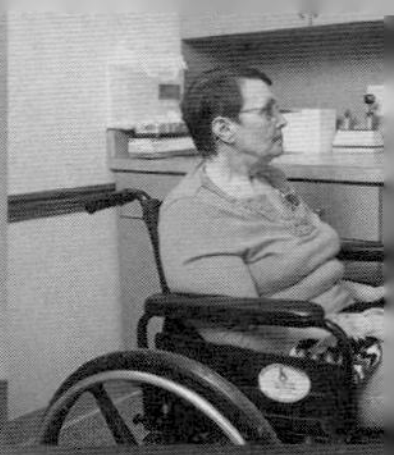

CHAPTER 46 Making the Transition: Student to Employee

Learning Outcomes

COG Cognitive Domain

1. Spell and define the key terms
2. Explain the purpose of the practicum experience
3. Understand the importance of the evaluation process
4. List your professional responsibilities during practicum
5. List personal and professional attributes necessary to ensure a successful practicum
6. Determine your best career direction based on your skills and strengths
7. Identify the steps necessary to apply for the right position and be able to accomplish those steps
8. Draft an appropriate cover letter
9. List the steps and guidelines in completing an employment application
10. List guidelines for an effective interview that will lead to employment
11. Identify the steps that you need to take to ensure proper career advancement
12. Explain the process for recertification of medical assisting credentials
13. Describe the importance of membership in a professional organization
14. Recognize elements of fundamental writing skills
15. List and discuss legal and illegal applicant interview questions
16. Discuss all levels of governmental legislation and regulation as they apply to medical assisting practice

PSY Psychomotor Domain

1. Write a résumé to properly communicate skills and strengths (Procedure 46-1)
2. Compose professional correspondence utilizing electronic technology (Procedure 46-1)

AFF Affective Domain

1. Apply local, state, and federal health care legislation
2. Recognize the impact of personal ethics and morals have on the delivery of health care

ABHES Competencies

1. Comply with federal, state, and local health laws and regulations.
2. Perform fundamental writing skills, including correct grammar, spelling, and formatting techniques when writing prescriptions, documenting medical records, etc.

Name: ______________________ Date: __________ Grade: __________

OG MULTIPLE CHOICE

1. Most practicums range from:
   a. 160 to 240 hours a semester.
   b. 80 to 160 hours a semester.
   c. 200 to 240 hours a semester.
   d. 240 to 300 hours a semester.
   e. 260 to 300 hours a semester.

2. Practicum site supervisors are typically:
   a. physicians.
   b. nurses.
   c. graduate medical assistants.
   d. academic instructors.
   e. other students.

3. When responding to a newspaper or online advertisement, you should:
   a. mail your résumé and a portfolio.
   b. send your résumé by e-mail.
   c. phone right away to inquire about the job.
   d. follow the instructions in the advertisement.
   e. call to schedule an interview.

4. A CMA wishing to recertify must either retake the examination or complete:
   a. 60 hours of continuing education credits.
   b. 50 hours of continuing education credits.
   c. 100 hours of continuing education credits.
   d. 30 hours of continuing education credits.
   e. 75 hours of continuing education credits.

5. Two standard ways of listing experience on a résumé are:
   a. functional and chronological.
   b. functional and alphabetical.
   c. alphabetical and chronological.
   d. chronological and referential.
   e. referential and alphabetical.

6. During your practicum, it is a good practice to arrive:
   a. a few minutes early.
   b. half an hour early.
   c. right on time.
   d. with enough time to beat traffic.
   e. as early as you can.

7. What is the appropriate length of a résumé?
   a. One page
   b. Two pages
   c. Three pages
   d. As long as it needs to be
   e. Check with the potential employer first

8. In addition to providing proof of general immunizations, what other vaccinations may be required before you begin your practicum?
   a. Vaccination for strep throat
   b. Vaccination for cancer
   c. Vaccination for hepatitis B
   d. Vaccination for hepatitis C
   e. Vaccination for HIV

9. During your practicum, you are expected to perform as:
   a. the student that you are; your site supervisor will teach you the same skills as in the classroom.
   b. an experienced professional; your site supervisor will expect you to perform every task perfectly.
   c. an entry-level employee; your site supervisor will expect you to perform at the level of a new employee in the field.
   d. a patient; you have to see what it feels like to be on the receiving end of treatment.
   e. independently as possible; your site supervisor will not have time to answer many questions.

10. Checking for telephone messages and arranging the day's appointments should be done:
    a. during your lunch break.
    b. at the close of the business day.
    c. after the office has opened.
    d. before the scheduled opening.
    e. between patients.

11. Fingernails should be kept short and clean to avoid:
    a. making your supervisor upset.
    b. accidentally scratching or harming a patient.
    c. transferring pathogens or ripping gloves.
    d. getting nail polish chips in lab samples.
    e. infecting sterile materials or surfaces.

12. Which document provides proof that tasks are performed and learning is taking place?
    a. Time sheet
    b. Journal
    c. Survey
    d. Evaluation
    e. Personal interview

13. Which document is used to improve performance and services offered to students?
    a. Time sheet
    b. Journal
    c. Survey
    d. Evaluation
    e. Personal interview

14. Membership in your professional medical assistant organization proves:
a. that you are an allied health student.
b. your level of professionalism and seriousness of purpose.
c. that you will become a medical professional in 2 years.
d. your willingness to network with other professionals.
e. your interest in the medical field.

15. Which question should you avoid asking during an interview?
a. Is there access to a 401(k) plan?
b. Is tuition reimbursement available?
c. How many weeks of vacation are available the first year?
d. Are uniforms or lab coats worn?
e. What are the responsibilities of this position?

16. If you decide to leave your job, it is a good idea to:
a. tell your employer the day before you plan to leave.
b. make sure your new job will pay more.
c. get contact information for all of the new friends you made.
d. finish all duties and tie up any loose ends.
e. criticize employees during an exit interview.

17. If you are having a problem performing your assigned job duties, it is best to:
a. volunteer for extra hours.
b. inform your preceptor and instructor.
c. ask for less challenging work.
d. ask for a different externship site.
e. switch your course of studies.

18. When anticipating calls from prospective employers, avoid:
a. leaving silly or cute messages on your answering machine.
b. telling family members or roommates that you are expecting important telephone calls.
c. keeping a pen near the telephone at all times.
d. checking messages on a regular basis.
e. calling them every day after submitting your résumé.

19. If bilingual applicants are encouraged to apply for a position you want, you should:
a. learn simple greetings and act as if you can speak several languages.
b. learn simple greetings and admit that you know a few words but are not fluent.
c. do nothing; being bilingual is not important.
d. avoid applying since you do not fluently speak another language.
e. learn how to answer possible interview questions in two different languages.

20. Being a lifelong learner is a must for all medical professionals because:
a. medical professionals have to recertify every 5 years.
b. medical professionals are widely respected.
c. changes in procedures, medical technologies, and legal issues occur frequently.
d. changes in medical technologies are decreasing the need for medical professionals.
e. medical professionals are required to change legal statutes once a year.

COG MATCHING

Grade: ______

Match the following key terms to their definitions.

Key Terms

21. ______ practicum
22. ______ networking
23. ______ portfolio
24. ______ site supervisor
25. ______ résumé

Definitions

a. someone who oversees another; one who gives direction, as in a technical matter
b. an educational course that allows the student to obtain hands-on experience
c. a system of personal and professional relationships through which to share information
d. a document summarizing an individual's work experience or professional qualifications
e. a portable case containing documents

COG SHORT ANSWER

Grade: ______

26. What is the purpose of a practicum?

______

______

______

______

27. List three responsibilities you will have during a practicum.

a. ______

b. ______

c. ______

28. How will the site supervisor assist you in your practicum?

______

______

______

______

29. List five traditional sources of information for job openings.

a. ______

b. ______

c. ______

d. ______

e. ______

AFF PSY REFLECTION

Grade: ______

30. Write a list of your strengths and weaknesses as discussed in the chapter. Critically evaluate what you are able to contribute to the job and address your weaknesses. How can you work with these weaknesses to make them strengths? Now evaluate what kind of medical assisting job would best work with what you are already good at and how you would like to continue to grow in your professional development. Identify for yourself what type of job would be ideal for you.

______

______

______

______

31. Practice interviewing with a fellow student. Make sure that you take turns asking questions so that you can both get to experience being on each side of the interview.

COG IDENTIFICATION

Grade: ____________

32. Below are items that could be included on a résumé. Circle all that are appropriate.

a. Contact information

b. Race

c. Relevant volunteer work

d. Birth date

e. Experience

f. Picture of yourself

g. List of professional goals

h. Education

i. Credit history

j. References

k. Date of high school graduation

Action Words

generates	ensures	implements and maintains	interviews	records	articulates
draws and collects	prepares	selects	measures	assists	composes

Choose a more accurate action word from the box to replace the words in bold.

33. **Helps** in examination and treatment of patients under the direction of a physician ____________

34. **Talks to** patients, **takes** vital signs (i.e., pulse rate, temperature, blood pressure, weight, and height), and **writes** information on patients' charts ____________

35. **Gets** blood samples from patients and prepare specimens for laboratory analysis ____________

36. **Sets up** treatment rooms for examination of patients ____________

37. Read each of the following tips for completing a job application. Circle all appropriate best practices for completing an application.

a. Read through the application completely before beginning.

b. Follow the instructions exactly.

c. In the line for wage or salary desired, write highest pay possible.

d. Answer every question. If the question does not apply to you, draw a line or write "N/A" so that the interviewer will know that you did not overlook the question.

e. Use your best cursive writing.

f. Highlight important information in red ink.

g. Ask for two applications. Use the first one for practice.

38. From the list of questions below, circle all that would be appropriate for a job applicant to ask a prospective employer.

a. What are the responsibilities of the position offered?

b. What is the benefit package? Is there access to a 401(k) plan or other retirement plan? Health insurance? Life insurance?

c. Is it acceptable to take 3 weeks off during the holiday season?

d. How does the facility feel about continuing education? Is time off offered to employees to upgrade their skills? Does the facility subsidize the expense?

e. Do I have to work with physicians who have bad attitudes?

f. How many potlucks and happy hours does this office usually have?

g. Is there a job performance or evaluation process?

COG EXPLANATION

Grade: __________

39. Explain what it means to be a lifelong learner.

____

____

____

____

40. How can you prepare for the process of recertification?

____

____

____

____

41. List two professional organizations you could join while you are a student.

a. ____

b. ____

AFF WHAT WOULD YOU DO?

Grade: ___________

42. The office manager at your practicum site does not allow CMAs to give injections. At an office meeting, the employees ask her why not. Her reply is, "it is illegal." The employees tell her that it is not illegal for medical assistants to give injections in the state where you are. She is surprised to hear this and asks the group to prove it to her. Because you are a student and have skills in researching topics, they ask you to find the legislation and bring it to the office manager. Choose all appropriate actions from the list below.

a. Go to the state Web site and search "general assembly."

b. Search for the information on the AAMA Web site by entering key words, "CMA scope of practice."

c. Search for the information in general statutes by entering key words, "health care legislation in [name of your state]."

d. Search for the information by entering key words, "unlicensed health personnel" under *general assembly* in your state.

e. Search for the information by entering key words, "practice of medicine."

43. While working as a practicum at a family care provider, you encounter an older adult patient who is uncomfortable with the fact that you as a student are participating in her care. What would you say to help her feel more comfortable?

____

____

____

____

44. There are multiple gaps in your work history, and your interviewer asks you to explain why. One of the gaps is from relocation, and other gaps are from taking time off to evaluate what you wanted to be doing. How would you explain this to your interviewer?

____

____

____

____

45. During an interview, you are asked to explain why your grades were low last semester. How would you answer this question honestly while still speaking about yourself fairly and objectively?

____

____

____

____

COG TRUE OR FALSE?

Grade: ____________

Determine whether the following statements are true or false. If false, explain why.

46. When you see dangerous practices, it is usually best to confront the employee first.

____

____

47. Problems encountered at a practicum site are best handled by site employees who have experience working with the office manager.

____

____

48. It is a good idea to include hobbies and personal interests on your résumé.

____

____

49. It is a good idea to write a long and detailed cover letter.

____

____

AFF CASE STUDY FOR CRITICAL THINKING

Grade: ____________

It is the first day of your medical assisting practicum.

50. Your practicum site supervisor has said that you cannot receive permission to draw blood and perform other phlebotomy procedures. However, you know this is an area that you are required to complete. Circle all of the appropriate actions from the list below.

a. Tell your practicum coordinator from your college at her next site visit.

b. Tell the site supervisor that you must perform these tasks and leave.

c. Call your practicum coordinator immediately.

d. Call a classmate and ask her what to do.

51. Your school will likely request that you fill out an evaluation form to determine if your practicum site was effective for training. This helps the school decide if it is a good site for future practicums. Review the list of questions below and circle all you should consider when filling out your site evaluation form on your practicum.

a. Was the overall experience positive or negative?

b. Was my site supervisor fun to be around?

c. Did the office have a good cafeteria or break room?

d. Were opportunities for learning abundant and freely offered or hard to obtain?

e. Was my site supervisor flexible about taking personal time during the day for phone calls and breaks?

f. Were staff personnel open and caring or unwelcoming?

g. Was the site supervisor available and easily approachable or preoccupied and distant?

52. Choose all appropriate ways to dress for your practicum from the list below.

a. Burgundy and navy scrubs along with a set of bangle bracelets, your favorite gemstone rings, and a pair of comfortable white clogs

b. The required scrubs with a pair of clean white sneakers. Dreadlocks placed in a neat ponytail above the shoulders

c. The required uniform and a pair of dark walking shoes. Hair with the tips of a spiked Mohawk dyed burgundy to match

d. The required uniform with white sneakers and college name tag

e. Street clothes with lab coat and required name tag

f. Long sleeves to cover the tattoo on your arm

PORTFOLIO

Grade: ___________

Design and compile a portfolio to present at your upcoming job interviews. Refer to Chapter 46 for a list of possible contents of the portfolio. Remember, the purpose of a portfolio is to impress an interviewer. You have worked hard to earn your medical assisting certificate, diploma, or degree. This is your opportunity to show off your professional skills, abilities, and accomplishments.

PSY PROCEDURE 46-1 Writing a Résumé

Name: ______________________ **Date:** __________ **Time:** __________ **Grade:** __________

EQUIPMENT/SUPPLIES: Word processor, paper, personal information

STANDARDS: Given the needed equipment and a place to work, the student will perform this skill with _____ % accuracy in a total of _____ minutes. *(Your instructor will tell you what the percentage and time limits will be before you begin practicing.)*

KEY: 4 = Satisfactory 0 = Unsatisfactory NA = This step is not counted

PROCEDURE STEPS	SELF	PARTNER	INSTRUCTOR
1. At the top of the page, center your name, address, and phone numbers.	❑	❑	❑
2. List your education starting with the most current and working back. List graduation dates and areas of study. It is not necessary to go all the way back to elementary school.	❑	❑	❑
3. Using the chronological format, list your prior related work experience with dates, responsibilities, company, and supervisor's name.	❑	❑	❑
4. List any volunteer work with dates and places.	❑	❑	❑
5. List skills you possess, including those acquired in your program and on your practicum.	❑	❑	❑
6. List any certifications or awards received.	❑	❑	❑
7. List any information relevant to a certain position (e.g., competence in spreadsheet applications for a job in a patient billing department).	❑	❑	❑
8. After obtaining permission and/or notifying the people, prepare a list of references with their addresses and phone contact information.	❑	❑	❑
9. Carefully proofread the résumé for accuracy and typographical errors.	❑	❑	❑
10. Have someone else proofread the résumé for errors other than content.	❑	❑	❑
11. Print the résumé on high-quality paper.	❑	❑	❑
12. AFF You had only one job before finishing your medical assisting program. Should you try to "pad" your résumé by listing some anyway? Why or why not?	❑	❑	❑

____

____

____

____

PROCEDURE 46-1 Writing a Résumé (continued)

CALCULATION

Total Possible Points: __________

Total Points Earned: __________ Multiplied by 100 = __________ Divided by Total Possible Points = __________ %

PASS ❑ **FAIL** ❑ **COMMENTS:**

Student's signature ____________________ Date __________

Partner's signature ____________________ Date __________

Instructor's signature ____________________ Date __________

CHAPTER 47

Capstone Activities: Applying What You Have Learned

Working in a medical office means dealing with situations as they arise in a professional, nonjudgmental manner. Your education and training has provided you with the information and tools to give you administrative competence as well as the clinical skills necessary to function in the medical office, but you must also use professional judgment and critical thinking when making decisions and interacting with patients, families, and staff. This chapter will provide opportunities for you to practice using professional judgment and critical thinking skills as would a practicing medical assistant in the physician office. Each section, containing documentation and active learning exercises, provides real-life scenarios followed by questions for you to think about and respond to according to directions from your instructor. Be sure to read carefully and, as usual, have fun!

COG PSY DOCUMENTATION

Grade: ___________

CHAPTER 1

Christopher Guest is waiting to see the physician, who has been called to the emergency room. You explain the situation to the patient, and he asks if you can perform his physical instead. You explain your scope of practice. Write a chart note to record the conversation.

____

____

____

____

CHAPTER 2

Your physician asks you to write a letter to Jean Mosley, a patient who has continued to be noncompliant. She wants to formally terminate the patient's care and refer her elsewhere. Write a note in the patient's chart documenting your actions.

____

____

____

____

CHAPTER 3

You are checking in a new patient who is obviously in acute pain. He is crying and pacing the floor. You take him to a private area to carry out the patient interview and help him complete his medical questionnaire. Write a note in the patient's chart documenting the fact that you assisted the patient with the questionnaire.

____

____

____

____

CHAPTER 4

Julia is an 8-year-old patient who has been diagnosed with juvenile diabetes. You supply the patient and her mother with educational materials about Julia's condition and how to manage her blood sugar. Write a chart note to document the conversation and actions.

____

____

____

____

CHAPTER 5

Megan O'Conner is a patient who was discharged from the hospital a few hours ago. She calls the office to report that she is now feeling woozy and nauseous. She thinks it might be a side effect of the pain medication she was given. Per your office protocol, she is advised to stop taking the medication, and you will have the doctor prescribe a different medication. Ms. O'Conner is obviously very upset. She is crying and says she just wants to go back to the hospital. You reassure her. Write a note about the conversation to be included in the chart.

CHAPTER 6

Mr. Sheffield did not show up for his appointment. You call him, and he says he forgot. You reschedule his appointment for the next day at 10:00 AM. Write a note to document this in the chart.

CHAPTER 7

The physician asks you to write a note to a patient, Nancy Chesnutt, informing her of her normal lab results. Construct the note that would be included as a copy in the patient's chart.

CHAPTER 8

A patient requests release of his records to another physician. What documentation is necessary for this release? Write a note to document the release in the patient's chart.

CHAPTER 9

You receive an e-mail from Mr. Hagler saying that his medication is working out well and is not causing any side effects. He will be in for this appointment next Tuesday. How do you document this information in Mr. Hagler's medical record?

____

____

____

____

CHAPTER 10

During a routine visit, Carlos Delgado, a 55-year-old male, slips in the exam room and strikes his right forearm on the exam table causing a small laceration. The physician examines the patient's arm and determines it is nothing significant, but he cleans and applies a sterile dressing to it. The patient is also given a tetanus booster and instructions to change the dressing and clean the wound again this evening and was told to contact the office if he has any further problems with it. Use the space below to record the incident in the chart.

____

____

____

____

CHAPTER 11

Theo Smith, a 7-year-old male patient, needs to have his tonsils removed ordered by Dr. Kyle Dunn. His father, Ted Smith, has a PPO insurance plan that has denied preauthorization for a tonsillectomy due to *lack of medical necessity*. The patient has had recurrent throat infections during the last 12 months (a total of eight) with six testing positive for a streptococcus infection. He has tonsil hypertrophy and obstructive sleep apnea. Write a letter to the insurance company appealing the preauthorization denial.

____

____

____

____

CHAPTER 12

An 18-year-old woman is seen for a college physical. While being examined, she tells the physician's assistant that her boyfriend is abusive on occasion. The visit becomes predominantly counseling for the next 20 minutes of her 30-minute visit. How would you document this in the chart so that the visit can be coded accurately?

____

____

____

____

CHAPTER 13

Laila Hildreath is a 4-year-old girl who needs to have tubes in her ears after failing conservative treatment for recurrent ear infections. Her father is a member of an HMO that requires preauthorization for surgery. You call the HMO and receive authorization for the inpatient procedure. You are given the following preauthorization number: 67034598 AB. Record your actions for the patient's financial record.

CHAPTER 14

Tonya Sushkin's insurance company paid $25.00 for an office visit on the 20th of last month. Your physician is a participating provider for this company. Your initial charge was $75.00 for the date of service on the 2nd of last month. Post the payment and adjustment on a blank daysheet. Ms. Sushkin's previous balance is $75.00.

CHAPTER 15

Ms. Bailey has a large balance, and she is in today to see the doctor. You have a conversation with her about her unpaid bill. She promises to send $50.00 on the fifth of each month beginning next month. Write a note to record this agreement for her financial record.

CHAPTER 16

A 40-year-old woman comes to talk to the physician because she would like to start a new exercise routine and change her diet to lose 15 pounds. She is currently 25 pounds overweight, so this is a great idea and a good move toward healthy living. The physician asks you to discuss exercise and diet changes with the patient. Write a narrative patient note describing your interaction with the patient to include in her chart.

CHAPTER 17

Although you always take care to protect yourself from exposure to biohazardous materials, you spill a tube of a patient's blood while performing hematology testing. You have a fresh cut on your hand that came into contact with the blood. Following your office's exposure control plan, you clean up and then document the incident. What information will you make sure to include in your report?

CHAPTER 18

You are interviewing a young patient during an assessment when you notice that he has three small burn marks on his arm. The burns are round and less than a centimeter in diameter. When you ask the patient about the burns, he suddenly turns solemn and avoids answering the question. You suspect that the patient has been abused. How should you document this interaction on the patient's chart?

CHAPTER 19

How should you record an axillary temperature, and why is it important to record it differently from other temperatures?

CHAPTER 20

A 45-year-old patient comes into the office for a routine physical examination. He has high blood pressure and is considerably overweight. The patient asks you for advice on healthy eating, and you provide him with several pamphlets and advise him to cut down on fatty foods. How would you document this interaction in the patient's chart?

CHAPTER 21

The autoclave in your office has not been working properly. It takes twice as long for the steam in the autoclave to reach an adequate temperature for sterilization. You realize that this may affect daily procedures within the office and could lead to bigger problems with the autoclave. You decide to have the autoclave serviced by a professional. What documentation will be needed in connection with this service request?

____

____

____

____

CHAPTER 22

A patient is recovering from a Caesarian section and returns to the office to have her staples removed. The physician asks you to remove the staples and apply adhesive skin closures over the incision site. The patient asks you when the strips should be removed, and you tell her that they should fall off on their own within 10 days. How would you document this interaction in the patient's chart?

____

____

____

____

CHAPTER 23

The physician has prescribed a patient 250 mg of amoxicillin for an ear infection. The patient should take this medication three times a day by mouth for 9 days. Write a note to document this in the patient's chart.

____

____

____

____

CHAPTER 24

The physician has asked you to prepare an administration of gr iii Haldol IM for a patient. The dispenser is labeled in milligrams. How do you convert this dosage to the metric system, and how many milligrams of Haldol should you dispense? Write the preparation as a chart note.

____

____

____

____

CHAPTER 25

You have just taken a chest x-ray to rule out pneumonia. Write a narrative note detailing this procedure to be included in the patient's chart.

CHAPTER 26

A patient received penicillin for a sexually transmitted infection, and this was the last event documented in the patient's chart. Fifteen minutes later, the patient began wheezing and gasping and within 5 minutes was clearly suffering anaphylactic shock. A first injection of epinephrine administered SC at that time was ineffective, and the patient was in respiratory arrest when EMS arrived. Mask-to-mouth respirations were given with supplemental oxygen at 15 L per minute for 2 minutes before EMS assumed care of the patient. How would you document this interaction in the patient's chart?

CHAPTER 27

Your patient is a 9-year-old girl who suffers from severe eczema. The physician has recommended that she wear bandages at night to protect against scratching. You demonstrate to the patient's mother how to apply the bandages. The patient's mother asks how often she should apply ointment to her daughter's skin, and you repeat the physician's instructions to use it twice a day. How would you document this interaction in the patient's chart?

CHAPTER 28

Your patient is an older adult man. The physician has determined that the patient requires an ambulatory assist device. You first attempt to teach the patient to use a cane. The patient is unsteady while using the cane, so you instead teach the patient to use a walker. The patient successfully learns how to use the walker and demonstrates stability and control. You explain to the patient how to use the aid safely, including how to maintain the aid and what changes the patient should make at home to operate the aid safely. The patient verbalizes that he is comfortable using the walker and that he understands his maintenance responsibilities. How would you document this interaction on the patient's chart?

CHAPTER 29

A patient has come in for ceruminosis treatment. Document the steps that were taken to complete this procedure as well as any complications that might have arisen during the procedure. Be sure to include any instructions that were given to the patient after the procedure.

CHAPTER 30

Write a patient care note for a patient recovering from bacterial pneumonia. Explain what her symptoms are as well as what remedies the physician recommends/prescribes. Also, indicate how these remedies are intended to combat specific elements of the disease. You do not need to explain the details of how a remedy works, only what it is intended to do (i.e., a glucocorticoid is prescribed to reduce inflammation).

CHAPTER 31

When interviewing a patient prior to a physical examination of the cardiovascular system, what should you ask the patient and document in his chart?

CHAPTER 32

A patient is being scheduled for a colonoscopy. You explain the preparation to him. Document your actions for inclusion in the patient's chart.

CHAPTER 33

A father brings in his 8-year-old daughter because she fell and hit her head while rollerblading. She was not wearing a helmet and seems to have lost consciousness for just a few seconds. The father is concerned about a possible traumatic brain injury. After a physical examination, the physician finds that the child has suffered a mild concussion. She is sent home, and you give her father instructions regarding her treatment. Write a narrative note documenting this visit for inclusion in the patient's chart.

____

____

____

____

CHAPTER 34

You have just spoken with a 20-year-old patient about cystitis and have given her tips on how to avoid cystitis in the future. Record what you would write on the woman's chart, and make a note of any handout materials you might give the patient.

____

____

____

____

CHAPTER 35

Ms. Molly Espinoza is a 43-year-old female patient. Dr. Cord ordered a routine screening mammogram for this patient. You confirm with her that she is not pregnant and explain the procedure. Then you prepare the patient, and two radiographs are taken of each breast, with repositioning the patient between each image. All four radiographs are developed and are readable and accurate. Record the incident in the chart.

____

____

____

____

CHAPTER 36

John Suiker is an athletic 38-year-old man scheduled for a routine visit. He arrives disoriented and appears to be drunk and unsteady on his feet. He presents with pale, moist skin; rapid, bounding pulse; and shallow breathing. You notify the physician, Dr. Burns, of the patient's condition, and she orders an immediate blood glucose test. The patient's blood glucose is 48 mg/dL. The patient is still conscious, so you provide him with fruit juice, which he accepts. Recovery is immediate. Record the incident in the chart.

____

____

____

____

CHAPTER 37

Rose Ryan is a 24-month-old girl visiting your office for a well-child visit. The physician directs you to obtain her length, weight, and head and chest circumference. You find the child measures 92 cm tall and weighs 15 kg. Her head circumference is 50 cm, and her chest circumference is 52 cm. Document these procedures. Use the space below to record the procedure in the chart. How would you document the above scenario on the child's chart? Be sure to document the interaction, as well as the education that was provided during her visit, and any scheduled follow-up appointments. How would you record the procedure in the chart?

____

____

____

____

CHAPTER 38

A 78-year-old patient visits the physician's office to ask about treatment for arthritis in his knees. While you are talking to the patient, you notice that his hearing has decreased considerably since the last time he was in the physician's office. How would you document this information in the patient's chart?

____

____

____

____

CHAPTER 39

How would you document the collection of a blood specimen and prepare it to be sent out for testing?

____

____

____

____

CHAPTER 40

You have just completed maintenance on the glucose meter. Document this maintenance as you would in the laboratory instrument maintenance log.

____

____

____

____

CHAPTER 41

Nicole Patton is a 35-year-old female inpatient receiving both a Lovenox injection and oral Coumadin. You are directed to obtain blood specimens by evacuated tube for platelet count, prothrombin time, and partial thromboplastin time tests. Document your collection as you would in the patient's chart. Include the type(s) of specimens you collected.

CHAPTER 42

You perform an ESR test on an older adult male patient with rheumatoid arthritis. You measure a rate of 16 mL/hour. How would you document the results of this test in the patient's chart?

CHAPTER 43

You instruct a patient how to perform a clean-catch midstream urine specimen. When you test the sample, you discover that the urine is cloudy, with a pH level of 7.5, and contains traces of red blood cells, nitrites, and leukocytes. Your office does not use laboratory report forms. How would you document this information in the patient's chart?

CHAPTER 44

The physician has ordered an influenza test on your patient. The influenza test requires a nasopharyngeal specimen. You collect the specimen. Document the collection as you would in a patient's chart.

CHAPTER 45

Dr. Ashanti asks you to perform a blood cholesterol test on a patient. The results are 282 mg/dL. Write a note to document this test and its results in the patient's chart as you would if your office does not use laboratory report forms.

____

____

____

____

CHAPTER 46

You just completed an interview with the office manager of a large family practice. Write a thank you note to the interviewer.

____

____

____

____

PSY ACTIVE LEARNING

CHAPTER 1

Talk with a grandparent or another older adult, and ask him or her to tell you about a medical discovery that he or she remembers well. Create a "before and after" chart, explaining what life was like before the discovery, and the changes and benefits that came about after the discovery.

CHAPTER 2

Go to the Health and Human Services Web site, http://www.hhs.gov/ocr/privacy. What is the mission statement of the Office for Civil Rights regarding the HIPAA Privacy Rule?

CHAPTER 3

Do a Web search for "anger management techniques." Are there suggestions that could help you communicate with an angry patient? Record your findings. Cite Web sites used.

CHAPTER 4

Go to the Council on Aging's Web site, http://www.ncoa.org. Describe the plan included in the *Falls Free Coalition* outlined in the Safety of Seniors Act of 2008.

CHAPTER 5

Go the Americans With Disabilities Web site, http://www.usdoj.gov/crt/ada. Go to the Primer for Small Businesses. Who is covered by the ADA?

CHAPTER 6

Memorize the days of the week in Spanish. Recite them for your classmates.

CHAPTER 7

When writing, it is important to know your audience. The way you write for a physician is different from the way you write for a patient. In the case of a physician, you can assume he or she understands medical terminology, but this is not so of a patient. Do some Internet research to better understand the possible digestive side effects of a common medication like simvastatin (Zocor) or esomeprazole (Nexium). Then, write two letters discussing the side effects, one to a physician and one to a patient. Think about what you must do differently when writing to a patient.

CHAPTER 8

If you were opening a new medical facility, consider whether you would want staff members using abbreviations in patient records. Then create a list of acceptable abbreviations that may be used in your new facility. Then create a "Do Not Use" list for abbreviations that may be confusing and should not be included in records. Visit the Web site for the Joint Commission (http://www.jointcommission.org) and include all of those abbreviations in addition to five other abbreviations of your own choice.

CHAPTER 9

Go to WebMD (http://www.webmd.com). Scroll down to the Symptom Checker. Think back to your last illness or pick an illness and answer the questions about the symptoms. What do you have?

CHAPTER 10

Prepare a list of emergency contacts in the area, including the contact information of local hospitals, poison control centers, and emergency medical services.

CHAPTER 11

Call two collection agencies in your local area. Compare services and fees. Record your findings.

CHAPTER 12

Research the banking services offered by your local bank. Gather brochures outlining the services. Share with classmates to compare services.

CHAPTER 13

When will/did ICD-10 CM codes go into effect? Search http://www.aapc.com/ICD-10 for the answer.

CHAPTER 14

Find the ICD-9-CM or ICD-10-CM codes for the following diseases:

a. Acute gastric ulcer with hemorrhage and perforation without obstruction ______________

b. Meningococcal pericarditis ______________

c. Impetigo ______________

d. Benign essential hypertension ______________

CHAPTER 15

Research the subject of Current Procedural Coding. Write a paragraph describing the origin of the CPT codes. What was the original purpose of CPT coding?

CHAPTER 16

The Centers for Disease Control (CDC) offers a body mass calculator on its Web site. Visit http://www.cdc.gov and search for the BMI calculator. Determine whether your BMI is within normal limits for your gender, age, and height. Describe at least three things you can do to either maintain your current weight or lose/gain weight if necessary.

CHAPTER 17

You have been asked to select the best hand soap for use throughout the urgent care center where you work. Do Internet research to identify different types of antibacterial agents that are commonly used in hand soaps. Cite any evidence you can find as to the effectiveness of the agents. Determine which soap you believe is best. Write a letter to the office manager that gives your recommendation, clearly explaining why you chose that soap.

CHAPTER 18

Conduct a patient interview with a family member or friend. Use a sample patient history form such as the one found in this chapter from your textbook. Be sure to perform the interview in person so that you can observe the physical and mental status of your patient. When you are finished, ask your patient for feedback, such as demeanor and professionalism or comfort level of the patient. Use his or her comments to set one goal for yourself regarding your skills conducting patient interviews.

CHAPTER 19

With a partner, practice taking body temperature measurements with all the types of thermometers you have access to. For those you cannot access, mime the process so that you at least have the steps down the first time you are faced with the real thermometer. For all methods, go through all the steps from picking up the thermometer to returning it to the disinfectant or returning the unit to the charging base.

CHAPTER 20

Even though the physician is the person who is responsible for using most of the instruments discussed in this chapter, you should still be familiar with how all the instruments are used. Working with a partner, access at least three of the following instruments: tongue depressor, percussion hammer, tuning fork, nasal speculum, otoscope, and stethoscope. If you do not have access to these instruments, ask your teacher if he or she can assist you. Once you have the instruments, identify the main use of those instruments during a physical exam.

CHAPTER 21

Using the library and the Internet, research the instruments and equipment commonly used by the following medical specialties: endocrinology, rheumatology, palliative care, and radiology. Add to the list found in Chapter 21 of your text with the information you find. Include images of some of the instruments and equipment.

CHAPTER 22

One of the most common minor surgeries performed in your office is the excision of skin lesions and moles, often related to the possibility of skin cancer. Skin cancer is prevalent today, and you feel that it's important to educate young people on the importance of taking proper precautions to protect skin from harmful sunrays. You have been asked to prepare a one-page patient education handout highlighting the dangers of skin cancer and prevention techniques designed especially for young adults.

- Do Internet research to identify the leading causes of skin cancer and the dangers associated with harmful sun exposure. Gather any statistics that are available from reputable Web sites.
- Outline steps that can be taken to protect the skin when outside.
- Highlight issues that are especially important to teens (e.g., summer jobs as lifeguards and outdoor sports practice during the day).
- Create a one-page handout to be given to teens in the office explaining how to protect their skin from the sun.

CHAPTER 23

You have just begun working in a medical office and are getting yourself acquainted with the types of medications that the physician frequently prescribes. You know that many medications interact with food; however, you don't know a lot about specific food–drug interactions. Choose 10 common drugs from different therapeutic classifications in Table 23-1 and then research any possible food interactions. Make a chart for patients showing how common drugs and foods interact with one another.

CHAPTER 24

Accidental needlesticks are one of the most frightening occupational hazards you will encounter as a medical assistant. The greatest fear is centered on human immunodeficiency virus (HIV) and hepatitis B (HBV). Research the incubation, signs and symptoms, treatment, and prognosis associated with these two diseases. Prepare a one-page handout on each.

CHAPTER 25

Research the current recommendations by the American Cancer Society for mammography. At what age does the ACS recommend that women get their first mammogram? What other important information do women need to know about breast cancer?

CHAPTER 26

Some medical professionals live on the front line of emergency medical care. Locate an EMT-Basic (EMT-B) textbook at a library, bookstore, or other source. Make a list of some basic emergency care that is expected of the EMT-B that may also be expected of the practicing medical assistant. Are there any skills that are similar? Different?

CHAPTER 27

Use the Internet to research the major causes of fungal infections and find out how they can be prevented. Produce a poster to display in the office, educating patients about the main types of fungal infection, how they are spread, and how patients can protect their families from outbreaks.

CHAPTER 28

School children, especially girls, are commonly screened for scoliosis. Research the methods used for this screening using the Internet or the library. Then, prepare a patient education pamphlet for school children who are about to undergo the screening. Explain the procedure in a way that will calm any anxieties. Include information about scoliosis as well as preventative measures the children can take and warning signs they should look for in the years following their school screening.

CHAPTER 29

The composer Beethoven was afflicted with hearing loss that left him completely deaf. Many music lovers today suffer from hearing loss as well, and they rely on the technology available to help them enjoy the subtle tones that are written into compositions. Research the new programs and software that are being installed in hearing aids that are specifically aimed toward listening to music. List differences between listening to music and listening to speech, and make a note of tips for listening to music that physicians can give to patients with hearing aids.

CHAPTER 30

Most people are aware of the dangers of smoking. However, it is still important to educate children about the long-term dangers of smoking. Create a pamphlet outlining the dangers of smoking to be presented to a group of middle school children.

CHAPTER 31

Pretend you are a patient who is keeping a Holter monitor diary. Create a diary based on experiences a patient is likely to have. What kinds of activities do you participate in during the day? How are these activities influencing your symptoms?

CHAPTER 32

One of the deadliest types of cancer is pancreatic cancer, which kills most patients within a year of diagnosis. Research the latest information about the suspected causes of pancreatic cancer on the Internet. Try to find out which treatments are proving the most effective and whether there have been any recent developments.

- Use the information you find to create an informational poster about pancreatic cancer, educating high-risk patients on how they can lower their chances of developing pancreatic cancer.
- Write a one-page leaflet for physicians, informing them of the latest treatments for pancreatic cancer.

CHAPTER 33

Safe use of car seats can reduce brain and spinal cord injuries in infants and young children. Research the guidelines for car seat use. Then research car seat ratings and find five car seats that receive high safety ratings in each category. Create a handout for parents of young children to promote car seat safety awareness.

CHAPTER 34

Prostate cancer is most common in men over age 50 years, and like many other cancers, it is best treated in the early stages. Testicular cancer is another form of cancer, but it occurs most often in younger men, ages 15 to 34 years. Go online and research more information about these diseases. Design a presentation to be educational for both your classmates and patients alike. Be sure to include information about the causes, the symptoms, the ways to diagnose them, and the treatments available.

CHAPTER 35

With so many prenatal tests, procedures, and appointments at the physician's office, a pregnant patient can feel overwhelmed. Create a packet that can be distributed to a patient during the first prenatal visit. Include the schedule of prenatal visits and the procedures that will be done at each of these visits. Also include important information for the patient to consult throughout the duration of the pregnancy: especially include a list of signs and symptoms that may indicate a problematic condition.

CHAPTER 36

Make a list of common foods for a diabetes sufferer to avoid. Then create a poster to display in the office highlighting your findings. Be sure to stress the importance of proper nutrition.

CHAPTER 37

The physician has asked that you make a poster for the waiting room that shows important hygienic tips for children, such as washing hands, covering the mouth while sneezing, etc. Come up with a list of five hygienic tips that could be illustrated and design the poster. Use visuals so that children who are too young to read can understand the concepts being displayed.

CHAPTER 38

Research the latest information about Alzheimer disease on the Internet. Produce an informative poster to display in a physician's waiting room, educating people about the early warning signs of Alzheimer disease. Include information about the stages of Alzheimer disease and what friends and families can expect if a loved one develops it.

CHAPTER 39

Patient confidentiality is always an important part of your job, but so is safety. Research your state's rules and regulations in regard to the rights of a patient and the rights of the public. For instance, is someone with HIV/AIDS required by law to report his or her condition to his or her employer? What about other illnesses? After you have run a test and found a patient who tested positive for a specific disease, what are the obligations of your office in dealing with this?

CHAPTER 40

You perform an HCG pregnancy test for your patient. She has a weak positive result, which fails the QC, so you must administer the test again. The second time, the test shows a positive result, and the QC is acceptable. Document the QC results as you would in the office QC log.

CHAPTER 41

Familiarize yourself with phlebotomy equipment and draw a diagram of your blood-drawing station; detail on your diagram where supplies are kept. Think, in terms of safety, about where your blood station should be positioned in the office. Think about how the organization of your station will assist you in phlebotomy procedures and minimize the likelihood of accidents.

CHAPTER 42

White blood cells are the body's defense against foreign substances and objects that enter the bloodstream. However, there are cancers, diseases, and other ailments that attack white blood cells and their production. Research one of these diseases. How many people are reported to have this disease? Is there current treatment or therapy? What are some of the cures that are being developed to stop these diseases and to rebuild the immune system? After you have gathered the information, prepare a report on this disease to present to the class.

CHAPTER 43

Identify common features that patients can take note of in their own urine (e.g., dark color = possible dehydration). Make a brochure to raise patients' awareness of how their physical health can be reflected in the color and clarity of their urine.

CHAPTER 44

Many soaps and cleaning products today are antibacterial, meaning that they work to kill bacteria. People use these antibacterial products to wash and sanitize their hands as well as their homes, especially the kitchen and bathroom. Some studies have shown that the rise in popularity of antibacterial products may be creating strains of bacteria that are resistant to antibiotics. Perform research on this topic and present it to the class.

CHAPTER 45

A new patient says there is a history of heart attacks in his family, and he wants to know what he can do to prevent it. He is middle aged and slightly overweight; however, he has a healthy diet and exercises regularly. Search the Internet and list Web sites that could contain credible information for the patient. Compile a brochure for the prevention of heart disease.

CHAPTER 46

Do an Internet search of medical assisting job opportunities in your area. Now broaden your search to check jobs in any large metropolitan area. What are the differences and similarities in your local opportunities and those in the other city?

PIMA MEDICAL INSTITUTE

Part (

Study Guide Addendum: Lab Skills

Medical Administrative Assistant and Medical Assistant

PIMA MEDICAL INSTITUTE

Medical Assistant
Medical Administrative Assistant
Professional Sequence I
MAA 100 Office Management
Lab Skills

Students must successfully complete the skills listed under each objective. Each listed skill is considered a required part of the mastery of the objective. Students unable to successfully perform the skills will be required to repeat the course.

Objective 1: Demonstrate an understanding of tasks related to human resources operations in the medical office.		
Skills	**Date Completed**	**Initials of Evaluator**
1. Describe how a job applicant should prepare and present herself/himself for a job interview in a medical office.		
2. Practice being interviewed for employment in a medical office.		
3. Describe the types of questions that are and are not allowed by law to be asked of a job applicant during an interview.		
4. Describe proper follow up to a job interview.		
5. Describe the role of policies and procedures manuals in dealing with various employee issues, including absenteeism, overtime, dress code, and sexual harassment.		

I certify that this student has successfully completed each of the listed skills for this objective.

Student:	
Evaluator:	**Date:**

PIMA MEDICAL INSTITUTE

Medical Assistant
Medical Administrative Assistant
Professional Sequence I
MAA 100 Office Management
Lab Skills

Objective 2: Demonstrate knowledge of the daily office tasks related to patient processing procedures.		
Skills	**Date Completed**	**Initials of Evaluator**
1. Describe procedures included in the daily opening of a medical office.		
2. List the key items that should be included in the reception area of a medical office.		
3. Demonstrate appropriate patient-processing procedures in various scenarios, including ways to manage difficult patients.		
4. Describe procedures included in preparing the medical office for the next day.		
5. Describe procedures included in closing the medical office for the day.		

I certify that this student has successfully completed each of the listed skills for this objective.

Student:	
Evaluator:	**Date:**

Objective 3: Demonstrate knowledge of scheduling appointments and referrals in a computer-based system.		
Skills	**Date Completed**	**Initials of Evaluator**
1. Schedule appointments based on given case studies/scenarios.		
2. Manage scheduling conflicts by rescheduling and cancelling appointments based on given case studies/scenarios.		
3. Prepare a daily list of appointments.		
4. Schedule referrals based on given case studies/scenarios.		

I certify that this student has successfully completed each of the listed skills for this objective.

Student:	
Evaluator:	**Date:**

PIMA MEDICAL INSTITUTE

Medical Assistant
Medical Administrative Assistant
Professional Sequence I
MAA 100 Office Management
Lab Skills

Objective 4: Demonstrate knowledge of effective medical records management.		
Skills	**Date Completed**	**Initials of Evaluator**
1. Explain how HIPAA affects the way medical records are created and maintained.		
2. Assemble a sample of a patient medical record.		
3. Demonstrate proper filing procedures for paper records (including alphabetizing).		
4. Demonstrate typing skills of 30 WPM with 95% accuracy.		
5. Demonstrate correct procedures for adding, correcting, and altering information, as well as releasing, transferring, and retaining patient medical records.		
6. Create a sample authorization form for release of records.		

I certify that this student has successfully completed each of the listed skills for this objective.

Student:	
Evaluator:	**Date:**

PIMA MEDICAL INSTITUTE

Medical Assistant
Medical Administrative Assistant
Professional Sequence I
MAA 100 Office Management
Lab Skills

Objective 5: Determine patient fees and post charges and payments manually and electronically.		
Skills	**Date Completed**	**Initials of Evaluator**
1. Complete a sample encounter form.		
2. Create a new patient account.		
3. Enter guarantor information about a new patient.		
4. Enter insurance policy information.		
5. Enter dependent information.		
6. Post patient payments.		
7. Explain and demonstrate how to print patient statements.		

I certify that this student has successfully completed each of the listed skills for this objective.

Student:	
Evaluator:	**Date:**

Objective 6: Demonstrate knowledge of various fee-collection techniques.		
Skills	**Date Completed**	**Initials of Evaluator**
1. Explain the process for collecting fees in special situations such as an estate, bankruptcy, or a "skip."		
2. In given scenarios, demonstrate how to create a sample payment plan with a patient.		
3. Create a document containing patient information that must be sent to a collection agency when releasing an account.		

I certify that this student has successfully completed each of the listed skills for this objective.

Student:	
Evaluator:	**Date:**

PIMA MEDICAL INSTITUTE

Medical Assistant
Medical Administrative Assistant
Professional Sequence I
MAA 100 Office Management
Lab Skills

Objective 7: Demonstrate knowledge of medical office banking procedures.		
Skills	**Date Completed**	**Initials of Evaluator**
1. Identify different types of checks, including traveler's check, certified check, voucher check, cashier's check, and money orders.		
2. Complete sample checks with information provided.		
3. Create a deposit slip with information provided.		

I certify that this student has successfully completed each of the listed skills for this objective.

Student:	
Evaluator:	**Date:**

Objective 8: Demonstrate how to complete accounting procedures for accounts payable, accounts receivable, and trial balance using the appropriate forms.		
Skills	**Date Completed**	**Initials of Evaluator**
1. Demonstrate accounts payable procedures.		
2. Demonstrate accounts receivable procedures.		
3. Demonstrate calculating a trial balance.		

I certify that this student has successfully completed each of the listed skills for this objective.

Student:	
Evaluator:	**Date:**

PIMA MEDICAL INSTITUTE

Medical Assistant
Medical Administrative Assistant
Professional Sequence I
MAA 100 Office Management
Lab Skills

Optional Objective

(Note: The portfolio will be completed in MAA 104 but can be started in MAA 100 if all other MAA 100 lab skills have been successfully completed.)

Optional Objective: Begin creating a professional portfolio consisting of sample documents.		
Skills	**Date Completed**	**Initials of Evaluator**
1. Create drafts of a sample business letter in full-block or modified-block style free of grammatical and spelling errors.		
2. Create drafts of a sample memorandum, free of grammatical and spelling errors.		
3. Create drafts of a résumé free of grammatical and spelling errors.		
4. Create drafts of a cover letter free of grammatical and spelling errors.		
5. Compose drafts of e-mail messages free of grammatical and spelling errors that follow etiquette guidelines for electronic mail.		

I certify that this student has successfully completed each of the listed skills for this objective.

Student:	
Evaluator:	**Date:**

PIMA MEDICAL INSTITUTE

Medical Assistant
Medical Administrative Assistant
Professional Sequence I
MAA 102 Introduction to Insurance and Coding
Lab Skills

Students must successfully complete the skills listed under each objective. Each listed skill is considered a required part of the mastery of the objective. Students unable to successfully perform the skills will be required to repeat the course.

Objective 1: Compare and contrast several types of health insurance.		
Skills	**Date Completed**	**Initials of Evaluator**
1. Describe the billing and payment process for a government insurance policy.		
2. Compare the billing and payment processes for an HMO with those of a PPO.		
3. Describe the billing and payment process for a person with dual coverage.		

I certify that this student has successfully completed each of the listed skills for this objective.

Student:	
Evaluator:	**Date:**

Objective 2: Verify insurance benefits using given information.		
Skills	**Date Completed**	**Initials of Evaluator**
1. Identify the plan member listed on a sample insurance card.		
2. Identify the insurance plan type on a sample insurance card.		
3. Locate the insurance company's contact information on a sample insurance card.		
4. Identify the preauthorization phone number listed on a sample insurance card.		
5. In role-play scenarios, practice calling an insurance company for pre-authorization.		
6. Complete a referral request to submit to an insurance company.		

I certify that this student has successfully completed each of the listed skills for this objective.

Student:	
Evaluator:	**Date:**

PIMA MEDICAL INSTITUTE

Medical Assistant
Medical Administrative Assistant
Professional Sequence I
MAA 102 Introduction to Insurance and Coding
Lab Skills

Objective 3: Demonstrate an understanding of how to select and assign codes to sample cases using the ICD-CM (current edition), CPT, and HCPCS Level II coding sets.		
Skills	**Date Completed**	**Initials of Evaluator**
1. Identify and assign codes from the current edition of the ICD-CM to case studies/examples.		
2. Complete Box 24 of the CMS-1500 form, using codes obtained from the current edition of the ICD-CM manual.		
3. Identify and assign CPT codes to case studies/examples.		
4. Identify and assign modifiers to case studies/examples using the CPT manual.		
5. Identify and assign E&M codes to case studies/examples using the CPT manual.		
6. Insert E&M codes in Box 24 of the CMS-1500 form based on a sample new and/or established patient's office visit.		
7. Identify and assign HCPCS Level II codes to selected case studies/examples.		

I certify that this student has successfully completed each of the listed skills for this objective.

Student:	
Evaluator:	**Date:**

Objective 4: Complete insurance billing tasks.		
Skills	**Date Completed**	**Initials of Evaluator**
1. Complete a paper copy of a CMS-1500 form using given information.		
2. Complete an electronic copy of a CMS-1500 form for a Medicaid patient using selected computer software/application.		
3. Complete an electronic copy of a CMS-1500 form for a Medicare patient using selected computer software/application.		
4. Role-play contacting an insurance company to verify benefits and check claim status.		
5. Explain how to complete an insurance tracking worksheet.		
6. Demonstrate how to post insurance payments using computer software or form provided.		

I certify that this student has successfully completed each of the listed skills for this objective.

Student:	
Evaluator:	**Date:**

PIMA MEDICAL INSTITUTE

Medical Assistant
Medical Administrative Assistant
Professional Sequence I
MAA 104 Business Writing and EHR
Lab Skills

Students must successfully complete the skills listed under each objective. Each listed skill is considered a required part of the mastery of the objective. Students unable to successfully perform the skills will be required to repeat the course.

Objective 1: Create properly formatted documents for a professional portfolio that contains samples of business letters, memos, résumés, cover letters, and other business-related correspondence.		
Skills	**Date Completed**	**Initials of Evaluator**
1. Create a properly formatted memorandum that is free of spelling and grammatical errors.		
2. Create a properly formatted business letter. The document may be full-block, semi-block, or modified-block style and must be free of spelling and grammatical errors.		
3. Create a properly formatted résumé and cover letter. The documents must be free of spelling and grammatical errors.		
4. Create other properly formatted documents as assigned that are free of spelling and grammatical errors.		

I certify that this student has successfully completed each of the listed skills for this objective.

Student:	
Evaluator:	**Date:**

PIMA MEDICAL INSTITUTE

Medical Assistant
Medical Administrative Assistant
Professional Sequence I
MAA 104 Business Writing and EHR
Lab Skills

Objective 2: Create an electronic patient medical record (EMR) for administrative tasks.		
Skills	**Date Completed**	**Initials of Evaluator**
1. Schedule a patient.		
2. Properly document a patient who misses his/her appointment.		
3. Enter a new patient's demographic information.		
4. Enter a patient's insurance information.		
5. Demonstrate the ability to track the patient while in the office (waiting room, exam room, etc.).		
6. Post charges and payments to patient account.		
7. Demonstrate the steps necessary to process a claim.		

I certify that this student has successfully completed each of the listed skills for this objective.

Student:	
Evaluator:	**Date:**

Objective 3: Create an EMR for clinical tasks.		
Skills	**Date Completed**	**Initials of Evaluator**
1. Record a patient history.		
2. Record vital signs.		
3. Record chief complaint.		
4. Record a progress note.		
5. Explain and/or demonstrate how to add an image to an EMR.		
6. Describe/demonstrate how to order labs, imaging items, or medical tests.		
7. Describe/demonstrate how to transmit and correctly document a prescription order.		

I certify that this student has successfully completed each of the listed skills for this objective.

Student:	
Evaluator:	**Date:**

PIMA MEDICAL INSTITUTE

Medical Administrative Assistant
Professional Sequence II
MAA 134 Vital Sign Basics
Lab Skills

Students will be tested on the skills listed under each objective. Each step is considered a required part of the mastery of the objective and will be evaluated using the following standards:

Pass: Able to perform skill in a laboratory setting in a safe, professional, and effective manner with distant supervision. Student should be able to perform the skill as an entry-level Medical Administrative Assistant.

Fail: Unable to perform skill in a laboratory setting in a safe, professional, and effective manner without constant cues and direct supervision. Student requires remedial training.

Students not able to perform the skills after the second attempt will receive a failing grade and will be required to repeat the course.

Objective 1: Demonstrate procedures to measure and document patient height and weight.

Skills	**Attempt 1**	**Attempt 2**
1. Wash hands.		
2. Greet and identify patient, explain procedure, and set patient at ease.		
3. Demonstrate proper skills in moving patient on/off scale.		
4. Measure and record a patient's height and correctly document results.		
5. Measure and record a patient's weight and correctly document results.		

I certify that this student has successfully completed each of the listed skills for this objective.

Student:	
Evaluator:	**Date:**

BRYAN MEDICAL INSTITUTE

Medical Administrative Assistant
Professional Sequence II
MAA 154 Vital Sign Basics
Lab Skill

Students will be tested on the skills listed under each objective. Each step is considered a critical part of the mastery of the objective and will be evaluated using the following standards:

Pass: Able to perform the skill in a laboratory setting in a safe, professional, and effective manner with distant supervision. Students should be able to perform these skills at an entry-level Medical Administrative Assistant.

Fail: Unable to perform skill in a laboratory setting in a safe, professional, and effective manner without continued and direct supervision. Student requires remedial training.

Students that fail to perform the skills on the second attempt will receive a failing grade and will be required to repeat the course.

Objective 1: Demonstrate procedures to measure and document patient height and weight		
Skills	Attempt 1	Attempt 2
1. Wash hands		
2. Greet and identify patient, explain procedure, and set patient at ease		
3. Demonstrate proper skills in balancing and zeroing scale		
4. Measure and record patient's height and correctly document results		
5. Measure and record patient's weight and correctly document results		

I certify that this student has successfully completed each of the listed skills for this objective.

Student:	
Evaluator:	Date:

PIMA MEDICAL INSTITUTE

Medical Administrative Assistant
Professional Sequence II
MAA 134 Vital Sign Basics
Lab Skills

Objective 2: Demonstrate procedures for taking and recording patient temperatures.		
Skills	**Attempt 1**	**Attempt 2**
1. Wash hands.		
2. Greet and identify patient, explain procedure, and set patient at ease.		
3. Obtain an **oral** temperature using a digital thermometer and correctly document results.		
4. Obtain an **aural** temperature using a tympanic thermometer and correctly document results.		
5. Obtain an **axillary** temperature and correctly document results.		
6. Obtain a **temporal** temperature and correctly document results.		

I certify that this student has successfully completed each of the listed skills for this objective.

Student:	
Evaluator:	**Date:**

Objective 3: Demonstrate procedures for obtaining and documenting pulse and respiration.		
Skills	**Attempt 1**	**Attempt 2**
1. Wash hands.		
2. Greet and identify patient, explain procedure, and set patient at ease.		
3. Obtain an **apical** pulse and correctly document results.		
4. Obtain a **radial** pulse and correctly document results.		
5. Determine patient's **respiratory rate** and correctly document results.		

I certify that this student has successfully completed each of the listed skills for this objective.

Student:	
Evaluator:	**Date:**

PIMA MEDICAL INSTITUTE

Medical Administrative Assistant
Professional Sequence II
MAA 134 Vital Sign Basics
Lab Skills

Objective 4: Use proper procedures to measure and document blood pressure.		
Skills	**Attempt 1**	**Attempt 2**
1. Wash hands.		
2. Greet and identify patient, explain procedure, and set patient at ease.		
3. Determine a patient's blood pressure and correctly document results.		

I certify that this student has successfully completed each of the listed skills for this objective.

Student:	
Evaluator:	**Date:**

PIMA MEDICAL INSTITUTE

Medical Administrative Assistant
Professional Sequence II
MAA 138 Medical Billing and Coding
Lab Skills

Students must successfully complete the skills listed under each objective. Each listed skill is considered a required part of the mastery of the objective. Students unable to successfully perform the skills will be required to repeat the course.

Objective 1: Demonstrate knowledge of how to process an insurance claim.		
Skills	**Date Completed**	**Evaluator's Initials**
1. Explain the purpose of the patient privacy notice relative to health insurance claims processing.		
2. Identify the information on a health insurance card that is needed to process an insurance claim.		
3. Record procedure and diagnostic codes from encounter form.		

I certify that this student has successfully completed each of the listed skills for this objective.

Student:	
Evaluator:	**Date:**

Objective 2: Demonstrate knowledge of how to determine the status of a health insurance claim and the actions that might be taken after confirming the claim's status.		
Skills	**Date Completed**	**Evaluator's Initials**
1. Verify and obtain required information from sample health insurance card.		
2. Identify the correct method of contacting a health insurance company to inquire on the status of a claim.		
3. Identify the correct steps to follow when appealing a denied claim (Medicare and/or other claims).		
4. Identify steps needed to re-bill a corrected claim.		

I certify that this student has successfully completed each of the listed skills for this objective.

Student:	
Evaluator:	**Date:**

PIMA MEDICAL INSTITUTE

Medical Administrative Assistant
Professional Sequence II
MAA 138 Medical Billing and Coding
Lab Skills

Objective 3: Complete insurance billing tasks.		
Skills	**Date Completed**	**Evaluator's Initials**
1. Complete a paper sample CMS 1500 form using specified information.		
2. Complete an insurance billing worksheet.		
3. Complete and print a sample CMS 1500 form for a patient with standard TRICARE coverage using computer software.		
4. Post insurance payments using computer software.		
5. Interpret a sample explanation of benefits (EOB): a. Define specified information (terminology) on the EOB		
b. Explain how to use the information to determine charges allowed by the carrier and why a service was reduced/denied		
6. Complete a patient collection letter for balance due.		

I certify that this student has successfully completed each of the listed skills for this objective.

Student:	
Evaluator:	**Date:**

Objective 4: Demonstrate knowledge of when and how to assign codes from commonly used coding sets for given examples.		
Skills	**Date Completed**	**Evaluator's Initials**
1. Identify and assign CPT codes for given examples.		
2. Identify and assign HCPCS level II codes for given examples.		
3. Identify and assign ICD-10-CM codes for given examples.		
4. Review completed forms and medical documentation and identify coding errors.		

I certify that this student has successfully completed each of the listed skills for this objective.

Student:	
Evaluator:	**Date:**

PIMA MEDICAL INSTITUTE

Medical Administrative Assistant
Professional Sequence II
MAA 138 Medical Billing and Coding
Lab Skills

Objective 5: Code sample E/M encounters.		
Skills	**Date Completed**	**Evaluator's Initials**
1. Identify place of service.		
2. Identify type of service.		
3. Determine patient status (as appropriate or required).		
4. Select the appropriate history, examination, and understand medical decision making (MDM) level.		
5. Determine if any contributing factors apply (as appropriate).		
6. Assign E/M codes for specified outpatient and inpatient services.		
7. Assign E/M codes for specified consultative services.		

I certify that this student has successfully completed each of the listed skills for this objective.

Student:	
Evaluator:	**Date:**

PIMA MEDICAL INSTITUTE

Medical Assistant
Professional Sequence II
MDA 111 Examination Techniques
Lab Skills

Students will be tested on the skills listed under each objective. Each step is considered a required part of the mastery of the objective and will be evaluated using the following standards:

Pass: Able to perform skill in a laboratory setting in a safe, professional, and effective manner with distant supervision. Student should be able to perform the skill as an entry-level Medical Assistant.

Fail: Unable to perform skill in a laboratory setting in a safe, professional, and effective manner without constant cues and direct supervision. Student requires remedial training.

Students not able to perform the skills after the second attempt will receive a failing grade and will be required to repeat the course.

Before final check-off, students must complete a minimum of 25 complete sets of vital signs including temperature, pulse, respiration, blood pressure, height, and weight.

Objective 1: Demonstrate procedures for preparing examination room, including identifying instruments, explaining which tests make up the vital signs component, and proper patient positioning.		
Skills	**Attempt 1**	**Attempt 2**
1. Wash hands.		
2. Prepare exam table.		
3. Check all medical equipment to be used to ensure proper working order and sterilization.		
4. Identify instruments used during various examinations.		
5. Identify and briefly explain vital signs.		
6. Demonstrate proper patient positioning for various examinations.		

I certify that this student has successfully completed each of the listed skills for this objective.

Student:	
Evaluator:	**Date:**

PIMA MEDICAL INSTITUTE

Medical Assistant
Professional Sequence II
MDA 111 Examination Techniques
Lab Skills

Objective 2: Demonstrate proper procedures to measure and document height and weight.		
Skills	**Attempt 1**	**Attempt 2**
1. Wash hands.		
2. Greet and identify patient. Explain the procedure and set patient at ease.		
3. Demonstrate proper skills in moving patient on/off scale.		
4. Measure a patient's height and correctly document results.		
5. Measure a patient's weight and correctly document results.		

I certify that this student has successfully completed each of the listed skills for this objective.

Student:	
Evaluator:	**Date:**

Objective 3: Demonstrate proper procedures to obtain and document temperatures.		
Skills	**Attempt 1**	**Attempt 2**
1. Wash hands.		
2. Greet and identify patient. Explain the procedure and set patient at ease.		
3. Obtain an **oral** temperature using a digital thermometer and correctly document results.		
4. Obtain a **tympanic** temperature using a tympanic thermometer and correctly document results.		
5. Obtain an **axillary** temperature and correctly document results.		
6. Obtain a **temporal** artery temperature and correctly document results.		
7. Demonstrate the procedure to obtain a **rectal** temperature and correctly document results.		

I certify that this student has successfully completed each of the listed skills for this objective.

Student:	
Evaluator:	**Date:**

PIMA MEDICAL INSTITUTE

Medical Assistant
Professional Sequence II
MDA 111 Examination Techniques
Lab Skills

Objective 4: Demonstrate proper procedures to obtain and document pulse and respiration.		
Skills	**Attempt 1**	**Attempt 2**
1. Wash hands.		
2. Greet and identify patient. Explain the procedure and set the patient at ease.		
3. Obtain an **apical** pulse and correctly document results.		
4. Obtain a **radial** pulse and correctly document results.		
5. Determine a patient's **respiratory rate** and correctly document results.		

I certify that this student has successfully completed each of the listed skills for this objective.

Student:	
Evaluator:	**Date:**

Objective 5: Demonstrate proper procedures to obtain and document blood pressure.		
Skills	**Attempt 1**	**Attempt 2**
1. Wash hands.		
2. Greet and identify patient. Explain the procedure and set the patient at ease.		
3. Determine a patient's blood pressure and correctly document results.		

I certify that this student has successfully completed each of the listed skills for this objective.

Student:	
Evaluator:	**Date:**

PIMA MEDICAL INSTITUTE

Medical Assistant
Professional Sequence II
MDA 111 Examination Techniques
Lab Skills

Objective 6: Demonstrate proper safety skills and body mechanics to assist mobility-challenged patients.		
Skills	**Attempt 1**	**Attempt 2**
1. Wash hands.		
2. Greet and identify patient. Explain the procedure and set the patient at ease.		
3. Assess patient mobility.		
4. Perform correct body mechanics during patient transfer to exam table/exam chair.		

I certify that this student has successfully completed each of the listed skills for this objective.

Student:	
Evaluator:	**Date:**

Objective 7: Perform vision and hearing tests and document results.		
Skills	**Attempt 1**	**Attempt 2**
1. Wash hands.		
2. Greet and identify patient. Explain the procedures and set the patient at ease.		
3. Perform visual acuity and color vision acuity tests and correctly document results.		
4. Perform auditory test and correctly document results.		

I certify that this student has successfully completed each of the listed skills for this objective.

Student:	
Evaluator:	**Date:**

Objective 8: Demonstrate the proper procedure and documentation for ear lavage (irrigation).		
Skills	**Attempt 1**	**Attempt 2**
1. Wash hands.		
2. Greet and identify patient. Explain the procedure and set the patient at ease.		
3. Demonstrate proper procedure for ear irrigation and correctly document results.		

I certify that this student has successfully completed each of the listed skills for this objective.

Student:	
Evaluator:	**Date:**

Objective 9: Demonstrate the proper procedure and documentation for eye irrigation.		
Skills	**Attempt 1**	**Attempt 2**
1. Wash hands.		
2. Greet and identify patient. Explain the procedure and set the patient at ease.		
3. Demonstrate proper procedure for eye irrigation and correctly document results.		

I certify that this student has successfully completed each of the listed skills for this objective.

Student:	
Evaluator:	**Date:**

PIMA MEDICAL INSTITUTE

Medical Assistant
Professional Sequence II
MDA 111 Examination Techniques
Lab Skills

Objective 10: Demonstrate the procedure and documentation for pulse oximetry.		
Skills	**Attempt 1**	**Attempt 2**
1. Wash hands.		
2. Greet and identify patient. Explain the procedure and set the patient at ease.		
3. Correctly apply sensor to patient.		
4. Demonstrate proper operation of pulse oximeter equipment for purpose of obtaining pulse ox and correctly document results.		

I certify that this student has successfully completed each of the listed skills for this objective.

Student:	
Evaluator:	**Date:**

FINAL CHECK-OFF

I certify that this student has successfully completed a minimum of 25 complete sets of vital signs including temperature, pulse, respiration, and blood pressure.

Student:	
Evaluator:	**Date:**

PIMA MEDICAL INSTITUTE

Medical Assistant
Professional Sequence II
MDA 111 Examination Techniques
Lab Skills

Optional Skills Practice

Demonstrate the procedure for diabetic foot examination.		
Skills	**Attempt 1**	**Attempt 2**
1. Wash hands.		
2. Greet patient, explain procedure, and set the patient at ease.		
3. Ask patient about the extent of any previous and current foot problems; ask patient to remove footwear and socks.		
4. Check patient's feet between toes for sores, calluses, infections, fissures, cracks, and deformities.		
5. Check each foot for pulses: posterior tibial pulse (behind ankle bone) and dorsalis pedis pulse (top of foot, just below ankle).		
6. Conduct monofilament exam.		
7. Correctly document results.		

I certify that this student has successfully completed each of the listed skills for this objective.

Student:	
Evaluator:	**Date:**

PIMA MEDICAL INSTITUTE

Medical Assistant
Professional Sequence II
MDA 121 Clinical Aspects of Coding and Billing
Lab Skills

Students must complete the skills listed under each objective. Each step is considered a required part of the mastery of the objective. Students not able to perform the skills will be required to repeat the course.

Objective 1: Use coding systems such as ICD-CM and CPT to assign codes to sample medical cases.		
Skills	**Date Completed**	**Evaluator's Initials**
1. Assign correct codes using the ICD-10-CM manual.		
2. Assign correct codes using the ICD-10-CM manual.		
3. Assign appropriate codes to laboratory paperwork.		
4. Assign procedural codes using the CPT manual.		
5. Assign E&M codes using the CPT manual.		
6. Complete a visit ticket patient encounter form.		

I certify that this student has successfully completed each of the listed skills for this objective.

Student:	
Evaluator:	**Date:**

Objective 2: Complete referral and preauthorization paperwork.		
Skills	**Date Completed**	**Evaluator's Initials**
1. Complete a referral for a patient to see a specialist.		
2. Role-play giving directions for a referral to a patient.		
3. Complete preauthorization paperwork for a procedure.		
4. Document in patient record the outcome of the referral and preauthorization.		

I certify that this student has successfully completed each of the listed skills for this objective.

Student:	
Evaluator:	**Date:**

PIMA MEDICAL INSTITUTE

Medical Assistant
Professional Sequence II
MDA 130 Surgical Procedures
Lab Skills

Students will be tested on the skills listed under each objective. Each step is considered a required part of the mastery of the objective and will be evaluated using the following standards:

Pass: Able to perform skill in a laboratory setting in a safe, professional, and effective manner with distant supervision. Student should be able to perform the skill as an entry-level Medical Assistant.
Fail: Unable to perform skill in a laboratory setting in a safe, professional, and effective manner without constant cues and direct supervision. Student requires remedial training.

Students not able to perform the skills after the second attempt will receive a failing grade and will be required to repeat the course.

Objective 1: Perform hand washing procedure.		
Skills	**Attempt 1**	**Attempt 2**
1. Remove hand and wrist jewelry.		
2. Stand so that you do not touch the sink.		
3. Turn on faucet with a clean paper towel.		
4. Wet hands under warm water.		
5. Apply soap to hands and work up a lather.		
6. Rub hands together to create friction.		
7. Remove debris under fingernails with an orange stick or similar device.		
8. Scrub everywhere, including between the fingers and around the knuckles, for at least 15 seconds.		
9. Rinse your hands in a downward motion from wrists to fingertips, making sure hands don't touch each other or the sink.		
10. Dry hands with a clean paper towel.		
11. Turn faucet off with another clean paper towel.		

I certify that this student has successfully completed each of the listed skills for this objective.

Student:	
Evaluator:	**Date:**

PIMA MEDICAL INSTITUTE

Medical Assistant
Professional Sequence II
MDA 130 Surgical Procedures
Lab Skills

Objective 2: Demonstrate surgical aseptic technique.		
Skills	**Attempt 1**	**Attempt 2**
1. Perform a surgical hand scrub.		
2. Demonstrate proper technique for applying and removing sterile gloves.		
3. Demonstrate proper technique for donning a sterile gown.		
4. Demonstrate proper technique for applying and removing surgical drape.		
5. Demonstrate proper technique for disposal of contaminated surgical materials.		

I certify that this student has successfully completed each of the listed skills for this objective.

Student:	
Evaluator:	**Date:**

Objective 3: Demonstrate techniques for preparing a sterile field.		
Skills	**Attempt 1**	**Attempt 2**
1. Identify instruments commonly used in minor surgery and the procedures for which they are used.		
2. Correctly wrap instruments for autoclave sterilization.		
3. Operate an autoclave using proper loading and unloading techniques.		
4. Properly open a sterile surgical pack.		
5. Add sterile solution to the sterile field.		
6. Identify supplies commonly used in minor surgery (drapes, bandages, sutures, antiseptics, anesthetics, etc.)		
7. Identify surgical tray preparation (sterile drapes, sterile packs and containers, sterile set-up, aseptic preparation)		

I certify that this student has successfully completed each of the listed skills for this objective.

Student:	
Evaluator:	**Date:**

PIMA MEDICAL INSTITUTE

Medical Assistant
Professional Sequence II
MDA 130 Surgical Procedures
Lab Skills

Objective 4: Demonstrate appropriate skin preparation for common office surgical procedures.		
Skills	**Attempt 1**	**Attempt 2**
1. Assemble the equipment using proper sterile technique.		
2. Greet and identify patient. Explain the procedure and set patient at ease.		
3. Perform surgical hand wash and apply gloves.		
4. Perform surgical skin preparation.		
5. Identify potential contamination sources.		
6. Apply antiseptic solution correctly to wound and dry.		

I certify that this student has successfully completed each of the listed skills for this objective.

Student:	
Evaluator:	**Date:**

Objective 5: Demonstrate applications of dressings and bandages.		
Skills	**Attempt 1**	**Attempt 2**
1. Greet and identify patient. Explain the procedure and set patient at ease.		
2. Wash hands and apply gloves.		
3. Demonstrate application of a sterile dressing (wet to dry, dry sterile and transparent).		
4. Demonstrate application of tubular gauze.		
5. Demonstrate application of a spiral bandage.		
6. Demonstrate application of a reverse spiral bandage.		
7. Demonstrate application of a figure eight bandage.		
8. Demonstrate changing an existing sterile bandage.		

I certify that this student has successfully completed each of the listed skills for this objective.

Student:	
Evaluator:	**Date:**

PIMA MEDICAL INSTITUTE

Medical Assistant
Professional Sequence II
MDA 130 Surgical Procedures
Lab Skills

Objective 6: Demonstrate removal of sutures and staples.		
Skills	**Attempt 1**	**Attempt 2**
1. Greet and identify patient. Explain the procedure and set patient at ease.		
2. Wash hands and apply gloves.		
3. Cleanse the wound with antiseptic.		
4. Lift, cut, and remove sutures from skin.		
5. Demonstrate removing staples from the skin with staple remover.		
6. Cleanse the site with antiseptic and cover with a sterile dressing.		

I certify that this student has successfully completed each of the listed skills for this objective.

Student:	
Evaluator:	**Date:**

Objective 7: Preparing and maintaining exam table and operative area.		
Skills	**Attempt 1**	**Attempt 2**
1. Identify equipment that must be discarded properly or sanitized.		
2. Demonstrate proper removal of paper sheets, table covers, and bio-hazardous materials,		
3. Describe/demonstrate wipe-down preparation of procedure area for next patient.		

I certify that this student has successfully completed each of the listed skills for this objective.

Student:	
Evaluator:	**Date:**

PIMA MEDICAL INSTITUTE

Medical Assistant
Professional Sequence III
MDA 120 Medical Office Laboratory Procedures
Lab Skills

Students will be tested on the skills listed under each objective. Each step is considered a required part of the mastery of the objective and will be evaluated using the following standards:

Pass: Able to perform skill in a laboratory setting in a safe, professional, and effective manner with distant supervision. Student should be able to perform the skill as an entry- level Medical Assistant.

Fail: Unable to perform skill in a laboratory setting in a safe, professional, and effective manner without constant cues and direct supervision. Student requires remedial training.

Students not able to perform the skills after the second attempt will receive a failing grade and will be required to repeat the course.

Before final check-off students must complete a minimum of 5 ECGs and 5 urinalysis tests.

Objective 1: Demonstrate the procedure for spirometry.		
Skills	**Attempt 1**	**Attempt 2**
1. Wash hands.		
2. Greet and identify patient. Explain the procedure and set the patient at ease.		
3. Confirm pre-test patient education (time of last meal, tobacco use, lips form tight seal on mouthpiece, maximum effort for accurate results)		
4. Allow patient to practice several times to become familiar with the machine and the feel of the testing.		
5. Enter patient demographic data as required by the spirometry program (include the patient's height, weight).		
6. Place nose clip on patient's nose to assure that all exhalation occurs via the oral airway.		
7. Place the disposable mouthpiece on the spirometer.		
8. Instruct patient that several readings may be needed to assure accurate test results for interpretation by provider.		
9. Remind the patient to exhale forcibly and rapidly until unable to exhale any more air.		
10. Coach patient during inhalation and exhalation to achieve maximum results. Instruct patient that to continue to exhale until instructed to stop; remind patient to remain upright.		
11. Be supportive and encouraging throughout the test. Attend to any special needs of the patient.		
12. Document results with proper notation & test results in patient's medical record; follow proper procedures for disposable & nondisposable equipment; wash hands.		

I certify that this student has successfully completed each of the listed skills for this objective.

Student:	
Evaluator:	**Date:**

PIMA MEDICAL INSTITUTE

Medical Assistant
Professional Sequence III
MDA 120 Medical Office Laboratory Procedures
Lab Skills

Objective 2: Demonstrate proper procedures for providing low dose of concentrated oxygen to a patient during periods of respiratory distress as well as how to instruct patient to properly operate the equipment.		
Skills	**Attempt 1**	**Attempt 2**
1. Wash hands.		
2. Greet and identify the patient. Explain the procedure set patient at ease.		
3. Demonstrate position of nasal prongs of cannula into nose, how to clear oxygen cylinder, and describe precautions.		
4. Demonstrate attachment of cannula/tubing to flowmeter adapter.		
5. Demonstrate proper checking of flow rate (3 times) according to provider's orders while ensuring oxygen flow through cannula.		
6. Demonstrate proper placement of nasal cannula, check patient comfort, and compare flow rate with provider's order. Adjust tubing as needed.		
7. Demonstrate proper instruction to patient to breathe slowly through nose.		
8. Demonstrate patient education about not smoking near patient.		
9. Complete proper documentation in patient's medical record.		

I certify that this student has successfully completed each of the listed skills for this objective.

Student:	
Evaluator:	**Date:**

Objective 3: Perform procedures required to assist with pulmonary function testing.		
Skills	**Attempt 1**	**Attempt 2**
1. Wash hands.		
2. Greet and identify the patient. Explain the procedure and set patient at ease.		
3. Demonstrate proper procedure for pulmonary function testing.		
4. Document as required in patient's medical record.		

I certify that this student has successfully completed each of the listed skills for this objective.

Student:	
Evaluator:	**Date:**

PIMA MEDICAL INSTITUTE

Medical Assistant
Professional Sequence III
MDA 120 Medical Office Laboratory Procedures
Lab Skills

Objective 4: Perform procedures required to assist with pulmonary medicine administration.		
Skills	**Attempt 1**	**Attempt 2**
1. Wash hands.		
2. Greet and identify the patient. Explain the procedure, set patient at ease.		
3. Instruct a patient on proper use of nebulizer for breathing treatment.		
4. Document as required in patient's medical record.		

I certify that this student has successfully completed each of the listed skills for this objective.

Student:	
Evaluator:	**Date:**

Objective 5: Identify procedures for electrocardiograph testing.		
Skills	**Attempt 1**	**Attempt 2**
1. Identify rhythm strip.		
2. Identify treadmill examination (exercise ECG).		
3. Prepare a patient for telemetry monitoring.		
4. Identify Holter monitor, apply electrodes to a patient, and verify patient understanding of Holter monitor procedures.		

I certify that this student has successfully completed each of the listed skills for this objective.

Student:	
Evaluator:	**Date:**

PIMA MEDICAL INSTITUTE

Medical Assistant
Professional Sequence III
MDA 120 Medical Office Laboratory Procedures
Lab Skills

Objective 6: Identify procedure for obtaining 12-lead electrocardiogram.		
Skills	**Attempt 1**	**Attempt 2**
1. Greet and identify patient. Explain procedure and set patient at ease.		
2. Wash hands.		
3. Apply ECG electrodes and leads to a patient.		
4. Identify leads and marking codes; perform standardization of ECG machine.		
5. Calculate patient heart rate from EKG tracing (eg, 6 second method, R to R, sequencing).		
6. Identify/resolve artifacts from the tracing (eg, wandering baseline, somatic, electrical).		
7. Identify cardiac cycle during electrocardiogram; verify leads recorded.		
8. Upload a completed EKG to a patient's electronic medical record.		
9. Mount a completed EKG for a patient's chart.		
10. Measure a patient's heart rhythm from the EKG tracing.		
11. Inspect the waveforms of a cardiac cycle for symmetry, direction, and amplitude (eg, P waves, QRS complexes, ST segments, T waves).		
12. Measure a patient's heart conduction from the EKG tracing (eg, PR-interval/PRI, QRS duration, QT interval).		
13. Identify major classifications of arrhythmias from an EKG tracing (eg, sinus, atrial, ventricular, junctional).		
14. Identify major variances to waveforms related to ischemia, injury, or infarction.)		
15. Verify EKG machine paper speed & machine sensitivity (eg, h, 1, 2).		
16. Recognize pacemaker spikes on EKG tracing.		

I certify that this student has successfully completed each of the listed skills for this objective.

Student:	
Evaluator:	**Date:**

PIMA MEDICAL INSTITUTE

Medical Assistant
Professional Sequence III
MDA 120 Medical Office Laboratory Procedures
Lab Skills

Objective 7: Demonstrate donning and removing personal protective equipment (PPE).		
Skills	**Attempt 1**	**Attempt 2**
A. Apply PPE		
1. Wash hands.		
2. Put on lab coat or gown and fasten buttons or ties appropriately.		
3. Apply goggles, face mask, or face shield. If applying mask, tie the mask on top, then on the bottom.		
4. Apply gloves over the cuffs of the lab coat or gown.		
B. Remove PPE		
1. Remove the first glove.		
2. Remove the second glove with the ungloved hand.		
3. Dispose of the gloves in a biohazardous waste container.		
4. Remove the face mask, goggles, or face shield. If wearing a mask, untie the top ties, then the bottom ties, and discard in a biohazardous waste container.		
5. Remove the gown or lab coat. If wearing a gown, turn inside out as it is removed and discard in a biohazardous waste container.		
6. Wash hands.		

I certify that this student has successfully completed each of the listed skills for this objective.

Student:	
Evaluator:	**Date:**

Objective 8: Perform proper procedures for removing biological spills.		
Skills	**Attempt 1**	**Attempt 2**
1. Describe/demonstrate donning personal protective equipment (PPE).		
2. Describe the steps necessary to cover a spill, disinfect the area, and properly dispose of waste materials.		
3. Describe/demonstrate removal of PPE.		
4. Wash hands.		

I certify that this student has successfully completed each of the listed skills for this objective.

Student:	
Evaluator:	**Date:**

PIMA MEDICAL INSTITUTE

Medical Assistant
Professional Sequence III
MDA 120 Medical Office Laboratory Procedures
Lab Skills

Objective 9: Perform procedures related to physical and chemical urinalysis.		
Skills	**Attempt 1**	**Attempt 2**
1. Greet and identify patient. Explain the procedure and set patient at ease.		
2. Wash hands.		
3. Instruct a patient in the collection of a 24-hour urine specimen.		
4. Instruct a patient in the collection of a clean-catch midstream urine specimen.		
5. Perform a urinalysis (chemical and physical); identify procedures for random, clean catch, timed, and drug screen.		
6. Prepare and mount a urine slide for microscopic exam.		
7. Prepare urine for lab.		
8. Instruct patient what happens next: getting dressed, checking out, when to expect results, what to do if they don't hear anything.		

I certify that this student has successfully completed each of the listed skills for this objective.

Student:	
Evaluator:	**Date:**

<u>Final Check Off:</u> I certify that this student has successfully completed a minimum of 5 ECGs and 5 urinalysis procedures:

Student:	
Evaluator:	**Date:**

PIMA MEDICAL INSTITUTE

Medical Assistant
Professional Sequence III
MDA 120 Medical Office Laboratory Procedures
Lab Skills

Optional Senior Practice (all on this page)

Demonstrate procedures for taking and recording patient temperatures.		
Skills	**Attempt 1**	**Attempt 2**
1. Wash hands.		
2. Greet and identify patient. Explain procedure; set patient at ease.		
3. Obtain an **oral** temperature using a digital thermometer and correctly document results.		
4. Obtain a **tympanic** temperature using a tympanic thermometer and correctly document results.		
5. Obtain an **axillary** temperature and correctly document results.		
6. Obtain a **temporal** artery temperature and correctly document results.		
7. Demonstrate the procedure to obtain a **rectal** temperature and correctly document results.		

Demonstrate procedures for taking and recording patient pulse and respiration.		
Skills	**Attempt 1**	**Attempt 2**
1. Wash hands.		
2. Greet and identify patient. Explain procedure; set patient at ease.		
3. Obtain an apical pulse and correctly document results.		
4. Obtain a radial pulse and correctly document results.		
5. Obtain patient's respiratory rate and correctly document results.		

Demonstrate proper procedures to measure and record blood pressure.		
Skills	**Attempt 1**	**Attempt 2**
1. Wash hands.		
2. Greet and identify patient. Explain the procedure; set patient at ease.		
3. Obtain patient's blood pressure and correctly document results.		

Demonstrate the procedures used to measure and record patient height and weight.		
Skills	**Attempt 1**	**Attempt 2**
1. Wash hands.		
2. Greet and identify patient. Explain procedure; set patient at ease.		
3. Demonstrate proper skills in moving patient on/off scale.		
4. Measure and record a patient's height and correctly document results.		
5. Measure and record a patient's weight and correctly document results.		

PIMA MEDICAL INSTITUTE

Medical Assistant
Professional Sequence IV
MDA 125 Medical Office Laboratory Procedures
Lab Skills

Students will be tested on the skills listed under each objective. Each step is considered a required part of the mastery of the objective and will be evaluated using the following standards:

Pass: Able to perform skill in a laboratory setting in a safe, professional, and effective manner with distant supervision. Student should be able to perform the skill as an entry-level Medical Assistant.
Fail: Unable to perform skill in a laboratory setting in a safe, professional, and effective manner without constant cues and direct supervision. Student requires remedial training.

Students not able to perform the skills after the second attempt will receive a failing grade and will be required to repeat the course.

Before final check-off students must complete a minimum of:

- 15 venous blood draws using an evacuated tube
- 5 butterfly blood draws
- 5 hematocrit procedures
- 5 glucose tests

(Note: Syringe draw appears after the final check-off page as an optional objective per state scope of practice.)

Objective 1: Perform tourniquet application & vein selection.		
Skills	**Attempt 1**	**Attempt 2**
1. Position arm correctly for vein selection.		
2. Select appropriate tourniquet application site.		
3. Place tourniquet in flat position behind arm.		
4. Smoothly position hands when crossing and tucking tourniquet.		
5. Fasten tourniquet at appropriate tightness (not folded into arm; loop & loose end do not interfere with puncture site).		
8. Ask patient to clench fist.		
9. Select antecubital area to palpate.		
10. Perform palpation using correct fingers.		
11. Palpate entire area or both arms if necessary.		
12. Check depth and direction of veins.		
13. Remove tourniquet smoothly and in a timely manner.		

I certify that this student has successfully completed each of the listed skills for this objective.

Student:	
Evaluator:	**Date:**

PIMA MEDICAL INSTITUTE

Medical Assistant
Professional Sequence IV
MDA 125 Medical Office Laboratory Procedures
Lab Skills

Objective 2: Perform a venipuncture using the winged infusion method (butterfly draws).		
Skills	**Attempt 1**	**Attempt 2**
1. Greet, identify patient; explain procedure; set patient at ease.		
2. Verify the lab tests ordered against the requisition.		
3. Ask if patient has any allergies or concerns re: blood draws.		
4. Wash hands and don PPE.		
5. Assemble equipment.		
6. Position arm correctly for vein selection.		
7. Apply the tourniquet around the wrist.		
8. Choose the puncture site and take off the tourniquet.		
9. Cleanse the site with alcohol wipe and allow to air dry.		
10. Reapply the tourniquet.		
11. Anchor the vein.		
12. Holding butterfly wings, insert the needle into the vein at the appropriate angle.		
13. Advance the needle until a flash of blood is observed.		
14. Collect the sample in accordance with the method being used (evacuated tubes or syringe).		
15. Release tourniquet, remove needle, apply safety over needle as it is removed		
16. Apply pressure to the site with gauze.		
17. Mix anticoagulated tubes if applicable.		
18. Discard needle and tubing into sharps container.		
19. If using syringe, use a transfer device to transfer blood to evacuated tubes.		
20. Label tubes with appropriate information.		
21. Check the site and apply bandage; thank patient.		
22. Dispose of used supplies and materials.		
23. Remove PPE and wash hands.		
24. Explain how to deliver specimens to appropriate departments.		

I certify that this student has successfully completed each of the listed skills for this objective.

Student:	
Evaluator:	**Date:**

PIMA MEDICAL INSTITUTE

Medical Assistant
Professional Sequence IV
MDA 125 Medical Office Laboratory Procedures
Lab Skills

Objective 3: Perform a venipuncture using the evacuated tube method.		
Skills	**Attempt 1**	**Attempt 2**
1. Greet, identify patient; explain procedure; set patient at ease.		
3. Verify the lab tests ordered against the requisition.		
4. Position/prepare the patient and explain procedure.		
6. Wash hands and don PPE.		
7. Assemble equipment.		
8. Apply the tourniquet.		
9. Palpate the vein and take off the tourniquet.		
10. Cleanse the site with alcohol wipe and allow to air dry.		
11. Reapply the tourniquet.		
12. Examine the needle.		
13. Anchor the vein.		
14. Insert the needle into vein at the appropriate angle.		
15. Advance and change tubes in appropriate order of draw.		
16. Release tourniquet, remove needle, apply safety over needle as it is removed.		
17. Mix anticoagulated tubes as they are removed from the adapter.		
18. Label tubes with appropriate information.		
19. Check the site and apply bandage; thank patient.		
21. Dispose of used supplies and materials.		
22. Remove PPE and wash hands.		
23. Explain how to deliver specimens to appropriate departments.		

I certify that this student has successfully completed each of the listed skills for this objective.

Student:	
Evaluator:	**Date:**

PIMA MEDICAL INSTITUTE

Medical Assistant
Professional Sequence IV
MDA 125 Medical Office Laboratory Procedures
Lab Skills

Objective 4: Perform hematocrit procedure.		
Skills	**Attempt 1**	**Attempt 2**
1. Wash hands and don PPE.		
2. Greet, identify patient; explain procedure; set patient at ease.		
3. Demonstrate proper steps for obtaining blood sample.		
4. Fill capillary tube 2/3-3/4 full with well-mixed, oxalated venous blood or fingertip blood (use heparinized tubes for fingertip blood & invert several times to mix).		
5. Seal one end of tube with clay; place filled tube into microhematocrit centrifuge with plugged end away from center of centrifuge.		
6. Centrifuge at preset of 10,000 to 12,000 rpm for 5 minutes. If hematocrit exceeds 50 percent, centrifuge for additional 3 minutes.		
7. Place tube in microhematocrit reader; follow manufacturer's guidelines.		
8. Document correctly in patient's medical record.		
9. Explain to patient when the test results will be available and what to do if for some reason they aren't notified.		
10. Prepare appropriate documentation for processing.		

I certify that this student has successfully completed each of the listed skills for this objective.

Student:	
Evaluator:	**Date:**

Objective 5: Perform glucose testing.		
Skills	**Attempt 1**	**Attempt 2**
1. Wash hands and don PPE.		
2. Greet, identify patient; explain procedure; set patient at ease.		
3. Place test trip into blood glucose meter.		
4. Choose location on side of patient's middle or ring fingertip and poke it with lancet device. Wait for drop of blood to form; if unsuccessful, gently squeeze finger until drop forms.		
5. Place drop of blood on/near test area of test strip. Wait until the right amount of blood has been drawn into test strip.		
6. Apply gauze/cotton ball to clean fingertip; hold until bleeding stops.		
7. Document blood sugar results correctly in patient's medical record.		

I certify that this student has successfully completed each of the listed skills for this objective.

Student:	
Evaluator:	**Date:**

PIMA MEDICAL INSTITUTE

Medical Assistant
Professional Sequence IV
MDA 125 Medical Office Laboratory Procedures
Lab Skills

FINAL CHECK-OFF: I certify that this student has successfully a minimum of:

- 15 venous blood draws using an evacuated tube
- 5 butterfly blood draws
- 5 hematocrit procedures
- 5 glucose tests

Student:	
Evaluator:	**Date:**

PIMA MEDICAL INSTITUTE

Medical Assistant
Professional Sequence IV
MDA 125 Medical Office Laboratory Procedures
Lab Skills

Optional Objective (per state scope of practice)

Venipuncture by syringe: Obtain venous blood acceptable for laboratory testing.		
Skills	**Attempt 1**	**Attempt 2**
1. Assemble supplies.		
2. Greet, identify patient; explain procedure; set patient at ease.		
3. Wash hands and don PPE.		
4. Open the sterile needle and sterile syringe packages; assemble if necessary. Pull plunger halfway out and push it all the way in again.		
5. Select the proper vacuum tubes for later transfer of the specimen; tap all tubes containing anticoagulants and check the expiration dates. Arrange them in a holding rack in proper order.		
6. Apply tourniquet and select a site. Ask the patient to close the hand; he/she must not pump the hand; place hand in a downward position.		
7. Select a vein, noting location and direction of the vein.		
8. Cleanse site with alcohol swab with one firm swipe. Avoid touching the site after cleansing.		
9. Draw skin taut with your thumb by placing it 1-2 inches below puncture site.		
10. Insert needle, bevel up, at appropriate angle.		
11. Release skin using same hand to pull back gently on plunger at same rate as syringe fills.		
12. When syringe is full, have patient open his/her hand. Remove tourniquet; place cotton/gauze over injection site and remove needle.		
13. Apply pressure to site for 2-3 minutes; patient can elevate arm but should be instructed not to bend the elbow.		
14. Aliquot blood into appropriate tubes in rack in proper order. During transfer, hold each tube at base only.		
15. Puncture vacuum tube through rubber stopper with syringe needle; allow blood to enter tube until flow stops. (Never push on plunger or force blood into tube.); implement safety mechanism immediately.		
16. Mix any anticoagulant tubes immediately.		
17. Discard used supplies in appropriate locations.		
18. Label all tubes correctly. If any special treatment is required for specimens, institute handling protocol immediately.		
19. Check patient's status. Document correctly in patient's medical record.		

Additional Practice (per instructor's discretion)

Perform procedures and professional interactions with atypical patient reactions.		
Skills	**Attempt 1**	**Attempt 2**
1. Role play drawing blood with patient prone to fainting.		
2. Role play drawing blood with a patient with weak or rolling veins.		

Additional SENIOR Practice (optional or per instructor's discretion)
Review objectives/skills in need of additional practice, including injections, blood draws, and equipment operation.

PIMA MEDICAL INSTITUTE

Medical Assistant
Professional Sequence IV
MDA 141 Medical Specialty Procedures
Lab Skills

Students will be tested on each skill listed under each objective. Each step is considered a required part of the mastery of the objective and will be evaluated using the following standards:

Pass: Able to perform skill in a laboratory setting in a safe, professional, and effective manner with distant supervision. Student should be able to perform the skill as an entry-level Medical Assistant

Fail: Unable to perform skill in a laboratory setting in a safe, professional, and effective manner without constant cues and direct supervision. Student requires remedial training.

Students not able to perform the skills after the second attempt will receive a failing grade and will be required to repeat the course.

Objective 1: Perform procedures required to assist with gynecologic and obstetric procedures.

Skills	**Attempt 1**	**Attempt 2**
1. Wash hands.		
2. Prepare a set-up tray for a pelvic exam/pap smear.		
3. Greet and identify the patient. Explain procedure; set patient at ease.		
4. Give a female patient instructions regarding positioning and draping for a gynecological exam.		

I certify that this student has successfully completed each of the listed skills for this objective.

Student:	
Evaluator:	**Date:**

Objective 2: Instruct patients on self-examination techniques.

Skills	**Attempt 1**	**Attempt 2**
1. Instruct a female patient on procedures for a self-breast exam.		
2. Instruct a male patient on procedures for a testicular self-exam.		

I certify that this student has successfully completed each of the listed skills for this objective.

Student:	
Evaluator:	**Date:**

PIMA MEDICAL INSTITUTE

Medical Assistant
Professional Sequence IV
MDA 141 Medical Specialty Procedures
Lab Skills

Objective 3: Perform procedures required to assist in pediatrics examinations.		
Skills	**Attempt 1**	**Attempt 2**
1. Wash hands.		
2. Identify the patient and greet patient and parent. Explain procedure; set patient at ease.		
3. Simulate procedure for proper restraining of infant/child.		
4. Perform the procedure for measuring an infant's head.		
5. Perform the procedure for measuring an infant's chest circumference.		
6. Perform the procedure for measuring an infant's length and weight.		
7. Simulate the procedure for applying a pediatric urinary collection device.		
8. Document measurements in patient medical record.		

I certify that this student has successfully completed each of the listed skills for this objective.

Student:	
Evaluator:	**Date:**

Optional Senior Practice (from this point forward):

Demonstrate proper procedures to measure and document height and weight.		
Skills	**Attempt 1**	**Attempt 2**
1. Wash hands.		
2. Greet and identify patient. Explain the procedure and set patient at ease.		
3. Demonstrate proper skills in moving patient on/off scale.		
4. Measure a patient's height and correctly document results.		
5. Measure a patient's weight and correctly document results.		

Optional Senior Practice (continued; all on this page)

Demonstrate proper procedures to obtain and document temperatures.		
Skills	**Attempt 1**	**Attempt 2**
1. Wash hands.		
2. Greet and identify patient. Explain the procedure and set patient at ease.		
3. Obtain an **oral** temperature using a digital thermometer and correctly document results.		
4. Obtain a **tympanic** temperature using a tympanic thermometer and correctly document results.		
5. Obtain an **axillary** temperature and correctly document results.		
6. Obtain a **temporal** artery temperature and correctly document results.		
7. Demonstrate the procedure to obtain a **rectal** temperature and correctly document results.		

Demonstrate proper procedures to obtain and document pulse and respiration.		
Skills	**Attempt 1**	**Attempt 2**
1. Wash hands.		
2. Greet and identify patient. Explain the procedure and set patient at ease.		
3. Obtain an **apical** pulse and correctly document results.		
4. Obtain a **radial** pulse and correctly document results.		
5. Determine a patient's **respiratory rate** and correctly document results.		

Demonstrate proper procedures to obtain and document blood pressure.		
Skills	**Attempt 1**	**Attempt 2**
1. Wash hands.		
2. Greet and identify patient. Explain the procedure and set patient at ease.		
3. Determine a patient's blood pressure and correctly document results.		